Preface

This **Laboratory Medicine pocket** is the first edition in English. There is a very successful sister version presently available in German which is available in its 4th edition. The purpose of the **Laboratory Medicine pocket** is to aid clinicians in their diagnostic decisions, as well as raise interest in the field of laboratory medicine. This pocket-sized reference guide is formatted to be an indispensable tool by health science students as well as internists, family medicine physicians, surgeons, pathologists, and any other professional who needs to make decisions based on laboratory findings. In addition, knowing this information can be essential to passing the boards in certain specialties (eg, pathology).

The German version has been very well received, and it is my hope that this version will be as well. I have presented the information as it appeals to me, and to assure continued improvement of the **Laboratory Medicine pocket**, any comments, criticisms, or additions would be greatly appreciated.

Please contact us at service@media4u.com.

Nicole Riddle, MD, FCAP
Asst. Professor and Asst. Residency Program Director, Department of Pathology, University of Texas Health Science Center

The authors and the publisher   January, 2016

Nicole D. Riddle, MD, FCAP

4 Contents

1 General Overview 11

1.1	**Laboratory Diagnostics**	**11**
1.2	**Pre-Analytical Phase**	**11**
1.2.1	Disinfection methods based on risk of infection	11
1.2.2	Sample types and extraction methods	12
1.2.3	Transport	16
1.2.4	Potential errors	16
1.3	**Analytical Phase**	**18**
1.3.1	Interpretation of laboratory values	18
1.3.2	Precision	18
1.3.3	Coefficient of variation	19
1.3.4	Standard deviation	19
1.3.5	Control	19
1.3.6	Quality assurance	19
1.4	**Postanalytical Phase/ Interpretation**	**21**
1.4.1	Reference ranges	21
1.4.2	Sensitivity	21
1.4.3	Specificity	22
1.4.4	Predictive value	23
1.4.5	Plausibility	23
1.4.6	Longitudinal evaluation	23
1.5	**Units**	**24**

2 Analytical Methods 26

2.1	**Optical Measurement Methods**	**26**
2.2	**Electrochemical Methods**	**27**
2.3	**Electrophoresis**	**28**
2.4	**Immunological Methods**	**30**
2.4.1	Direct antigen and antibody detection	30
2.4.2	Indirect antigen and antibody detection	31
2.4.3	Flow cytometry	34
2.5	**Chromatographic Separation Processes**	**34**
2.6	**Osmotic Pressure**	**36**
2.7	**Molecular Diagnostics**	**36**

3 Proteins, Metabolites 38

3.1	**Total Protein**	**38**
3.2	**Serum Protein Electrophoresis (SPEP)**	**39**
3.3	**Albumin**	**41**
3.4	**Alpha-1-Globulins**	**42**
3.5	**Alpha-2-Globulins**	**43**
3.6	**Beta-Globulin**	**44**
3.7	**Gamma Globulins**	**46**
3.8	**Total Complement Activity (CH50)**	**47**
3.9	**Complement Factor C1-inh**	**47**
3.10	**Hyperimmunoglobulinemia**	**48**
3.11	**Hypoimmunoglobulinemia**	**49**
3.12	**Soluble Transferrin-Receptor (sTfR)**	**50**
3.13	**Transferrin Saturation**	**50**
3.14	**Carbohydrate-Deficient Transferrin (CDT)**	**50**
3.15	**Ferritin**	**51**
3.16	**Iron (Fe)**	**51**
3.17	**Deferoxamine Test**	**52**
3.18	**Procalcitonin (PCT)**	**52**
3.19	**Neopterin**	**53**
3.20	**Acute Phase Reactants**	**53**
3.21	**"Negative" Acute-Phase Reactants**	**53**
3.22	**Ammonia (NH$_3$)**	**54**
3.23	**Urea**	**54**
3.24	**Uric Acid**	**55**
3.25	**Homocysteine**	**56**
3.26	**Granulocyte Elastase**	**57**
3.27	**Lysozyme**	**58**
3.28	**Myoglobin**	**58**
3.29	**Cardiac Troponins (C, T and I)**	**59**
3.30	**Atrial Natriuretic Peptide (ANP)**	**60**
3.31	**B-type Natriuretic Peptide (BNP) /NT-proBNP**	**60**
3.32	**Vasoactive Intestinal Polypeptide (VIP)**	**61**
3.33	**Hereditary Amino Acid Disorders**	**61**
3.33.1	Phenylketonuria (PKU)	61
3.33.2	Maple syrup urine disease (MSUD)	62

4	Tumor Markers	63
4.1	Clinically Relevant Tumor Markers	63
4.2	Sensitivities for (Selected) Solid Tumors	71

5	Lipids	75
5.1	Cholesterol	76
5.2	Triglycerides	78
5.3	Fredrickson Classification	79
5.4	Refrigerated Standing Plasma Test	80
5.5	Lipoprotein Electrophoresis	80
5.6	The Main Lipoproteins	80
5.7	Lipoprotein(a) [Lp(a)]	81

6	Carbohydrate	82
6.1	Diabetes Mellitus	82
6.2	Diagnosis of Diabetes	83
6.3	Glucose in the Blood	83
6.4	Hyperglycemia	84
6.5	Hypoglycemia	84
6.6	Mellituria	85
6.7	Glycosuria	85
6.8	Oral Glucose Tolerance Test (OGTT)	85
6.9	Ketone Bodies	86
6.10	Hemoglobin A1c (HbA1c)	87
6.11	Fructosamine	89
6.12	Insulin	90
6.13	C-peptide (Connecting Peptide)	90
6.14	Lactate	91
6.15	Glucagon	92
6.16	Glucagon Test	93
6.17	Congenital Disorders	94
6.17.1	Fructosuria	94
6.17.2	Galactosemia	94
6.17.3	Other urinary saccharides	94
6.17.4	Lactose intolerance	95
6.17.5	Glycogen storage disorders	95
6.18	Common Mono- and Disaccharides	96

7	Enzymes	97
7.1	Alkaline Phosphatase	97
7.2	Leukocyte Alkaline Phosphatase (LAP)	97
7.3	Alpha-Amylase	98
7.4	Cholinesterase (ChE)	98
7.5	Creatinine Kinase (CK)	99
7.6	Creatine Kinase of Cardiac Muscle (CK-MB)	100
7.7	Macro-CK	100
7.8	Gamma Glutamyl Transferase (GGT)	101
7.9	Glucose-6-Phosphate-Dehydrogenase (G6PD)	101
7.10	Pyruvate Kinase (PK)	102
7.11	Transaminases	103
7.11.1	Aspartate aminotransferase (AST)	103
7.11.2	Alanine aminotransferase (ALT)	103
7.12	AST/ALT Ratio	104
7.13	Glutamate Dehydrogenase (GLDH)	104
7.14	(AST + ALT) – GLDH	104
7.15	Lactate Dehydrogenase (LDH)	105
7.16	Hydroxybutyrate Dehydrogenase (HBDH)	106
7.17	LDH/AST Ratio	106
7.18	Lipase	106
7.19	Acid Phosphatase (AP)	107
7.20	Leucine Aminopeptidases (LAP)	107
7.21	Enzyme Localization	107
7.22	Laboratory Findings in Specific Diagnoses	108
7.23	Half-Lives of Enzymes	108
7.24	Cardiac Markers	108

6 Contents

8 Hematology 110

8.1	Erythrocyte Morphology	111
8.2	Erythrocyte Sedimentation Rate (ESR)	113
8.3	Anemia	114
8.3.1	Disorders of erythropoiesis	114
8.3.2	Blood loss	115
8.3.3	Increased red blood cell destruction	116
8.4	Diagnosis by Morphological Criteria	121
8.5	Polycythemia	123
8.6	Reticulocyte	123
8.7	Osmotic Resistance	124
8.8	Hemoglobin	124
8.9	Hematocrit	125
8.10	Methemoglobin	125
8.11	Hemoglobin Electrophoresis	126
8.12	Hemoglobin F (Fetal)	126
8.13	Thalassemia	127
8.14	Sickle Cell Anemia (HbS)	129
8.15	Hemoglobin C (HbC)	130
8.16	Hemoglobin E	130
8.17	Porphyrins	131
8.18	Complete Blood Count (CBC)	133
8.19	Hematopoiesis	135
8.20	Erythropoietin (EPO)	138
8.21	Delta–Aminolevulinic Acid	139
8.22	Bilirubin	139
8.23	Leukocytosis	141
8.24	Leukopenia/Leukocytopenia	141
8.25	Granulocytosis	142
8.26	Agranulocytosis	142
8.27	Neutrophilia	143
8.28	Neutropenia	143
8.29	Eosinophilia	143
8.30	Basophilia	143
8.31	Monocytosis	144
8.32	Monocytopenia	144
8.33	Lymphocytosis	144
8.34	Lymphocytopenia	144
8.35	Thrombocytosis/Thrombocythemia	145
8.36	Thrombocytopenia	145
8.37	Infections	145
8.38	Granulocyte Pathomorphology	145
8.39	Lymphocyte Pathomorphology	146
8.40	Leukemia	146
8.41	Acute Leukemia	146
8.41.1	Acute lymphoblastic leukemia (ALL)	147
8.41.2	Acute myeloid/myelogenous leukemia (AML)	149
8.42	Chronic Leukemia	152
8.42.1	Chronic lymphocytic leukemia (CLL)	152
8.42.2	Chronic myeloid/myelogenous leukemia (CML)	153
8.43	Myeloproliferative Syndromes (MPS)	155
8.44	Myelodysplastic Syndromes (MDS)	157
8.45	Plasma Cell Disorders	160
8.45.1	Plasma cell myeloma	160
8.45.2	Monoclonal gammopathy of undetermined significance (MGUS)	161
8.45.3	Asymptomatic "smoldering" myeloma	162
8.45.4	Solitary plasmacytoma	162
8.45.5	Waldenström's macroglobulinemia	162
8.45.6	Systemic amyloidosis	162
8.45.7	POEMS syndrome	163

9 Hemostasis 164

9.1	Primary Hemostasis	164
9.2	Secondary Hemostasis	165
9.3	Global Coagulation Tests	165
9.4	Phase Specific Coagulation Tests	166
9.5	Factor Specific Tests	166
9.6	Stages of Blood Loss	166
9.7	Bleeding Time	166
9.8	Coagulation Activation as a Result of Vascular Injury	168
9.9	Clotting Factors	168
9.10	Coagulation Inhibitors	169
9.11	Coagulation Cascade	170

9.12 Prothrombin Time (PT) 171
9.13 Activated Partial Thromboplastin Time (aPTT) 172
9.14 Thrombin Time (TT) 174
9.15 Reptilase Time (RT) 174
9.16 Recalcification Time 174
9.17 Fibrinogen 175
9.18 Fibrin Split Products (FSPs) 175
9.19 Hyperfibrinolysis 176
9.20 Platelet Function Tests (PFTs) 177
9.21 Antithrombin (AT) 178
9.22 Protein C 178
9.23 Protein S 179
9.24 Activated Protein C-Resistant/ Factor V Leiden 180
9.25 Spontaneous Clot Lysis Time 181
9.26 Euglobulin Lysis Time (ELT) 181
9.27 Plasmin 181
9.28 Platelet Disorders 182
9.29 Heparin 184
9.30 Anti-Xa Activity 185
9.31 Coumarins (Warfarin) 186
9.32 Specific Coagulation Factor Deficiencies 187
9.33 Hemophilia 189
9.34 Factor-Inhibitor Induced Hemophilia 190
9.35 Von Willebrand Factor 191
9.36 Thrombocytopenias 193
9.37 Hemorrhagic Disease 199
9.38 Disseminated Intravascular Coagulation (DIC) 201
9.39 Thrombophilia 204
9.40 Overview of Coagulation Testing 205

10 Transfusion Medicine 207
10.1 Blood Group Systems 207
10.2 Transfusion Medicine Testing 212
10.3 Transfusion Planning Timeline 217

11 Water and Electrolytes 220
11.1 Disorders of Water Balance 220
11.2 Extracellular Space 220
11.3 Intracellular Space 220
11.4 Oncotic Pressure 220
11.5 Volume Status Evaluation 220
11.6 Hypervolemia 220
11.7 Euvolemic and Isotonic 221
11.8 Hypovolemia/Dehydration 221
11.9 Osmolarity 221
11.10 Osmolality 221
11.11 Increased Serum Osmolality 222
11.12 Osmotic Gap 222
11.13 Anion Gap 222
11.14 Sodium (Na$^+$) 223
11.15 Potassium (K$^+$) 225
11.16 Chloride (Cl$^-$) 227
11.17 Calcium (Ca^{2+}) 228
11.18 Phosphate (PO$_4^{3-}$) 230
11.19 Diagnose Water/Electrolyte Imbalance 231

12 Urinary System 232
12.1 Urinalysis 232
12.2 Macroscopic Assessment 232
12.3 Urine Dipstick Evaluation 233
12.4 Microscopic Examination 234
12.5 Urine pH 235
12.6 Glucose 235
12.7 Protein 236
12.8 Bence-Jones Proteins 238
12.9 Erythrocytes 238
12.10 Myoglobin 239
12.11 Hemoglobin 239
12.12 Leukocytes 240
12.13 Ketones 240
12.14 Bilirubin 240
12.15 Urobilinogen 241
12.16 Nitrite 242
12.17 Amylase 242

8   Contents

12.18 Phenylketones	243
12.19 Cysteine and Homocysteine	243
12.20 Sulfite	243
12.21 Urine Concentration	243
12.22 Clearance	244
12.23 Glomerular Filtration Rate (GFR)	244
12.24 Renal Blood Flow	245
12.25 Creatinine	245
12.26 Creatinine Clearance	245
12.27 Calculation of GFR	247
12.28 Cystatin C	247
12.29 Phosphate Clearance	248
12.30 Urea (BUN)	249
12.31 Calculi (Stones)	249

13   Gastrointestinal Tract   250

13.1 Gastric Secretions	**250**
13.1.1 Analysis	250
13.1.2 Gastrin	250
13.1.3 Zollinger-Ellison syndrome (ZES) and gastrinoma	251
13.1.4 Secretin provocation test	252
13.1.5 Pentagastrin stimulation test	252
13.2 Exocrine Pancreas Function	**253**
13.2.1 Stool examination	253
13.2.2 Chymotrypsin	253
13.2.3 Pancreatic elastase	254
13.2.4 Pancreoauryl test	254
13.2.5 N-Benzoyl-L-Tyrosyl-p-Aminobenzoic-acid-test	255
13.2.6 Pancreatic enzyme secretion test	255
13.3 Small Intestine Function	**256**
13.3.1 Xylose tolerance test	257
13.3.2 Lactose-load test	257
13.3.3 Schilling test	258
13.4 Fecal Occult Blood Test	**258**
13.5 Meconium Albumin Testing	**259**

14   Cerebrospinal Fluid (CSF)   260

14.1 Macroscopic Examination	260
14.2 Cells in the CSF	260
14.3 Normal CSF Differentials	261
14.4 Meningitis CSF Differentials	261
14.5 CSF Protein	262
14.6 CSF Glucose	265
14.7 CSF in Nasal Secretions	265
14.8 Contraindications to Lumbar Puncture (LP)	266

15   Pleural, Peritoneal and Synovial Fluid   267

15.1 Pleural Effusion	267
15.2 Ascites	269
15.3 Synovial Fluid	269

16   Musculoskeletal System   271

16.1 Bone Matrix	**271**
16.2 Bone Formation Markers	**271**
16.2.1 Alkaline phosphatase (AP)	271
16.2.2 Bone specific alkaline phosphatase	273
16.2.3 Osteocalcin	273
16.2.4 Procollagens I (PICP, PINP)	274
16.3 Bone Resorption Markers	**275**
16.3.1 Pyridinium crosslinks (PyD, DPyD)	275
16.3.2 Hydroxyproline (OH-proline)	276
16.3.3 Tartrate resistant acid phosphatase (TRAP)	276
16.3.4 Type-I collagen telopeptide (CTx)	277
16.4 Laboratory Findings	**277**

17 Hormones 278

17.1 Thyroid and Parathyroid 278
17.1.1 Thyroid stimulating hormone (TSH, Thyrotropin) 278
17.1.2 Thyroxine (T4) 279
17.1.3 Triiodothyronine (T3) 279
17.1.4 Free thyroid hormone (fT3, fT4) 280
17.1.5 Thyroid binding globulin (TBG) 280
17.1.6 Thyroid releasing hormone (TRH) 281
17.1.7 Calcitonin 282
17.1.8 Parathyroid hormone (PTH) 283
17.2 Adrenal Cortex 284
17.2.1 Cortisol 284
17.2.2 Adrenocorticotropic hormone (ACTH, Corticotropin) 286
17.2.3 Dexamethasone suppression test 286
17.2.4 Corticotropin releasing hormone test 287
17.2.5 ACTH test 288
17.2.6 Adrenal androgens (DHEA, ANDRO) 289
17.2.7 17-Hydroxyprogesterone 289
17.2.8 11-Deoxycortisol (Cortodoxone) 290
17.3 RAAS and ADH 290
17.3.1 Renin (Angiotensinogenase) 290
17.3.2 Aldosterone 291
17.3.3 Angiotensin converting enzyme (ACE) 292
17.3.4 Renin-aldosterone-orthostatic-test 293
17.3.5 Captopril test 294
17.3.6 Antidiuretic hormone 295
17.3.7 Water deprivation test 296
17.3.8 Desmopressin test (DDAVP test) 296
17.3.9 Salt loading test 297
17.4 Growth Hormone 297
17.4.1 Growth hormone (GH, Somatotropic hormone) 297
17.4.2 Growth hormone releasing hormone (GHRH Test) 298
17.4.3 Oral glucose challenge 298
17.4.4 Insulin hypoglycemia test (IHT) 299
17.4.5 Arginine loading test 299

17.5 Prolactin 300
17.5.1 Prolactin 300
17.5.2 Metoclopramide test 300
17.5.3 TSH releasing hormone test (TRH test) 301
17.6 Sex Hormones 301
17.6.1 17-Beta-estradiol (E2) 301
17.6.2 Progesterone 302
17.6.3 Luteinizing hormone (LH) 302
17.6.4 Follicle stimulating hormone (FSH) 303
17.6.5 Gonadotropin releasing hormone test (GnRH Test) 304
17.6.6 Human chorionic gonadotropin (HCG) 305
17.6.7 Alpha-fetoprotein (AFP) 305
17.6.8 Testosterone 306
17.6.9 Sex hormone binding globulin (SHBG) 307
17.6.10 HCG test 307
17.7 Catecholamines, Serotonin, and Metabolites 308
17.7.1 Plasma catecholamines 308
17.7.2 Urine catecholamines 308
17.7.3 Urine catecholamine metabolites 309
17.7.4 Clonidine test 309
17.7.5 5-Hydroxyindoleacetic acid (5-HIAA) 309
17.7.6 Serotonin (5-hydroxytryptamine, 5 HT) 310
17.7.7 5-Hydroxytryptophane (5 HTP) 310

18 Blood Gas Analysis 311

18.1 Pulse Oximetry 311
18.2 Arterial Blood Gas Analysis 312
18.3 Acid-Base Disorders 315

19 Antibodies 321

19.1 Antibodies in Detail 324
19.2 Human Leukocyte Antigen (HLA) 342
19.3 Hepatitis 342
19.4 Syphilis 345

10   Contents

20	**Vitamins**	**348**
20.1	Vitamin A	348
20.2	Beta Carotene	349
20.3	Vitamin B1 (Thiamine)	350
20.4	Vitamin B2 (Riboflavin)	351
20.5	Vitamin B3 (Niacin, Nicotinic Acid)	352
20.6	Vitamin B5 (Pantothenic Acid)	352
20.7	Vitamin B6 (Pyridoxine)	353
20.8	Vitamin B7 (Biotin, Vitamin H)	353
20.9	Vitamin B9 (Folic Acid)	354
20.10	Vitamin B12 (Cobalamin)	355
20.11	Vitamin C (Ascorbic Acid/Ascorbate)	356
20.12	Vitamin D (Calciferol)	356
20.13	Vitamin E (Tocopherol)	357
20.14	Vitamin K	358

21	**Minerals**	**359**
21.1	Calcium (Ca)	359
21.2	Magnesium (Mg)	360
21.3	Cobalt (Co)	361
21.4	Copper (Cu)	362
21.5	Chromium (Cr)	363
21.6	Manganese (Mn)	363
21.7	Selenium (Se)	364
21.8	Zinc (Zn)	364

22	**Therapeutic & Toxicological Analyses**	**366**
22.1	Basic Concepts	366
22.2	Therapeutic Drug Monitoring	366
22.3	Drugs of Abuse	367
22.4	Poisoning/Overdose	372
22.5	Targeted Testing of Blood and Urine	376

23	**Prenatal Testing**	**377**
23.1	Human Chorionic Gonadotropin (hCG)	377
23.2	Prenatal Screening	378
23.3	Preterm Delivery Risk Evaluation	379
23.3.1	Fetal fibronectin (FFN)	379
23.4	Fetal Lung Maturity Methods	380
23.4.1	Lecithin: Sphingomyelin ratio (L:S)	380
23.4.2	Other methods	380
23.5	Fetal Hemolysis and Bilirubin Levels	381
23.6	Effect of Pregnancy on Certain Laboratory Tests	381

24	**Appendix**	**382**
24.1	Abbreviations	382

25	**Index**	**392**

1   General Overview

1.1   Laboratory Diagnostics

A prerequisite of a rational diagnosis is the targeted use of diagnostic methods. Laboratory investigations should not be used in a vacuum, but rather must be evaluated within the clinical context, history, and physical examination. One should have a "working hypothesis" and order tests appropriately so that the information gleaned from the results will have meaning. Therefore, it is important to understand what you are trying to accomplish by ordering each test, and you should already know how each possible answer (positive/negative, low/high) will effect the clinical decision.

Diagnostic steps:
Step-by-step ordering of tests can be considered based on the differential diagnosis:
- **Basic studies:** Often ordered for first evaluation in order to help formulate the differential diagnosis and avoid the cost associated with more specific and expensive tests
- **Further studies:** For the purpose of confirmation or exclusion of a suspected disorder; usually require a higher effort and higher costs

The benefit of the multiple-step approach is the cost savings obtained by the more targeted use of more expensive tests. However, the first priority is patient care. If a delayed diagnosis would adversely affect the patient outcome, the stepwise process should be used with caution. This process should be avoided in acutely dangerous, treatable diseases (such as the DDx of the acute abdomen) and when there is a high diagnostic probability based on clinical findings.

1.2   Pre-Analytical Phase

1.2.1   Disinfection methods based on risk of infection

- **Low risk of infection:** Venous blood draws: Use disinfectant (typically alcohol) - wipe thoroughly, from center outward in circular motion, at least 2x. Do not touch area afterwards unless you also disinfected your fingertip. (Note: allowing some drying time allows bacteria to die, decreases puncture pain, and decreases introduction of alcohol into the system)
- **Intermediate risk of infection:** (Intravenous catheters, blood cultures to prevent a contamination): Use disinfectant (typically alcohol, but may be betadine or chlorhexidine) - wipe thoroughly, from center outward in circular motion, at least 3x. Do not touch afterwards

- **High risk of infection:** Joints, spine, and other body cavities: Clean and shave skin, then use disinfectant (typically betadine or chlorhexadine) - wipe thoroughly, from center outward in circular motion, at least 3x. Do not touch afterwards; wear sterile gloves and face mask

1.2.2   Sample types and extraction methods

Def:
- **Specimen:** sample, what was extracted/obtained
- **Analyte:** the component to be measured or identified

Met:
- **Qualitative** procedures ascertain whether substance is present or not, but cannot determine the exact amount
- **Semi-quantitative** procedures give a range of quantity, concentration or activity of an analyte, but do not give an accurate measurement of the amount
- **Quantitative** procedures give the specific quantity, concentration, or activity of the substance as a relative or absolute numeric value

Blood: **General:**

Draw blood into the appropriate color-coded test tube. For serum or plasma, draw ~2.5 times the needed volume. When filling a tube with an anticoagulant or preservative, try to fill completely to avoid dilution and immediately mix by gently inverting the tube 5+ times. Be cognizant of the test being ordered and the specifics recommended: sometimes a tourniquet is not recommended due to the stress it causes, the patient's position (sitting/lying), or the time of day may all be a factor

Whole blood: The plasma with the red and white blood cells

Blood draw: Usually venous, arterial for blood gases, small gauge needle (often 18 for adults, 23 or 25 for babies, 16 for longer IV access) Collect whole blood according to the instructions of the individual test. Typically in a tube with an added preservative, gently invert ~8 times (less for light-blue top, sodium-citrate). Keep at room temperature, or on refrigerator temp. cool packs, do not place tubes in direct contact with cool packs; do not freeze unless part of the test's specific instructions

Capillary: When only small amount of blood is needed, i.e glucose monitoring. Finger stick, typically on the distal lateral ring finger - least painful. Usually wipe away first blood with sterile gauze, then squeeze gently. Apply droplet to test surface or capillary filling tube as indicated by test instructions. Typically use heel in newborns

Plasma:
Pale yellow, ~55% of blood volume, the liquid that blood cells are suspended in: 92%-94% water, 6%-8% plasma proteins (albumin, globulins, fibrinogen, etc.), glucose, clotting factors, electrolytes (Na^+, Ca^{2+}, Mg^{2+}, HCO_3^-, Cl^-, etc), hormones and carbon dioxide
Use an anticoagulant (EDTA, Na-citrate, Na-/NH4/Li-Heparin or NaF), draw 12 mL of blood for each 5 mL of plasma needed into an appropriate anticoagulant tube and gently swish to distribute evenly, centrifuge for 10-15 min @ 2,200-2,500 rpm, and the supernatant is equivalent to the plasma

Advantages:
Coagulation does not have to be waited for (saves 30-60 min), 10%-20% higher material yield, avoid changes caused by blood clotting, no re-clotting of centrifuged material

Disadvantages:
Contamination with cations, reaction of metal with EDTA and citrate (inhibition of AP, and amylase-activity), serum electrophorese only after pre-treatment

Serum:
- Plasma without the clotting factors/fibrinogen
- May use a tube without anticoagulant and wait for clotting to occur; place tube upright, equilibrate 30-60 min, then centrifuge 10-15 min @ 2,200-2,500 rpm; or may use a serum-separator tube with coagulation promoting additives (invert 5-8x), after blood clot forms (~30 min) centrifuge for 10-15 min @ 2,200-2,500 rpm
- Do not use serum separating tubes for drug level monitoring or toxicology as the material in these extracts lipophilic substances (most drugs) and will give falsely low concentrations

Anticoagulants/additives
- **EDTA (ethylenediamine tetraacetic acid):** Purple/lavender. Binds Ca^{2+} needed for coagulation (factors V and VIII, and fibrin polymerization). Will also bind other divalent metals (Mg^{2+}, Cu^{2+}, Fe^{2+}, Hg^{2+}, Pb^{2+}) as well as divalent ions (AP and amylase). Most common; CBCs, lipoprotein analysis.

- **Citrate (sodium-citrate):** Light-blue. Binds Ca^{2+}, reversible anticoagulant, used for coagulation testing, appropriate citrate: blood ratio is 1:10 to avoid dilution, tests should be done within 2 h. When testing the ESR, the citrate: blood ratio is 1:5
- **Heparin:** Green. Inhibits activation of prothrombin to thrombin, the cleavage of fibrinogen to fibrin, and helps stabilize platelets; used in most chemistry analysis (electrolytes, enzymes, blood gases), except ammonia and acid phosphatase
- **Fluoride:** An antiglycolytic agent, used when glucose analysis is needed, forms flourophosphate and binds with Mg^{2+} to complex and inactivate enolase, ie, blocks the glycolysis pathway. Usually combined with an anticoagulant

Top-color codes for blood collection tubes:

- **Red glass:** Contains no additives, for antibodies and drugs
- **Light yellow:** Sodium polyanethol sulfonate (SPS), for blood culture or acid-citrate-dextrose (ACD), for HLA phenotyping, DNA, and paternity

Containing coagulants:

- **Gold or red/black 'tiger':** Clot activator and gel, used for serum
- **Orange or grey/yellow 'tiger':** Thrombin, a rapid clot activator, for STAT serum testing

Red plastic: Clot activator and silicone coated, used for serum

Containing anticoagulants:

- **Black:** Buffered Na-citrate, used for erythrocyte sedimentation rate (ESR)
- **Dark blue:** May contain EDTA or have no additive, used for trace metal analysis
- **Green:** Sodium heparin or lithium heparin used for plasma (eg, urea and electrolytes)
- **Grey:** Potassium oxalate/NaF, NaF/Na_2EDTA, or NaF; for determining glucose; fluoride is antiglycolytic agent, oxalate/EDTA as anticoagulant
- **Light blue:** Na-citrate or citrate/theophylline/adenosine/ dipyridamole (CTAD); citrate is a reversible anticoagulant; used for coagulation and platelet function tests. Because the liquid citrate dilutes the blood, it is important the tube is filled

- **Light green or green/gray 'tiger':** Lithium heparin and gel, used for plasma
- **Pink:** Spray-coated K2EDTA plastic tubes, similar to purple tops; designed with special blood cross-match label as required by AABB
- **Purple or lavender:** EDTA (potassium salt: liquid K3EDTA-glass, spray-coated K2EDTA-plastic), generally used when whole blood needed (CBC, peripheral smears), can be used for blood type and screen (but not cross-matches)
- **Tan (glass or plastic):** Sodium heparin (glass) or K2EDTA (plastic), certified to contain no lead, for lead determinations

Special considerations:
- **Fibrin split products (FSP):** To prevent in vitro split product formation complete coagulation is required
- **Transport >1 h or longer storage:** Need to separate serum/plasma and blood cells
- **Blood grouping:** Venous whole blood, pink-top tube if cross-match
- **Protein electrophoresis:** Need serum, fibrinogen removed
- **Lipoprotein electrophoresis:** Do not use heparin, sequesters lipoproteins

Urine:
- **Random:** Mostly for routine urinalysis
- **Mid-stream urine:** To test for bacteria, last urination should be at least 3 h prior, first morning controversial some say best due to bacterial growth time, some say will give false positives due to the stagnant nature. **Procedure:** Patient washes the hands, then cleans area with wipes 2-3 times, one swipe each in same direction, first part of urine allowed to fall, then collect in sterile cup until ~half full, patient can then finish into toilet as normal
- **Catheter:** Tube directly inserted through urethra into bladder, care must be taken to insert under sterile conditions to avoid introducing bacteria, especially in women considering proximity of normal vaginal and rectal flora, only use when clinically indicated
- **24 hour urine:** For quantitative studies, patient can choose time, but often 8 am to 8 am the next day; begin by emptying bladder and discarding urine, for the next 24 h urinate into a container and then transfer to a storage container, store urine in fridge immediately after each addition, last sample will be at 24 h, then turn in container as instructed

CSF: **Cerebrospinal fluid (CSF):**
Largely water with 0.3% plasma proteins, clear, acellular. Typically obtained by lumbar puncture: patient lies on side in fetal position, or sitting-up leans far forward (knees to chest), to open the posterior spine; area is cleaned in sterile manner, needle is inserted, opening pressure may be measured, first 5 drops discarded, fluid slowly flows/drips out and is collected in sterile container. Adults: 5-10 mL, children: 3-5 mL. Should be evaluated within 2 h to avoid cellular degeneration (if cells present)
Alternative sites are cisternal (through occipital bone), with fluoroscopy, or ventricular (hole drilled in skull). These sites are rarely, if ever, used, but may be necessary if there is significant need for CSF and there is a back deformity or infection

Body sites: Abdomen, pleural cavity, joint spaces, bone marrow. Not routinely performed unless obvious clinical indication. Sterile conditions required. Usually needle inserted and fluid removed with syringe. Individual techniques will vary

Feces: May be done in the hospital or at home. Stool is made in a container/bed pan, and then scooped into a provided container with provided spatula

1.2.3 Transport

All human materials must be considered infectious and require stable transport in leak-proof containers. If samples are being mailed, container must be shatter proof, usually opaque, and packed in absorbent material. Cool packs provided if necessary for sample preservation

1.2.4 Potential errors

Laboratory errors may be thought of as preanalytical, analytical, and postanalytical. Preanalytical would include incorrect test, incorrect patient, and circumstances that effect the integrity of the specimen. Analytical refers to systematic and random errors (discussed below). Postanalytical include errors in/delayed reporting, miscommunication, and inappropriate reaction. Most errors are pre- and postanalytical

- **Collection (preanalytical):** Variable and preventable. Sources include patient preparation, sampling itself, storage and transport. Inappropriate cleaning. Order of draw. Drawing downstream of IV input. Lack of attention to timing (cardiac enzymes after suspected MI, circadian rhythms-cortisone). Artificial hemolysis due to delayed transport or insufficient mixing of tube. Dilution in additives (not enough blood). Other tests are affected by eating/fasting, recent physical activity/immobilization, stress, drugs (including prescription, smoking, alcohol, and illicit), diseases. Must know the nuances of the test you are ordering

- **Physiologic (preanalytical):** Considered invariable and are not preventable, but must be taken into account. Age, gender, weight/BMI, ethnic origin, menstrual cycle/pregnancy, and if necessary, climate, muscle mass, socio-economic status and lifestyle
- **Interference:** Some tests will be effected by other components in the sample. Hemolysis, jaundice (hyperbilirubinemia), and hyperlipidemia are common examples. Antibodies/antigens. Also, many drugs affect testing pathways

Common examples of lab result interference:
- Physical activity: CK ↑
- Immobilization: creatinine ↓, CK ↓, urine Ca^{2+}, ammonia, phosphate, Na^+ and Cl^- ↑; catecholamines ↓
- Resuscitation: CK ↑, CK-MB ↑, myoglobin ↑
- Rectal palpation: PSA ↑
- Thyroid palpation: thyroglobulin ↑
- Mechanical heart valve: hemolysis
- Stress/mental stress: adrenaline ↑ → glycogenolysis and cortisol ↑
- Long-standing stasis: cholesterol levels ↑
- Light exposure of the samples: rapid destruction of bilirubin and vitamin D
- Vegetarians: significant reduction of age-related cholesterol levels
- Alcohol abuse: AST ↑, ALT ↑, MCV ↑, B12 ↓; AST/ALT >2
- Smoking: CEA ↑, CO ↑ → total hemoglobin ↑, cholesterol ↑, antinuclear antibodies ↓
- Lack of sun exposure (eg, winter): vitamin D ↓

1.3 Analytical Phase

1.3.1 Interpretation of laboratory values

The analytical phase is the actual testing that is performed, often by laboratory equipment, but sometimes by hand/personnel. Errors can occur if the machine is not set up or cared for properly, the reagents are expired or inappropriate, etc. **Systematic variability** (analytical bias) is when there is a set issue that is affecting all of the results. They may be constant (slope of line similar but intercepts vary, ie, parallel lines, all results are lower or higher than they should be) or proportional (slope differs, ie, lines cross, results at one end will be higher/lower, and the other end will be opposite)

There are rules in laboratory medicine to try and limit these errors to ensure that the 'target value' and the 'actual value' are consistent

The **accuracy** is how close the result is to the actual value (ie, how close you get to the bulls-eye). This is determined by using control samples: samples of a known quantity/value. If the target value is specified, there are rules on the variation of the results. By calibrating the test accordingly, the laboratory test can be safely used for patient samples

1.3.2 Precision

Precision describes the reproducibility of repeated measurements, their dispersion around the mean (ie, how close all your results are to each other, regardless of how accurate they are). These differences are due to the inherent random variability of the testing process. There is precision within a specific run that is based on analyte concentration (higher generally equals better). And there is day-to-day precision: the same sample is run several times on different days and the results are analyzed to see how much variability there is. These differences may be due to environmental factors (temperature) or the technologist performing the test. The best test is both precise and accurate.

Accuracy	Good	Good	Bad
Precision	Good	Bad	Good
Assessment	Optimal	Random error	Systematic error

1.3.3 Coefficient of variation

Coefficient of variation (CV) is the term used to express precision and is the standard deviation (SD) of the results expressed as a percentage of the mean

$$CV = SD/mean \times 100$$

CV varies with analyte concentration

1.3.4 Standard deviation

The mean is the mathematical average of a set of data. The **median** is literally the number in the middle when you line them all up in numerical order. In a normal Gaussian distribution (data makes a symmetric bell-shaped curve), the mean equals the median. The **standard deviation (SD)** describes the average deviation of each of the measured values (x_i) compared to the mean

$$SD = \sqrt{[\sum(x_i - mean)^2/(n - 1)]}$$

where "n" is the number of data points

1.3.5 Control

A test is **under control if no systematic** (reagent [lot change, deterioration]), calibration, temperature, gradual deterioration of equipment) or no extreme **random** (bubbles [in reagent or equipment], improper set-up, technician variation) error is present (typically values within 2-3 standard deviations around the mean). The method to test control is to plot the SD around the mean (Levey-Jennings chart) and then utilize the **Westgard rules**. If any of the below conditions are met, the run was 'out-of-order' and the results must be discarded.

1:3s - if 1 value is +/- 3 SD from the mean (random)
2:2s - if 2 consecutive values are located >2 SD on the same side of the mean (systematic)
R: 4s - if 2 values within the same run are located >4 SD from each other (random)
4:1s - if 4 consecutive values are located >1 SD on the same side of the mean (systematic)
10: mean - if 10 consecutive values are on the same side of the mean (systematic)

1.3.6 Quality assurance

Quality assurance (QA) refers to the activities implemented in a laboratory to ensure the quality of product/service. It involves systematic measurements, comparison to the standard, constant monitoring of processes, and an appropriate response pathway for error notification and prevention. The principles of QA include: 1) Is the test suitable for the intended purpose? and 2) Mistakes should be evaluated and eliminated. It includes the quality of the materials, equipment, personnel, and inspection. Determined by users, not by general public, and is not related to cost.

Laboratory organization:

Typical laboratory errors occur when dividing the original samples, performing serial measurements, and/or error in the evaluation or transfer of data. Laboratories today strive for organization (and therefore error reduction) by creating primary sample identification by using automatically printed and scan-able labels, measuring instruments, and automatic computerized data.

- **Internal quality controls** are based on the constant review of accuracy and precision of the analytical methods based on control samples
- **External quality controls** are represented by the so-called interlaboratory tests: the same sample is sent to different laboratories and the results are compared to ensure quality not only in your lab (that your values are not off), but to ensure consistent care between institutions (so that laboratory data can be transmitted and useful from New York to California). Participation in external QC is required by law

1.4   Postanalytical Phase/Interpretation

1.4.1   Reference ranges

For laboratory purposes, these are the 'normal values', ie, the range of values for healthy individuals (samples often obtained from laboratory staff or volunteers). For testing purposes, in a Gaussian/parametric distribution (bell-shaped curve) this is the middle 95% (+/- 2 SD). That implies that 5% of individuals may be healthy, but will have abnormal values (2.5% high, 2.5% low). A non-parametric approach may be used for a test where the values are skewed or has an asymmetric tail (eg, where '0' is normal)

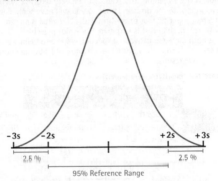

95% Reference Range

1.4.2   Sensitivity

The sensitivity is the probability of a test to accurately identify a positive result, ie, if the disease/analyte is present, will the test be positive. False negatives (type II error) are when the disease/analyte is present, but the test was negative, ie, didn't 'catch it'.

Sensitivity = True positives/(True positives + False negatives) × 100

High sensitivity is good for a screening test, very few false negatives means few people with the disease will be missed. This is especially important in diseases that are very aggressive and/or easily treatable. Sensitivity will be limited by the levels of possible detection (the smallest concentration detectable - analyte sensitivity). A very sensitive test may give false positives and therefore may be followed up with a more specific, but more expensive, test.

1.4.3   Specificity

The specificity is a probability of a test to accurately identify a negative result, ie, if the disease/analyte is absent will the test be negative. False positives (type I error) are when the disease/analyte is absent, but the test was positive.

Specificity = True negatives/(True negatives + False positives) × 100

A high specificity is good to confirm a disease/analyte is absent. They are often used to confirm a result after a less expensive, but more sensitive, screening test. A low specificity leads to many false positive results, hence, not a good screening tool.

A good example is HIV screening. You want it to be very sensitive to ensure that you 'catch' everyone with the disease, knowing you will have some false positives. You then get a more specific test to confirm if the HIV virus is present. If the confirmatory (more specific) test is negative, HIV is not present.

The best test is both highly sensitive and specific, while also being inexpensive, very few of these exist. You also want a limited amount of overlap between the positive and negative results.

Punnett square for sensitivity and specificity:

	Disease/analyte present	Disease/analyte absent	
Test positive	True positive (TP)	False positive (FP)	PPV = TP(TP+FP)
Test negative	False negative (FN)	True negative (TN)	NPV = TN/(TN+FN)
	Sensitivity = TP/(TP+FN)	Specificity = TN/(TN+FP)	

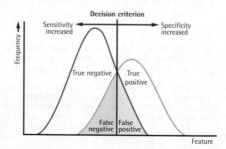

1.4.4 Predictive value

While sensitivity and specificity are from the perspective of the disease/analyte, the predictive value is based on a test result perspective. It is akin to saying how accurate the test is. Predictive value is effected by the pretest probability based on the prevalence of a disease, whereas sensitivity and specificity are not. This means that when the prevalence is low, the PPV of a test ↓ and the NPV ↑; and vice versa.

Positive predictive value:

Positive predictive value (PPV) is the probability that the disease is present when there is a positive test result, ie, if the test is positive, how likely is it that you have the disease

$$PPV = True\ positives/(True\ positives + False\ positives) \times 100$$

A high PPV is good for ruling in a certain disease, especially important when the treatment is expensive and/or toxic and not to be taken lightly

Negative predictive value:

Analogous to the PPV, the negative predictive value (NPV) is the probability that the disease is absent when there is a negative test result, ie, if the test is negative, how likely is it that you don't have the disease

$$NPV = True\ negatives/(True\ negatives + False\ negatives) \times 100$$

A high NPV is good when you want to be sure you have ruled out a disease, especially important when a disease is aggressive and/or easily treated, and can now be taken off the differential diagnosis

1.4.5 Plausibility

Lab results should always be considered for plausibility; that is, always be cognizant of the possibility of an error, particularly if the findings are much different than expected given the clinical history and/or other laboratory findings. Each lab needs to be addressed as part of the whole picture, not in isolation. This is particularly useful for catching random errors. If the results seem erroneous, follow-up with the laboratory and work together to ensure that the test is accurate. Remember to address the issue with respect for those involved.

1.4.6 Longitudinal evaluation

This refers to the comparison of the results with those previously obtained from that individual. Be wary of any results that vary widely from previous. This works concurrently with plausibility in reference to errors and is important for assessment of disease progression and response.

1.5   Units

- **Volume:** How much space a substance takes up. In the laboratory the base unit is the **liter (L)**, commonly used subunits are dL and mL. Small amounts are measured in the **cubic centimeter (cc–cm^3)**, which is equivalent to 1 **milliliter (mL)**
- **Weight:** The base unit of mass is the **gram (g)**, commonly used units are kg, mg, µg
- **Length:** The base unit is the **meter (m)**, commonly used subunits are cm and mm
- **Concentration:** The particle count per volume of a liquid; g/dL, g/mL, µg/L
- **Pressure:** Pressure is the vertical force acting on a surface divided by the area. Typically reported in pounds per square inch (PSI) or millimeters of mercury (mmHg)
- **Partial pressure:** The partial pressure is the measurement of a specific gaseous component in reference to the pressure in the total gaseous system
- **Density:** The ratio of the mass to volume of a solid; kg/L, g/dL. Dependence on ambient pressure and temperature
- **Mole:** A unit of measurement used to express amount of a substance as defined by the amount particles as there are atoms in 12 g of pure carbon. This corresponds to the Avogadro's number, 6.022×10^{23}
- **Enzyme activity:** The mass concentrations (g/L) of enzymes in the blood are very low and with the exception of few enzyme-specific tests, not measurable. One (1) **International enzyme unit** (IU) is the amount that releases 1 µmol of substrate per minute

Prefixes in the SI-system:

Yotta Y x10^{24} = 1 000 000 000 000 000 000 000 000 (septillion)
Zetta Z x10^{21} = 1 000 000 000 000 000 000 000 (sextillion)
Exa E x10^{18} = 1 000 000 000 000 000 000 (quintillion)
Peta P x10^{15} = 1 000 000 000 000 000 (quadrillion)
Tera T x10^{12} = 1 000 000 000 000 (trillion)
Giga G x10^{9} = 1 000 000 000 (billion)
Mega M x10^{6} = 1 000 000 (1 million)
Kilo k x10^{3} = 1 000
Hecto- h x10^{2} = 1 00
Deka D x10^{1} = 10
Deci d x10^{-1} = 0.1 (tenth)
Centi c x10^{-2} = 0.01 (hundredth)
Milli m 10^{-3} = 0.001 (thousandth)
Micro µ 10^{-6} = 0.000 001 (millionth)
Nano n 10^{-9} = 0.000 000 001 (billionth)
Pico p 10^{-12} = 0.000 000 000 001 (trillionth)
Femto f 10^{-15} = 0.000 000 000 000 001 (quadrillionth)
Atto a 10^{-18} = 0.000 000 000 000 000 001 (quintillionth)
Zepto z 10^{-21} = 0.000 000 000 000 000 000 001 (sextillionth)
Yocto y 10^{-24} = 0.000 000 000 000 000 000 000 001 (septillionth)

2   Analytical Methods

2.1   Optical Measurement Methods

- **Spectrophotometry:**
  Photometry is a quantitative measurement of the reflection or transmission of wavelengths through a material. It is used to measure the concentration of particles in solution. Using light of a certain wavelength, the amount absorbed in the material (the difference between the course and what is present after passing through) is measured. Substance-specific wavelengths with the strongest absorption rates are used

- **Fluorophotometry:**
  Fluorophotometry is measurement of the light emitted by a fluorescent substance (typically fluorescein) in order to evaluate the integrity of the retinal vasculature, commonly done in diabetics

- **Turbidimetry:**
  The process of measuring the loss of intensity of a transmitted light through a substance due to scattering effect of the suspended particles. Used for concentrations of liquids and gases, or to count the number of cells in a solution. The stronger the turbidity, the higher the concentration

- **Nephelometry:**
  Related to turbidimetry. The process of measuring the concentrations of particles in a fluid. Typically in immunology (immunonephelometry) to determine levels of plasma proteins (immunoglobulins). May detect antigens or antibodies, but is usually run with antibody as the agent and searching for the patient's unknown antigen. Light is passed through a sample and the amount of scatter is measured for a given angle (usually 30 and 90 degrees). Antibody and antigens are mixed and small aggregates are formed that do not quickly settle to the bottom, but will effect the light scatter

- **Luminescence:**
  The emission of light, not resulting from heat, but from some sort of reaction. In laboratory medicine, this is typically the result of chemiluminescence - the emission of light and production of a new substance as a result of a chemical reaction. Often used for enzyme immunoassays. Another example is the glow of Luminal when it interacts with the iron in blood

- **Fluorescence anisotropy/spectroscopy:**
  Based on the theory that light emitted by a fluorescent molecule has different intensities along different axes. When a molecule emits energy (typically by losing a photon), it occurs along a certain axis. When polarized light is applied to a group of randomly oriented fluorescent molecules, the ones that gain energy will be oriented at a particular angle to the light. Due to random rotation, the light given off when the molecule loses energy will be in a different plane. A smaller molecule will rotate faster than a larger one, and a bound pair even slower, therefore, by slowly adding a substrate (titrating) and measuring the light given off, you can measure the amount of a specific substance in a solution. This method is used with proteins or RNA to study the dynamics of folding, and in signaling cascades to detect binding of molecules to certain cues.

- **Flame emission spectrometry (Photometry):**
  When molecules are heated they emit energy in the form of light, analysis of the wavelength of light emitted can be used to identify a substance/compound, and even the amount present. The emissions are measured using a calibrated spectroscope. Particularly suitable for Na^+, K^+, Ca^{2+}, Mg^{2+}, and Li^+. A cheap, but less accurate method is performed without a monochromatic measuring device (flame photometry)

- **Atomic absorption spectroscopy (AAS):**
  The quantitation of a substance by way of light absorption by free atoms in a gaseous state. Used for determining the concentration of a specific element in a steam form. Over 70 elements possible, but best for Ca^{2+}, Mg^{2+}, and Fe^{2+}.

2.2   Electrochemical Methods

A group of analytical techniques which study an analyte by measuring the volts (potential) and amperes (current). They are broken down based on which aspects are controlled and what is actually measured

- **Potentiometry:**
  Measurement of potential difference in an electrode in an electrolyte solution, measured in volts. The potential is related to the concentration of one or more analytes in the solution. The electrode is actually 2 electrodes, indicator and reference, and may be selectively sensitive for the analyte in question. pH is the most common application

- **Voltammetry:**
  Measurement of current output while actively applying a constant or variable potential, revealing the reduction potential of an analyte. Specific electrodes can be used for high sensitivity, similar to potentiometry. One subclass is **polarimetry/polarography**, which uses a mercury electrode. This method is not often used due to the toxicity of mercury. Another subclass is **amperometry**, in which the electrode is held at a constant potential for varying lengths of time. Historically this was different from voltammetry based on the variability of the potential, but today the terms are practically interchangeable. The one difference is that amperometry uses an average reading over time, while in voltammetry each reading is read independently at specific time intervals. This makes amperometry more precise.

- **Coulometry:**
  Measuring a current over time, unit: coulomb (C). Uses an applied current to change an analyte's oxidative state and the total current used is measured to determine the number of electrons present, and through that, the concentration. Or similarly, an analyte (eg, Ag^+) can be added that binds an analyte (eg, Cl^-) in the solution, an insoluble salt will form, and the amount of free analyte (in this case, Ag^+) can be measured. By titrating the additive analyte, you can calculate the concentration of the original analyte in the solution (in this case, Cl^-).

2.3   Electrophoresis

The motion of particles through a viscous suspension in response to an applied voltage. The particle movement is effected by charge and size (smaller particles move farther) and their relative position can be used for identification. Results are dependent on the applied voltage and the viscosity of the suspension. Cataphoresis - positively charged particles (cations), anaphoresis - negative charged particles (anions)

- **Serum protein electrophoresis (SPEP):**
  Examines the specific proteins in blood serum, largely globulins: albumin, $\alpha1$, $\alpha2$, β, and γ. Using a special paper treated with agarose gel, an electrical current (~200 V) is applied for a set amount of time (~20 min). The amount of particles in each location can then be measured and the amount of those proteins can be inferred.

- **Gel electrophoresis:**
  Used for separating DNA (Southern blot), RNA (Northern blot), and proteins (Western blot). Particles are placed in a gel and a current is applied to cause migration based on size and charge. Typically the substance is amplified by PCR prior to testing. There are several gel types: agarose - most common, easy to make/store, inexpensive, used for DNA or proteins larger than 200 kDa; polyacrylamide - good for smaller particles (5-2,000 kDa), proteins, small DNA fragments, acrylamide is a neurotoxin; partially hydrolyzed potato starch - more opaque, used for proteins. Often combined with **electroblotting**, a method used to transfer proteins or nucleic acids from the gel onto a membrane allowing further analysis using probes such as specific antibodies or stains.

- **Isoelectric focusing (IEF):**
  AKA electrofocusing. Used to separate molecules by their isoelectric point (pI), best for proteins as their charge varies based on the surrounding pH. The analyte solution is added to an immobilized pH gradient gel, an acrylamide gel co-polymerized with a pH gradient, and a current is applied creating a 'positive' anode (acidic) end and a 'negative' cathode (alkaline) end. When a protein is in a region below its pI, it will be positively charged and will migrate towards the cathode. When it reaches its pI there is no net charge and the protein becomes stationary and can be identified.

- **Isotachophoresis:**
  Uses a discontinuous electrical field to create sharp delineations of particles. Particularly useful for proteins and lipoproteins. Typically performed in a capillary tube, the sample is placed between a fast leading electrolyte and a slow terminating electrolyte at a specific pH. When a potential is applied, the particles separate based on charge and size.

- **Capillary electrophoresis:**
  Used to separate particles by their ionic charge, frictional forces, and hydrodynamic radius. Voltage is applied to the ends and separation occurs based on the size-to-charge ratio of individual particles to the interior of a small capillary tube filled with an electrolyte.

2.4   Immunological Methods

2.4.1   Direct antigen and antibody detection

- **Agglutination:**
  In general, the clumping of particles, Latin agglutinare = 'to glue.' In immunology, the clumping of bacteria or red blood cells in the presence of an antibody.
- **Immunodiffusion:**
  The diffusion of antigens and antibodies (immunoglobulins) through a gel.
  - **Simple/Radial immunodiffusion (Mancini method):** Used in immunology to determine the quantity of an antigen. An antigen is added to an agar gel containing a suspended antibody. The resultant circle of precipitant can be measured and corresponds to the original concentration of the antigen. Measurements are more accurate of larger circles than of smaller circles, so it is best to adjust the concentration of antibody and the quantity of antigen accordingly.
  - **Ouchterlony double immunodiffusion:** AKA agar gel immunodiffusion or passive double immunodiffusion. Used to detect, identify, and quantify antibodies and antigens. A sample and purified antibodies are each placed in separate wells (holes) in a gel. Over time, the antigens from the sample and the antibodies will diffuse through the gel. If the appropriate antigen is present for the given antibody, the two meet and a precipitant will form (immune complex) that can be visualized. This can be performed with multiple known antibodies at once in a clock-like pattern around a sample, therefore identifying the presences of multiple antigens at once.
- **Immunoelectrophoresis**:
  A general name for several methods of separation and identification of proteins using gel electrophoresis and antibody reaction. In the classic method, proteins are separated by electrophoresis, antibodies are then applied and the presence of immunoprecipitates is evaluated. Not widely used because it is work intensive, and it requires skill and require large amounts of antibody. Variations of this include **crossed immunoelectrophoresis** (also called two-dimensional quantitative immunoelectrophoresis) - proteins are first separated using electrophoresis, then the proteins are electrophoresed into an antibody-containing gel; **rocket immunoelectrophoresis** - one-dimensional method used for quantitation of serum proteins before automated methods became available; **affinity immunoelectrophoresis** - based on changes in the electrophoretic pattern of proteins through interaction with other ligands; used for estimation of binding constants similar to affinity chromatography, but uses mobilized ligands.

- **Immunofixation electrophoresis:**
  Similar to immunoelectrophoresis. Used to detect and type monoclonal antibodies (immunoglobulins) in serum or urine. The sample is placed in a gel and the proteins dispersed, then antigens are added for the target antibody and precipitation is measured. Good for diagnosing myeloma and Waldenstrom macroglobulinemia. Often replaces protein electrophoresis because it is quicker (~3 h), more sensitive, and more easily performed and interpreted, but is more expensive and only works for antibodies.

- **Immunoturbidimetry:**
  The process of performing turbidimetry (measuring light absorption/scatter changes; see turbidimetry above) based on immunocomplex formation in order to quantify antigen in serum/urine.

- **Immunonephelometry:**
  The process of performing nephelometry (measuring light scatter; see nephelometry above) based on immune complex formation in order to quantify antigen or antibody.

2.4.2 Indirect antigen and antibody detection

- **Latex agglutination (Direct):**
  An immunochemical detection method for the presence of an antibody or antigen in various body fluids (blood, CSF, saliva, urine). The sample is added to tiny latex beads coated with a specific antibody or antigen; clumping occurs if immunocomplexes are formed giving a positive result. Common uses: rapid strep test (throat swab), rheumatoid factor (blood), pregnancy tests (urine).

- **Direct antiglobulin test (Direct Coombs):**
  Used to detect antibodies or complement proteins bound to the surface of RBCs in vivo. A blood sample is washed in saline (to remove the patient's plasma) and then the RBCs are incubated with a specific antihuman globulin (Coombs reagent). If agglutination occurs, this is a positive test, ie, the antibody/protein was present on the RBC surface. Commonly used to look for immune-mediated hemolytic anemias.

- **Indirect antiglobulin test (Indirect Coombs):**
  Used to detect in vitro antibody-antigen reactions in order to detect very low concentrations of antibodies present unbound in a patient's plasma. This is a two-stage test: The patient's serum is added to washed RBCs with known antigens (ie, RBCs with known reference values from other patient samples), if the serum has the specific antibodies they will bind to the RBC surface. Then the RBCs are washed again with saline and incubated with antihuman globulin (Coombs reagent).

If agglutination occurs, this is a positive result, ie, the antibody was present in the serum. Commonly used in prenatal testing (looking for antibodies that could cause hemolytic disease of the newborn), and in blood transfusion testing.

- **Complement fixation test:**
Serological testing method used to detect the presence of a specific antibody or antigen. Compliment factors are serum proteins that react with immunocomplexes and if a reaction occurs on the surface of a cell, a trans-membrane pore is formed and hemolysis ensues. A patient's serum is heated appropriately to destroy any complement proteins, but none of the antibodies. Then a known amount of standard complement is added, followed by the antigen of interest. The mixture is then added to sheep RBCs (sRBC) which have pre-bound anti-sRBC. If the solution turns pink (hemolysis present), the test is negative, ie, no antibodies were present in the patient's serum. This is because if the patient's serum contains antibody to the antigen of interest, they will form immunocomplexes that will activate the complement factor, depleting it all. Therefore, if there is complement left to hemolyze the sRBC, there was no antibody-antigen reaction prior. May be used to quantify the amount of antibody by setting up multiple dilutions of the patient's serum and determining the highest dilution factor that will yield a positive result. Used to diagnose infectious agents, particularly those not easily cultured; and rheumatic diseases, but has been largely replaced by other methods such as ELISA and PCR.

- **Hemagglutination assay (HA):**
Used to quantify viruses or bacteria based on surface proteins that will agglutinate RBCs, forming a 'lattice.' The virus/bacteria is titrated (tested at multiple dilutions) to see where the last viable 'lattice' is formed, thereby quantify the amount of infectious particles present. The related hemagglutination inhibition assay is used specifically for influenza virus antibody levels in the serum. Here titrated serum antibodies will interfere with virus attachment to RBCs, and the concentration can be ascertained by inhibition of hemagglutination.

- **Immunofluorescence:**
Method for the detection of antigens in cells and tissues by using specific antibodies tagged with a fluorescent dye.
  - **Direct immunofluorescence:** A single (primary) fluorescent-labeled antibody binding directly to the target antigen. Commonly used in autoimmune disorders/transplant rejection or in virus detection in cell cultures. Few steps, limited background signal, less antibody cross-reactivity; but since less antibody is bound there is a smaller signal, therefore it is less sensitive.

- **Indirect immunofluorescence:** Uses two antibodies; the first (primary) unlabeled antibody binds the target antigen, and the secondary fluorescent-labeled antibody binds to the first antibody. Since many secondary antibodies (or even a variety of secondary antibodies) can bind to one primary antibody there is signal amplification, hence higher sensitivity. However, there are more steps and therefore more time consuming, and there is a greater possibility of cross-reactions and background staining.

- **Radioimmunoassay (RIA):**
  A very sensitive and specific method for determining the concentration of an antigen by using antibodies (The inverse of a **radiobinding assay** which quantifies antibody using antigens). Though it requires special equipment, training, and licensing for the radioactive substances, it is still the least expensive method available, but more recently has been replaced with ELISA, a more expensive, but less difficult procedure. The test is done by making a known quantity of antigen radioactive, then mixing it with a known amount of antibody forming immunocomplexes. This is added to the patient's serum containing an unknown quantity of the same antigen. The unlabeled (cold) antigen will compete with the labeled (hot) antigen for antibody binding. As the concentration of the unlabeled antigen is increased it will displace more of the labeled antigen. The unbound antigens are then separated and tested for the amount of radioactivity present. The amount of antigen in the patient's serum can then be derived using known binding curves. Examples of this test include blood hormone levels and radioallergosorbent test (RAST) for allergens.

- **Enzyme immunoassay (EIA):**
  A similar method to RIA, where the reaction between the antigen and specific antibodies with bound enzyme. This enzyme then causes a visible color change indicative of a positive result. Almost as sensitive as the RIA, but without the radioactivity.
  - **Enzyme-linked immunosorbent assay (ELISA):** "heterogenous" EIA. Uses antibodies and color change for antigen identification purposes via solid-phase EIA and colorimetry (color change). Antigens from the sample are attached to a solid surface, then specific antibody (with bound enzyme) is added, after washing, the enzymes substrate is added and if enzyme is present (ie, antibody bound to antigen) then a color change occurs.
  - **Enzyme multiplied immunoassay technique (EMIT):** "homogeneous" EIA. Used to identify and quantify drugs and their metabolites in serum/urine, for both drugs of abuse and therapeutic monitoring. Because of social and legal implications, drugs of abuse may be confirmed with mass spectroscopy.

It is similar to ELISA, but has the ability to detect antigen-antibody binding without cumbersome washing. This is done by combining a sample that may contain the drug of interest with a solution containing a known concentration of antibody and enzyme substrate, after allowing a short time for binding a conjugate consisting of the drug bound to enzyme is added, the rate of color change can then be correlated with known concentration curves and the original amount of drug can be quantified.

- **Fluorescence/luminescence enzyme immunoassay**:
  Analogous to RIA and EIA, but the reaction emits fluorescence/light.
- **Immunoblotting (Western blot)**:
  Used to detect proteins in serum using electrophoresis and then transferring the dispersed proteins to a membrane (nitrocellulose or PVDF) and staining with antibody

2.4.3   Flow cytometry

A laser based test used for cell counting, sorting, and biomarker detection. Cells are suspended in a liquid and passed single-file through a laser-based detection device. The scatter of the light is then read and through this measurement, the size of the cell, as well as the presence and amount of specific markers, can be detected. Most commonly used in leukemias/lymphomas

2.5   Chromatographic Separation Processes

- **Chromatography**:
  A method for separating out analyte mixtures. The sample is dissolved into fluid form (mobile phase) and is passed through a stationary phase. As various components of the mixture travel at different speeds, separation occurs. Can be used for purification or analysis. There are two main types, absorbtion and distribution; and variations exist based on the stationary phase (solid, liquid, material, structure) and the mobile phase (gas, liquid).
- **Column chromatography**:
  A separation technique in which the stationary bed is within a tube and the particles of the stationary phase may fill the whole inside volume (packed column) or be concentrated along the inside tube wall leaving a path for the mobile phase (open tubular column). Differences in rates of movement through the medium are then measured. A modified version, **flash column chromatography**, has a solvent driven through the column by applying positive pressure, decreasing the time required (~20 min). **Expanded bed adsorption** uses a fluidized bed, rather than a solid phase, allowing the omission of initial clearing steps (centrifugation, filtration). **Phosphocellulose chromatography** utilizes the binding affinity of many DNA-binding proteins for phosphocellulose.

- **Planar chromatography:**
  A stationary phase is present as a plane. Can be paper (**paper chromatography**) or a layer of solid adsorbent (silica, alumina, or cellulose) spread on a inert support such as a glass plate (**thin layer chromatography**). Compared to paper, TLC is faster and gives better separation.

- **Displacement chromatography:**
  A molecule with a high affinity for the chromatography matrix (the displacer) competes for binding sites, thus displacing molecules with lesser affinities.

- **Gas chromatography:**
  A separation technique in which the mobile phase is a gas. Gas chromatography is always performed in a column, which is typically "packed" or "open."

- **Liquid chromatography:**
  A separation technique in which the mobile phase is a liquid. Can be performed in a column or on a plane. High performance liquid chromatography uses very small packing particles and high pressure to push the mobile phase through.

- **Affinity chromatography:**
  Based on selective non-covalent interaction between an analyte and specific molecules (tag). Often used for the purification of proteins. The 'tagged' proteins are labeled with compounds that bind to the stationary phase. Afterward, the 'tag' is removed and the pure protein is obtained.

- **Ion exchange chromatography:**
  Uses an ion exchange mechanism to separate analytes based on their charges. Usually performed in columns but can be done on planes. A charged stationary phase is used, typically an ion exchange resin. The mobile phase then separates based on the charge of the individual molecules. Commonly used for purification.

- **Gel permeation chromatography:**
  AKA gel filtration chromatography. Separates molecules according to their size (ie, hydrodynamic diameter or volume). Smaller molecules are able to enter the pores of the media and get 'trapped', effectively being removed from the mobile phase. Commonly used as final step in purification, or to determine the tertiary or quaternary structure of a protein.

2.6   Osmotic Pressure

Related to the movement of a solution through a semi-permeable membrane and is dependent on the number of dissolved particles per unit volume (osmotic concentration [osm/L], AKA **osmolarity**), and is independent of the particle size. Similar to **molarity**, the number of moles per unit volume (M/L), and **osmolality**, the number of particles per kg of solvent (osm/kg). Osmolarity and molarity are temperature dependent due to water volume changes, whereas osmolality will remain constant. Often used in reference to blood plasma as a measure of the electrolyte/water balance. Measured by osmometers - increased particles decreases the freezing.

Oncotic pressure:
AKA colloid osmotic pressure. A form of osmotic pressure exerted by macromolecules (proteins, most notably albumin [80%]), used in discussion of blood plasma (~28 mmHg). Dissolved particles have osmotic pressure, but as large proteins cannot cross the vessel walls, their effect on this pressure is constant and helps balance out the tendency for fluid to leak (hydrostatic pressure). High oncotic pressure pulls water into the vasculature. If there is protein loss (proteinuria or malnutrition), the reduction in oncotic pressure leads to fluid loss into the extracellular space resulting in edema.

2.7   Molecular Diagnostics

- **Polymerase chain reaction (PCR):**
  When performing genetic testing or during the detection of microorganisms, there is often insufficient quantity of the target DNA. PCR amplifies the DNA in vitro prior to testing. The process takes several hours and generates thousands to millions of copies. The method relies on thermal cycling; repeated heating and cooling, to denature the DNA, make new double strands using a DNA primer, a bath of free nucleotides, and a thermostable DNA polymerase such as Taq polymerase. As the process continues, the new strands are then themselves used as a template for replication, resulting in exponential amplification.
  The test tube should contain the target DNA, free nucleotides, the primers (3'-5' and 5'-3', must be complements of each other), and a thermostable DNA polymerase such as Taq polymerase.
  The three phases:
  1. Denaturing: Sample is heated to >90°C in order to denature (separate) the double-stranded DNA. This step is reversible (ie, bands could re-unite)

2. Primer-binding/Annealing: Sample is cooled to ~ 50°C allowing the primers to bind the single-stranded DNA. When the primers are in surplus, they will bind their complementary sequences before the strands renaturalize.

3. DNA-synthesis: Sample then reheated to 70°C to allow the free nucleotides to elongate the complementary DNA strand. Polymerization stops when the temperature again reaches 90°C and the process begins again. The process can be continued until the primers or nucleotides are exhausted.

A similar method can be used to amplify RNA. **Reverse transcription polymerase chain reaction (RT-PCR)** is variant of PCR used in molecular biology to detect the presence of RNA by transcribing it into cDNA via reverse transcription. This cDNA product can then be amplified as above. RT-PCR is often confused with **real-time polymerase chain reaction (qPCR)** which quantitatively measures the amplification of DNA using fluorescent probes.

- **Gene probes and nucleic acid hybridization:**
  A method of molecular genetic diagnosis where a specific DNA or RNA fragment is used as a probe to identify if a target is present in the sample.
  - **Southern blot:** A method used to detect specific DNA sequences in a sample. The sample is first separated via gel electrophoresis and transferred to a membrane, then subjected to probe hybridization. If the probe adheres, then the target was present, yielding a positive result. **Northern blot** is a similar method performed with RNA.
  - **Dot blot:** Used for the detection of immobilized antigens on a membrane. A mixture containing the antigen to be detected is directly applied to a membrane as a 'dot.' The sample is then applied. If hybridization occurs, the antigen is present (ie, a positive result). As opposed to Southern, Western, and Northern blotting, no separation by electrophoresis is performed, therefore takes much less time. But there is no way to decipher if 2 or more different molecules are present, and can only be used for molecules that can be detected by DNA probes or antibody. The development of hybridization can be measured by enzymatic color change or radioactivity.
  - **In-situ hybridization:** A type of hybridization that utilizes a labeled DNA or RNA marked probe to identify a specific sequence in tissue cells. Fluorescent ISH (**FISH**) is a commonly used variant using fluorescent markers.

3   Proteins, Metabolites

3.1   Total Protein

A measurement of the total protein in blood plasma/serum.

Ind: Proteinuria, edema, polyuria, chronic kidney disease, chronic liver disease, chronic diarrhea, malignancy, bone pain, lymphomas, bleeding, pregnancy, trauma, shock

Norm: (May vary slightly by institution)
  Serum/plasma:
  - 60-85 g/L (6.5-8.5 g/dL) (children/adults)
  - 45-75 g/L (4.5-7.5 g/dL) (for neonates and infants)

  Urine:
  - ≤10 mg/dL (random)   - ≤150 mg (24 h)

  CSF:
  - 0.15 -0.50 g/dL 15-50 mg/dL (children/adults)
  - ≤150 mg/dL (newborns ≤1 months)
  - ≤100 mg/dL (1-2 months)
  - ≤80 mg/dL (2-3 months)

Path: Dysproteinemias: qualitative and/or quantitative changes of proteins in the serum

↑ **Hyperproteinemia** (↑ protein concentration):
  • **Absolute:** Immunoglobulinemia
    - Chronic infections (rarely >90 g/L)
    - Monoclonal gammopathy (up to 140 g/L) eg, multiple myeloma or Waldenstrom's macroglobulinemia
  • **Relative:** Pseudohyperproteinemia
    - Reduction in plasma volume; eg, diabetes insipidus, diarrhea, extreme dehydration

↓ **Hypoproteinemia** (decreased protein concentration):
  • **Absolute:** Loss or synthesis/storage disorders gamma-globulin reduction
    - Renal (nephrotic syndrome, glomerulonephritis)
    - Exudative enteropathy (Crohn's disease, ulcerative colitis)
    - Burns (loss through the skin)
    - Ascites/pleural effusion
    - Acute viral hepatitis
    - Exocrine pancreatic insufficiency

↓ | • **Relative**: Pseudohypoproteinemia
- Increase in fluid component of plasma volume, ie, infusions, after blood loss, pregnancy

Mat: Serum, plasma, urine, CSF, body fluids

Met: **Serum/fluids:**
- **Biuret-method:** Used to detect peptide bonds. When present, a bright violet forms when Cu- ions are added in an alkaline pH. The color intensity ratio (as measured by light absorption at 540 nm) is directly proportional to the concentration. Despite the name, does not actually contain 'biuret' ($(H_2N-CO-)_2NH$)
- **Kjeldahl method:** Quantitative measurement of the nitrogen content

Cerebrospinal fluid and urine:
- **Coomassie-method:** Coomassie Brilliant Blue is the name of 2 similar dyes original used in the textile industry, now used for staining proteins. Can be used with electrophoresis for staining and identification purposes, or via measuring light absorption (595 nm) using the Bradford assay for quantification
- **Turbidimetry method:** Proteins in solution are denatured using trichloroacetic acid, light scatter is measured, resulting in concentration

3.2   Serum Protein Electrophoresis (SPEP)

Electrophoresis performed on blood serum for the purposes of identifying and quantifying albumin and globulins (α1, α2, β, γ), performed at pH 8.6. Similar test can be performed on urine (UPEP) for identification of proteins lost though the kidneys (should be none) and CSF. Often followed by **immunofixation electrophoresis, immunoelectrophoresis, or immunotyping** in order to specify a monoclonal band.

Func: • Quantitative measure of dysproteinemia
• Great importance for the follow-up of various diseases

Ind: Evaluation of elevated or decreased protein levels (inflammation, kidney/liver disease, malignancy, monoclonal gammopathy, antibody)

Norm: May vary by institution.

3.8-5 g/dL	55%–69%	Albumin
0.1-0.4 g/dL	2%–6%	Alpha-1-globulins
0.3-1 g/dL	6%–1%	Alpha-2-globulins
0.7-1.4 g/dL	8%–14%	Beta-globulins
0.7-1.6 g/dL	11%–18%	Gamma-globulins

Mat: Serum

Met: Perform electrophoresis on a serum sample. Proteins will separate based on size and charge. Albumin is the major component and is normally the largest peak, closest to the positive electrode. See figure below for schematic representation. The area under the curve corresponds to the quantity present

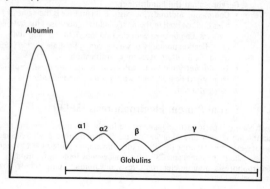

3.3　Albumin

The main protein in the albumin family, a group of proteins that are water-soluble, moderately-soluble in salt solutions, and are not glycosylated

Func:
- Maintains the colloid osmotic (oncotic) pressure within vasculature (80% of plasma protein)
- Important transport molecule, especially for substances with low water solubility (free fatty acids, bilirubin, some hormones and acidic drugs)

Ind:　Any illness associated with protein or fluid loss/dysregulation

Prod:　Liver, approximately 14 g/day

Norm:　**Serum:**　3.5-5 g/dL (≥3 years)
　　　　　　　　　　2.9-5.5 g/dL (<3 years)
　　　　Urine: up to 20 mg/L
　　　　CSF: 110-350 mg/L

↑　Almost always from dehydration, but may be seen in vitamin A deficiency (water enters cells, decreasing vascular volume)

↓　Similarly to general hypoproteinemia
- ↑ vascular permeability ("capillary leakage", sepsis, shock)
- Liver disease (decreased production)
- Ascites, edema
- Increased loss (burns, enteropathy, glomerulonephrosis)
- Malabsorption/malnutrition
- Late pregnancy
- Acute-phase response (negative acute-phase protein!)

Mat:　Serum, urine, CSF

Met:
- **Serum:**
  Same as for general protein. Dye methods, light scatter, turbidimetry/nephelometry, electrophoresis (SPEP). Heterozygous individuals may have 2 albumin bands on SPEP, not associated with disease. ↑ mobility results from binding of bilirubin, fatty acids, penicillin, and ASA possibly leading to a falsely low albumin and a falsely high α1 or α2
- **Cerebrospinal fluid and urine:**
  Same as for general protein. Turbidimetry/nephelometry

- **Prealbumin:**
Transthyretin/Thyroxine-binding prealbumin; the fastest migrating protein on SPEP, however, low concentration, so usually not seen; transports T3 (triiodothyronine), T4 (thyroxine), and RBG/vitamin A complex; The **amyloid precursor** in senile cardiac amyloidosis; and it's short half-life (48 h) makes it especially useful for **nutritional status**; A **negative acute phase reactant**

3.4 Alpha-1-Globulins

Alpha-1-antitrypsin (A1AT): AKA α1-proteinase inhibitor; largest constituent of α1 band (~90%)

Func:	The most important protease inhibitor in plasma; protects tissues from enzymes of inflammatory cells (especially neutrophil elastase → mutation leads to emphysema and cirrhosis)
Ind:	Prolonged icterus in infants, unclear liver disease in children, emphysema in early adulthood, greatly ↑ by smoking
Prod:	Liver and monocytes
Norm:	150-350 mg/dL (1.5-3.5 g/L)
↑	Acute phase reactant, malignancy
↓	Hereditary Alpha-1-antitrypsin deficiency (A1AD) - 10%-20% cirrhosis, 50%-60% emphysema, more than 75 variants known, PiMM: 100% (normal), PiMS: 80%, PiSS: 60%, PiMZ: 60%, PiSZ: 40%, PiZZ: 10%-15% (50% cirrhosis)

- **Alpha-1-antichymotrypsin:** Glycoprotein that inhibits certain proteases (eg, cathepsin G in neutrophils, chymases in mast cells); produced in liver; positive acute phase reactant (increases during inflammation); has been associated with Parkinson disease, COPD, and Alzheimer's disease
- **Orosomucoid:** AKA alpha-1-acid glycoprotein; glycoprotein; 0.6-1.2 mg/mL; carrier of basic and neutrally charged drugs, steroids, and protease inhibitors; produced in liver; positive acute phase reactant; increases in obstructive jaundice and decreases in hepatocellular jaundice; useful for monitoring intestinal disorders (ulcerative colitis)
- **Inter-alpha-trypsin-inhibitor:** protease inhibitors, high concentrations in rheumatoid arthritis
- **Alpha-1-microglobulin:** degrades heme and other free radicals; immune regulator via partial suppression of lymphocytes and neutrophils; produced in all cells, particularly liver; used as indicator of proteinuria (>0.7 mg/mmol creatinine)

- **Alpha-1-lipoprotein:** high-density lipoprotein (HDL); "good" cholesterol; smallest of the lipoproteins; transports cholesterol and triglycerides; removes them from atheroma and returns them to liver for excretion/reutilization; higher levels >40 mg/dL are beneficial; variant ApoA1 Milano gives low measured HDL levels, but also low rates of cardiovascular events
- **Transcobalamin:** vitamin B12 (cobalamin) transport protein
- **Retinol binding globulin:** vitamin A transport protein
- **Transcortin:** cortisol-binding protein (CBG); produced by liver, regulated by estrogens; ↓ in cirrhosis, ↑ in pregnancy
- **Factors II, VII, IX, X, and complement:** removed from serum; would be present if done on plasma

Albumin–alpha-1 interzone:

HDL: Leads to even staining in this area. A sharp band in this location may be from high levels of alpha-fetoproteins (AFP): elevated in hepatocellular carcinoma and germ cell (yolk sac) tumors

Alpha-1–alpha-2 interzone:
- **Thyroid binding globulin (TBG):** One of 3 proteins that carries thyroxine (T4) and triiodothyronine (T3) (along with transthyretin and albumin); lowest concentration of the 3, but highest affinity, and only single binding site for T3/T4; produced in liver
- **Haptoglobin/hemoglobin complexes:** migrate more cathodally than unbound haptoglobin, typically seen as a broadening of the alpha-2 zone

3.5   Alpha-2-Globulins

Note: A normal alpha-2 zone and an elevated alpha-1 zone is a typical pattern in hepatic metastasis and cirrhosis
- **Alpha-2-macroglobulin:** plasmin inhibitor

Func:	One of main constituents of alpha-2 band (along with haptoglobin); protease inhibitor (inhibits fibrinolysis- plasmin, kallikrein, coagulation- thrombin); also binds growth factors and cytokines (eg, PDGF, TGF-β, insulin)
Prod:	Produced mainly in liver, but also macrophages, fibroblasts, and adrenal cortex
Norm:	100-280 mg/dL

↑   Children, elderly, and pregnancy/OCPs; markedly raised in nephrotic syndrome (very large and retained while smaller proteins, and water, are lost), diabetes, and malignancy

↓   Gluten-sensitive enteropathy, cirrhosis, sepsis, and fibrinolytic therapy

- **Alpha-2-antiplasmin:** plasmin inhibitor
- **Haptoglobin:** positive; decreased in acute hemolytic anemia

Func: Binds free hemoglobin, then removed by phagocytes, protects from free radical damage

Ind: Evaluation of hemolytic disease

Prod: Liver

Norm: 30–200 mg/dL

↑   Acute phase reactant

↓   Intra-vascular hemolysis

- **Alpha-2-lipoptotien/pre-beta-lipoprotein:** very low-density lipoprotein (VLDL); transports cholesterol, triglycerides, and phospholipids; produced in liver; converted to LDL in blood stream
- **Ceruloplasmin:**

Func: Copper transport, 95% of serum copper bound, 8 atoms per molecule; antioxidant (particularly Fe^{2+} to Fe^{3+})

Prod: Liver

Norm: 15–60 mg/dL

↑   Inflammation (positive acute phase reactant), pregnancy, cholestasis

↓   Wilson disease, liver failure, malnutrition, Menke syndrome

- **Protein C:** Autoprothrombin IIA/factor XIV; removed from serum; would be present if done on plasma

3.6   Beta-Globulin

- **Transferrin:**

Func: Ferric iron (Fe^{3+}) transport glycoprotein, when not bound to iron called apotransferrin

Ind: DD of iron deficiency, suspected hemochromatosis

Prod: Liver

Norm: 220–370 mg/dL, ~25% saturated

↑   Iron deficiency anemia, pregnancy/estrogen therapy, chronic inflammatory states

↓   Acute inflammation (**negative acute phase reactant**) neoplasm, nephrotic syndrome, liver disease, hemochromatosis, thalassemia

- **Fibrinogen: Factor I;** typically removed from serum; would be present if done on plasma; 200-400 mg/dL; converted by thrombin into fibrin during clot formation; produced in liver; acute phase reactant; can be present in serum in dysfibrinogenemia, liver disease, vitamin K deficiency, or heparin use

- **Beta-2-microglobulin:**

Func: Part of MHC class I, present on all nucleated cells; also works with HFE protein to regulate iron concentration via hepcidin/ferroportin; loss of function causes hemochromatosis

Norm: Serum/plasma: 0.8-2.4 mg/L
       Random urine: ≤300 µg/L
       24 h urine: 33-360 µg

↑   Lymphoma, myeloma, tubulo-interstitial nephrosis, rejection following bone marrow transplant, rheumatic diseases, HIV; in long-term hemodialysis increased amounts may lead to aggregation into amyloid fibers, dialysis-related amyloidosis

- **Beta-lipoprotein:** Low-density lipoprotein (LDL); "bad" cholesterol; second smallest lipoprotein; transports cholesterol and triglycerides from liver to cells.

- **Complement factors:** Part of the innate immune system that "complements" the function of antibodies and phagocytes; when the complement system is activated the end result is cell destruction by the membrane attack complex; positive acute phase reactants
  - **C2:**
    - **Normal:** 2.2-3.4 mg/dL
    - ↑: Inflammation
    - ↓: Hereditary disorders, malnutrition
  - **C3:**
    - **Normal:** 55-120 mg/dL
    - ↑: Inflammation
    - ↓: Autoimmune and immune complex disorders eg, lupus, cryoglobulinemia, glomerulonephritis

- **Hemopexin:**

Func: Transport protein; binds heme with highest affinity; protects from free radical oxidative damage; helps preserve iron stores, no acute phase response

Ind: Assessment of the extent of the intravascular hemolysis, along with haptoglobin

Prod: Liver

Norm: 50-115 mg/dL

↑ Melanoma

↓ Hemolysis, myoglobulinemia, chronic hepatitis, porphyria, malnutrition

- **Beta-gamma interzone:**
  - **IgA:** Critical role in mucosal immunity, in mucous/secretions; poor activator of complement system and opsonization; ↑ in **cirrhosis**, respiratory infection, skin diseases, and rheumatoid arthritis
  - **C-reactive protein (CRP):** Sometimes considered a gamma zone constituent; see below

3.7 Gamma Globulins

- **Immunoglobulins:** IgG, IgM, IgE, IgD, IgA (may be in beta-gamma interzone), kappa and lambda; produced in B-cells, part of the immune system that binds and removes 'foreign' antigens; a 'spike' may mean monoclonal gammopathy and specification (IFE, IT) required; broad elevation may mean polyclonal gammopathy, typically non-neoplastic (severe infection, liver disease, autoimmune disorders); decrease is normal in infants or may represent immunoglobulin deficiency

- **C-reactive protein (CRP):** Often in beta-gamma interzone, cause of β-γ bridging

Func: The most important **acute phase protein** (fast response [8-10 h], extreme increase [up to 2,000 fold], short half-life [24 h]), degree of increase correlates with extent of inflammation, strongest reaction to bacterial infections; little response to viral infections; binds phosphocholine on surface of dying cells and some bacteria to activate the complement system. Named for binding capacity of the C-polysaccharide in the wall of *Streptococcus -pneumoniae*

Ind: Evaluate inflammation, assess activity of rheumatic diseases, evaluate antibiotic effectiveness

Prod: Liver

Norm: Usually <3 mg/L, but some healthy individuals up to 10 mg/L

↑   **3-10 mg/L** - May indicate cardiac event; **>10 mg/L** - infection (bacterial>viral), trauma, collagen vascular disease, surgery (6 h after surgery: >10 mg/L, 48 h: peaks (rare >150 mg/L), 7-10 days: returns to normal if no further trauma/infection

3.8   Total Complement Activity (CH50)

Func: Measures the level of functionality of the complement system, does not identify which component may be involved in dysfunction

Norm: 19-60 mg/dL

↑   Inflammation, malignancy (acute phase reactant)

↓   Immune/genetic deficiency, consumption in immune complex/autoimmune disorders, infection/sepsis

3.9   Complement Factor C1-inh

C1-INH: C1 esterase inhibitor

Func: Protease inhibitor of the complement system to prevent spontaneous activation; also inhibits proteases of the fibrinolytic, clotting, and kinin pathways (most important inhibitor of kallikrein, Factors XIa and XIIa)

Norm: 16-33 mg/dL
       Enzymatic activity: 70%-130%

↑   Inflammation (acute phase reactant)

↓   **Hereditary angioneurotic edema:** ↓C1-inh → ↑kallikrein activation → ↑bradykinin → vascular leakage; type 1 - 85%, levels are low; type 2 - 15%, levels are normal, but protein dysfunctional
    Acquired angioedema: Autoantibody to C1-inh, sometimes associated with B-cell lymphomas

3.10   Hyperimmunoglobulinemia

Polyclonal hyperimmunoglobulinemia:
Immune response to infections (rarely more than 90 g/L)
- Bacterial infections - especially IgG
- Early infection - especially IgM
- Allergic reactions, parasitosis - especially IgE

Monoclonal hyperimmunoglobulinemia:
Multiple myeloma [(MM)/MGUS/plasmacytoma]
MM 2nd most common hematologic malignancy in US (after non-Hodgkin lymphoma). Elderly, M>F, African Americans>Caucasians
Neoplasms of plasma cells leading to extremely high production of monoclonal antibody (paraprotein). Can produce any Ig, but most common is IgG-kappa, followed by IgA and IgM. IgD and IgE are very rare. Ig-kappa>Ig-lambda, and isolated heavy or light chains are possible. Specific antibody identified by SPEP/UPEP and IFE. Paraprotein often leads to kidney damage. Rarely involves lymph nodes or spleen.
The criteria vary per diagnosis:
MM: (all 3 required)
- >10% clonal plasma cells on bone marrow biopsy
- A monoclonal antibody (paraprotein) in serum/urine (except in cases of true non-secretory myeloma)

Evidence of end-organ damage thought to be related to the plasma cell disorder (related organ or tissue impairment (ROTI), "CRAB" - Hyper**C**alcemia, **R**enal insufficiency, **A**nemia, **B**one lesions

Asymptomatic (smoldering) myeloma:
- Serum paraprotein >30 g/L and/or
- >10% clonal plasma cells on bone marrow biopsy and
- No myeloma-related organ or tissue impairment

Monoclonal gammopathy of undetermined significance (MGUS):
- Serum paraprotein <30 g/L
- <10% clonal plasma cells on bone marrow biopsy and
- No myeloma-related organ or tissue impairment

Solitary plasmacytoma: A single tumor of plasma cells
Plasma cell dyscrasia: Where only the antibodies produce symptoms, eg, AL amyloidosis

POEMS syndrome: **P**eripheral neuropathy, **O**rganomegaly, **E**ndocrinopathy, **M**onoclonal plasma cell disorder, **S**kin changes

Waldenstrom's macroglobulinemia: AKA lymphoplasmacytic lymphoma

Rare, ~1,500 cases/yr in US, indolent course. Malignant B-cell proliferation leading to overproduction of IgM. Expansion of B-cells in bone marrow leads to anemia, and extremely high IgM levels lead to ↑ blood viscosity.

Symptoms include fatigue, weight loss, chronic oozing of blood from the nose and gums, peripheral neuropathy (10%), lymphadenopathy/hepatosplenomegaly (30%), blurring or loss of vision, headache, and rarely stroke or coma.

5 year survival rate stratification based on 5 criteria: age >65 years, hemoglobin ≤11.5 g/dL, platelet count ≤100×10³/mm³, β-2 microglobulin >3 mg/L, and serum monoclonal protein concentration >70 g/L.

Low (87%): ≤1 adverse variable except age
Intermediate (68%): 2 adverse characteristics or age >65 years
High (36%): >2 adverse characteristics

3.11   Hypoimmunoglobulinemia

Reduction of circulating antibodies, can be congenital or acquired; the most common are listed below:

Common variable (primary) immunodeficiency (CVID):

Congenital defect in B-lymphocytes; over 150 types, defect/absence of immunoglobulins, susceptible to bacterial and viral infections

X-linked agammaglobulinemia: AKA Bruton syndrome; tyrosine

kinase mutation; patients do not generate mature B cells, leading to a complete lack of antibodies in the blood, therefore are prone to develop serious and even fatal infections, in particular with extracellular, encapsulated bacteria

Severe combined immunodeficiency (SCID):

Absence of functional T-lymphocytes leading to lack of activation of B-cells, agamaglobulinemia, and a practically non-existent immune system. Patients are affected by severe bacterial, viral, and fungal infections early in life and often present with interstitial lung disease, chronic diarrhea, and failure to thrive. Usually die within 1 year without stem cell transplant

Acquired (secondary) immunoglobulin deficiency:

Hematologic disorders, immunosuppression, infectious diseases, malnutrition, burns, HIV

3.12   Soluble Transferrin-Receptor (sTfR)

Func: A transmembrane protein used to internalize iron bound to transferrin, portion is cleaved off into the blood stream

Ind: Evaluation of suspected iron deficiency in patients who may have inflammation, infection, or chronic disease in which ferritin (a positive acute phase reactant) concentration does not correlate with iron status (ie, CF, diabetics). sTfR is inversely proportional to the total iron

Norm: 1.8-4.6 mg/L

↑   Iron deficiency anemia

3.13   Transferrin Saturation

Form: The ratio of serum iron to total iron-binding capacity (TIBC) expressed as a percentage, ie, of the transferrin that is available, how much serum iron is actually bound

$$\%Saturation = Serum\ iron/TIBC \times 100$$

Ind: Suspected lack of function or iron overload

Norm: Serum iron: 60-170 µg/dL
TIBC: 240-450 µg/dL
Saturation: 15%-50%

↑   **Iron overload:** Hemochromatosis, primary or acquired (eg, multiple blood transfusions, hemoglobinopathies, ineffective erythropoiesis), hemolysis, anemias (hemolytic, sideroblastic, megaloblastic), porphyria, iron poisoning

↓   Iron deficiency or decreased iron availability: chronic inflammation, infection, tumors, liver disease, uremia

3.14   Carbohydrate-Deficient Transferrin (CDT)

Transferrin is a polypeptide with two N-linked polysaccharide chains branched with sialic acid (a monosaccharide carbohydrate). Various forms of transferrin exist, with differing levels of sialylation (most common is 4). In persons who consume ≥4-5 drinks/day, the amount of sialic acid chains is decreased (CDT) .

Ind: Used with other tests (AST, ALT), can be useful in identifying alcohol abuse, follow-up in treatment of alcoholism

Norm: <1.7% when alcohol <40 g/day (95th percentile for social drinkers)

↑ Alcoholism (returns to normal after ~14-day abstinence), also rarely in primary biliary cirrhosis, active hepatitis, carbohydrate-deficient - glycoprotein- (CDG) -syndrome, genetic transferrin variants

3.15 Ferritin

Func: Ubiquitous intracellular protein that stores iron, keeping it soluble and non-toxic (each molecule stores ~4,000 Fe^{3+} ions). Ferritin not bound to iron is called apoferritin. Also present in the serum in minute amounts, where it reflects iron stores

Ind: Iron deficiency or iron overload conditions

Prod: All cells, especially in jejunal mucosa, liver, and reticuloendothelial system

Norm: 10-330 µg/L

↑ Hemochromatosis (>1,000 µg/L), acute hepatitis, Gaucher disease, malignancy, inflammation (positive acute phase reactant); may be increased or normal in anemia of chronic disease and thalassemia

↓ Iron deficiency

3.16 Iron (Fe)

A chemical element (Fe from Latin: *ferrum*) with wide range of oxidation states, -2 to +6, however +2 and +3 are most common

Func: Form complexes with hemoglobin and myoglobin to transport oxygen

Ind: Evaluate iron stores, used in transferrin saturation calculation

Norm: 40-150 µg/dL

↑ Hemolysis, hemochromatosis (primary or acquired), ineffective erythropoiesis, porphyria, iron poisoning, liver damage

↓ Blood loss (hemorrhage, menstruation), malnutrition, malabsorption (after gastrectomy/ duodenectomy), dialysis, pregnancy

Note **A low serum iron does not prove iron deficiency.**
- Assessment only in connection with transferrin and ferritin
- Significant circadian rhythm with peaks in the first half day
- Significant intra-individual variability
- Dependent on food intake, can change within 10 min

3.17 Deferoxamine Test

Deferoxamine (AKA desferrioxamine or Desferal) is a bacterial siderophore produced by the actinobacteria *Streptomyces pilosus*. Acts as a chelating agent used to remove excess iron by enhancing urine elimination, thereby reducing damage. Used to treat iron overload, especially in small children or hemochromatosis.

Ind:	Suspicion of iron overload
Norm:	Iron excretion <2 mg/6 h
↑	Iron excretion >3 mg/6 h >10 mg/6 h implies hemochromatosis
Proc:	1. Empty the bladder 2. Dosing of deferoxamine 3. Collect urine over 6 h

3.18 Procalcitonin (PCT)

Func:	A protein precursor of calcitonin (involved in calcium homeostasis→ ↑Ca^{2+}). Extreme rise in bacterial infections, but not viral, may help reduce unnecessary antibiotic use (decreasing healthcare costs and drug resistance)
Ind:	Diagnosis and follow-up of bacterial infections
Prod:	Parafollicular (C-) cells of thyroid, and neuroendocrine cells of lung and intestine
Norm:	<0.5 µg/L; half-life: 25 h
↑	Inflammation, especially bacterial infection, may rise to 100 µg/L (minimal rise in viral and non-infectious inflammation); ↑ procalcitonin in response to inflammation does not lead to ↑ calcitonin or Ca^{2+} levels

3.19   Neopterin

A catabolic product of GTP

Func: Direct marker of macrophage activity and indirect marker of
T-lymphocyte activity, and therefore, the cellular immune system. Also
associated with increased production of oxygen radicals, so may
estimate the extent of oxidative stress by the immune system

Prod: Macrophages, upon stimulation by IFN-γ

Stand.:   Serum/urine: <2.5 ng/mL

CSF: <1.0 ng/mL

↑   Infections, cardiovascular disease, autoimmune diseases, malignancy,
transplant rejection

3.20   Acute Phase Reactants

Plasma proteins formed in the liver; stimulation by IL-6; ↑ in acute
inflammation and chronic relapsing conditions
• C-reactive protein
• Serum-amyloid -A
• Fibrinogen
• Alpha-1-antitrypsin
• Complement factors (C1s, C2-C5, C9)
• Haptoglobin
• Ceruloplasmin

3.21   "Negative" Acute-Phase Reactants

Decrease In Inflammation
• Transferrin
• Albumin
• Prealbumin
• Alpha-lipoprotein (HDL)

3.22 Ammonia (NH$_3$)

Func: Byproduct of protein metabolism

Ind: Cerebral or neuromuscular disorders, liver disease, chemotherapy, valproic acid

Prod: Formed from the metabolism of nitrogen products (proteins), converted to urea in the liver (urea cycle) and excreted in the urine

Norm: 20–90 µg/dL, may be higher in newborns, especially premies

↑ Cirrhosis/marked liver damage (acute viral hepatitis, necrosis), urea cycle disorders/enzyme defects

Met: **Enzymatic:** Ammonia, NADPH, glutamine, and 2-oxoglutarate react to form glutamate, NADP$^+$, and water. The decrease in NADPH can be measured by light absorption at 340 nm and correlates with the ammonia concentration

L-glutamine + 2-oxoglutarate + NADPH + H+ 12 L-glutamate + NADP+ + H$_2$O

Ammonia-specific electrode: Ammonium (NH$_4$$^+$) is added to an alkaline solution (NaOH, KOH) resulting in ammonia, this ammonia diffuses through a permeable membrane, and the resultant pH change is measured

Colorimetric: Indophenol blue or phenate (blue dyes) will have color change when oxidizing agent (hypochlorite) is present. Light absorbance performed and can estimate ammonia concentration

3.23 Urea

AKA carbamine, CO(NH$_2$)$_2$

Func: The final product of protein metabolism; ammonia is toxic in high levels and is transformed to non-toxic urea by the urea cycle, then excreted in the urine. After filtered through the glomeruli, some urea is reabsorbed in the inner medullary collecting ducts, thus raising the osmolarity in the ascending loop of Henle, which causes water to be reabsorbed. By action of the urea transporter 2, some of this reabsorbed urea will be transported back into the urine. This mechanism is controlled by antidiuretic hormone, allows the body to create hyperosmotic urine, and is important to prevent excessive water loss and balance electrolytes

Ind: Diagnosis and follow-up in renal insufficiency

Prod: In the mitochondria of hepatocytes

Norm: Will vary depending on protein intake
Serum: 10-50 mg/dL
Urine: 20-35 g/24 h

↑ **Prerenal:** Decreased renal perfusion - circulatory disruption (shock, cardiac insufficiency); ↑ nitrogen production/↑ proteolysis (fever, necrosis, tumors, cytotoxic agents, cell breakdown (starvation, malnutrition, excessive exercise)
Renal: Disruption of glomerular filtration (glomerulonephritis, pyelonephritis), GFR of 50% or less; a good measure of kidney function is blood urea nitrogen
Postrenal: Kidney/bladder stones may impede urine output leading to restriction of filtration
Uremia: Associated with symptomatic kidney failure, creatinine typically also elevated
Azotemia: Also refers to high levels of urea and creatinine, but asymptomatic

↓ Acute liver failure, anorexia/starvation, pregnancy

Met: **Urease method:** Urea is split by urease into ammonia and carbon dioxide, the ammonia can then be measured as described above

3.24 Uric Acid

$C_5H_4N_4O_3$; forms salts known as **urates**; high blood concentrations can lead to gout and kidney stones

Func: Product of purine metabolism. Purines are components of nucleic acids and coenzymes; may be synthesized in the body or ingested (eg, liver, sweetbreads) ~75% excreted in the urine; ~25% secreted into the GI tract

Ind: Diagnosis, treatment and/or monitoring of renal failure, gout, leukemia, psoriasis, starvation, or patients receiving cytotoxic drugs

Norm: May be lower in children
Serum: 3.7-7.8 mg/dL (Men)
2.7 -6.5 mg/dL (Women)
Urine: 350-2,000 mg/24 h

↑   **Primary Hyperuricemia (Gout):**
           Idiopathic
           Lesch–Nyhan syndrome (X-linked recessive; hypoxanthine-guanine-
           phosphoribosyltransferase [HGPRT] total defect; gout, kidney disease,
           and neuropsychiatric symptoms (eg, mental retardation, self-mutilation)
           Kelley–Seegmiller syndrome (partial HGPRT defect; have gout and
           kidney disease, but fewer neurological issues)
           Secondary hyperuricemia:
           Renal insufficiency, ↑ synthesis, excess intake, malignancy/ leukemia,
           polycythemia, cytotoxic drugs/therapies (thiazides, TB drugs, chemo,
           radiation), total parenteral nutrition (TPN)

↓   Allopurinol, severe liver disease (decreased production), defective renal
           reabsorption. Methyldopa, deferoxamine and calcium dobesilate cause
           falsely decreased levels.

Met: **Uric acid method:** Uric acid (absorption at 293 nm) is oxidized by
           urease into allantoin (no absorption at 293 nm). The difference is
           proportional to the quantity

           $$Uric\ acid + 2H_2O + O_2 \rightarrow Allantoin + H_2O_2 + CO_2$$
           (absorbs at 293 nm)   (no absorption at 293 nm)

           Catalase method: Continuation of the uric acid method. The hydrogen
           peroxide then reacts with a peroxidase and a dye. The color formed is
           proportional to the uric acid concentration (colorimetry)

3.25 Homocysteine

Func: A homologue of cysteine; an intermediary amino acid in the sulfur-
           amino acid metabolism pathway. Breakdown is dependent on vitamins
           B6 (pyridoxine), B12 (cobalamin), and folic acid

Ind: Methionine metabolism disorders, vitamin deficiency. Also, possibly
           useful in patients with atherosclerotic vascular diseases as indicator of
           increased risk of cardiac event

Prod: Produced by demethylation of methionine

Norm: Fasting levels:
           Serum: ≤12 μmol/L
           Urine: ≤9 μmol/g creatinine

↑   **Moderate** (12-30 µmol/L): Vitamin deficiency (B6, B12, folic acid),
         MTHFR mutation, renal insufficiency, thyroid dysfunction, psoriasis,
         rheumatoid arthritis, leukemia, drugs, smoking, coffee, alcohol
         Intermediate (30-100 µmol/L): Inborn errors of metabolism
         (heterozygous mutation; cystathionine-beta -synthase, methionine
         synthetase, etc), renal insufficiency, severe vitamin deficiency
         (contributing factor in the pathogenesis of neural tube defects in folate
         deficiency)
         Severe (>100 µmol/L): Inborn errors of metabolism (homozygote
         mutation)
         Homocystinuria: Autosomal-recessive defect in methionine metabolism
         due to a lack of the cystathionine-beta-synthetase (CBS). Methionine is
         normally converted to homocysteine, then to cysteine by CBS. Lack of
         enzyme leads to accumulation of methionine and homocysteine.
         Symptoms: Marfanoid habitus, long limbs, high-arched feet, knock
         knees (genu valgum), mental disability, seizures, ocular lens issues,
         glaucoma, retinal detachment, vascular disease (atherosclerosis,
         thrombosis)
         Ind: Universal neonatal screening

Mat: Must be immediately packed on ice and centrifuged within 30 min or
         may lead to false elevation (hemolysis, insufficient cooling, late
         centrifugation)

3.26   Granulocyte Elastase

Func: Lysosomal proteolytic enzyme involved in fighting infection,
         inflammation and necrosis; breaks down membranes of gram negative
         bacteria. Regulated by circulating proteinase inhibitors to reduce tissue
         destruction

Ind: Inflammation (early detection and monitoring - short half-life, 1 h)

Prod: Neutrophils, macrophages, endothelial cells

Norm: Heavily dependent on a homogeneous enzyme immunoassay
         12-32 µg/L
         Newborns can be up to 75 µg/L

↑　　　Infection (post-operative/trauma monitoring), sepsis, shock, chronic joint disorders (synovial fluid), meningitis (cerebrospinal fluid), acute pancreatitis, Crohn's/UC, rheumatoid arthritis, cause of bullous formation in certain skin diseases
Falsely high: Late separation of plasma and cellular component (leaks from degraded leukocytes

Mat:　Sample must be processed within 2 h to avoid false elevation

3.27 Lysozyme

AKA Muramidase/ N-acetylmuramide glycanhydrolase

Func:　Glycoside hydrolase: low molecular weight bacteriolysis protein in the lysosomes of cells. Also abundant in secretions (tears, saliva, human milk, mucus)

Ind:　Renal damage, leukemia, meningitis, UTI, sepsis, inflammatory disease

Prod:　Mainly from neutrophils, but also macrophages, and small amount in lymphocytes

Norm:　Serum:　　　2.7-9.4 mg/L
　　　　24 h Urine:　<1.5 mg/L
　　　　CSF:　　　　<0.5 mg/L

↑　　　Serum: Granulocytic/monocytic leukemias/proliferative disorders, sepsis, distinction between bacterial and non-bacterial meningitis, Crohn's/UC
Urine: Renal transplant rejection/tubular damage, UTI, leukemias
CSF: Bacterial meningitis (>1.5 mg/L), much less in viral and tuberculous

↓　　　Associated with bronchopulmonary dysplasia of newborns and infant diarrhea from gram-positive bacteria

3.28 Myoglobin

Func:　Iron- and oxygen-binding protein (similar to hemoglobin) present in skeletal and cardiac muscle, (accounts for red color). A small molecule readily filtered by kidney. Of note, higher concentrations of myoglobin in muscle cells allow organisms to hold their breaths longer (skin-divers, whales, seals)

Ind:　Diagnosis and follow-up of infarction, injury evaluation, sports performance and training, suspected prerenal proteinuria

Prod: Skeletal and cardiac muscle, typically non-detectable in serum/urine, unless muscle injury (trauma, disease, exercise). Correlates with muscle concentration (body builders) and severity of damage

Norm: Serum: <110 µg/L
Urine: <50 µg/L
      <17 µg/g creatinine

↑ Muscle injury (trauma, rhabdomyolysis, myopathy, infarction)
Myocardial infarction: Sensitive marker, early detection, rapidly drops (short half-life, 5.5 h) good for accessing severity of damage and monitoring progression

3.29   Cardiac Troponins (C, T and I)

Func: Myofibrillary regulatory proteins integral to contraction of skeletal and cardiac muscle. Attached to tropomyosin and lies in between actin filaments, blocking contraction in relaxed state. When calcium rises troponin transformation takes place, moving tropomyosin out of the way, allowing myosin-actin binding, leading to contraction. **Troponin C** binds to calcium ions to produce a conformational change; **Troponin T** binds to tropomyosin, interlocking them to form a troponin-tropomyosin complex; **Troponin I** binds to actin to hold the troponin-tropomyosin complex in place
Troponin T and I have **cardiac specific isoforms**, and the subunit concentration can be determined individually. Due to long half-life, can be used to diagnose myocardial infarction for 1-2 weeks afterwards

Ind: Suspected **myocardial infarction (MI)**, assessment of thrombolytic therapy

Norm: Troponin T: <0.01 ng/mL
Troponin I: <0.04 ng/mL

↑ **Cardiac specific:** MI (higher levels), angina (lower levels), myocarditis, supraventricular tachycardia, cardiomyopathy, amyloidosis, contusion, defibrillation, cardiac surgery/transplant, toxins/drugs, sepsis, pulmonary hypertension/COPD (right ventricular strain and ischemia)
Non-cardiac conditions: Sepsis, end-stage renal disease, strenuous exercise (marathons/triathlons), myositis, rhabdomyolysis, preeclampsia

3.30   Atrial Natriuretic Peptide (ANP)

Func: A powerful vasodilator released in response to hypertension to reduce water, sodium, and potassium, decreasing the load on the circulatory system
Target organs: Blood vessels (dilation) and kidney (natriuresis and diuresis; opposite effect of aldosterone)

Prod: Cardiac atria cells

3.31   B-type Natriuretic Peptide (BNP)/NT-proBNP

AKA Brain natriuretic peptide

Func: Natriuretic peptides are a family of structurally closely related peptide hormones (ANP, BNP, CNP, urodilatin. BNP and NT-proBNP have the greatest importance for the assessment of **congestive heart failure (CHF)**. Whereas ANP reflects atrial overload, BNP ↑ in ventricular overload

Ind: Congestive heart failure: diagnosis, staging, and anticoagulant monitoring

Prod: Stored and secreted primarily in membrane granules of cardiac ventricular muscle as NT-proBNP. Once released, the N-terminal (NT) piece (76 aa) is cleaved by to release the active BNP (32 aa)

Norm: NT-proBNP is routinely ordered as it is more stable for testing purposes. Both peptides will be in the blood in ventricular dysfunction (NT-proBNP ~2-3 days, BNP ~12 h).
Varies widely with age; basic numbers below

	NT/BNP	
	<100 pg/mL	Men (maximum)
	<40 pg/mL	Men <50
	<150 pg/mL	Women (maximum)
	<75 pg/mL	Women <50

↑ **CHF:** <200 pg/mL: compensated, 200-400 pg/mL: moderate, >400 pg/mL: moderate-to-severe
Unstable angina, ventricular dysfunction, ventricular hypertrophy, atrial fibrillation, hypertension, renal failure, cirrhosis, right heart failure (200-500 pg/mL), pulmonary hypertension (300-500 pg/mL), acute pulmonary embolism (150-500 pg/mL)
Note: A normal value makes CHF unlikely; the negative predictive value is ~96%

3.32   Vasoactive Intestinal Polypeptide (VIP)

Func: A neuropeptide hormone (28 aa) which belongs to glucagon/secretin superfamily. Acts on smooth muscle causing ↑ contractility in the heart, vasodilation, and relaxes the muscles of the trachea, GE junction, stomach, and gallbladder. Also stimulates secretion of water into pancreatic juice, intestinal secretions, and bile, inhibits gastrin (gastric acid secretion), stimulates pepsinogen secretion, and ↑ glycogenolysis. In the brain it is crucial for maintaining circadian rhythms

Ind: Suspicion of **VIPoma**

Prod: Numerous tissues including GI tract, pancreas, hypothalamus. Increased production in certain tumors (VIPoma) of the pancreas or hypothalamus Inactivation occurs in the liver; half-life ~2 mins

Norm: <75 pg/mL

↑ VIPoma (assoc. w/ MEN type 1 symptoms: watery diarrhea, hypokalemia, achlorhydria)

3.33   Hereditary Amino Acid Disorders

3.33.1 Phenylketonuria (PKU)

Gen: Autosomal recessive metabolic disorder characterized by **phenylalanine hydroxylase (PAH) gene mutation**, decreased/absent conversion of phenylalanine to tyrosine. Most common amino acid storage disorder, incidence of ~1:8,000

Symp: Reduced PAH activity leads to accumulation of phenyl alanine, converted to phenylpyruvate, detected in blood and urine: if left untreated leads to **mental disability, delayed physical development and neurological symptoms** such as seizures

Treat: With early diagnosis and strict phenylalanine-restricted diet, largely normal development possible. Children of mothers with PKU often have birth defects

Ind: Part of universal neonatal screening

3.33.2 Maple syrup urine disease (MSUD)

Gen: AKA branched-chain ketoaciduria. Rare autosomal-recessive metabolic disorder caused by a deficiency of the branched-chain alpha-keto acid dehydrogenase complex (BCKDC-consisting of 4 subunits) leading to excessively **increased concentrations of branched-chain amino acids (leucine, isoleucine, and valine)** and their metabolites in blood and urine

Symp: Classically, infants seem healthy at first, then progress to poor feeding, vomiting, lethargy, seizures, hypoglycemia, ketoacidosis, pancreatitis, coma and death. Variant forms will lead to varying timeline. Sotolone is the compound responsible for the sweet (maple syrup) smell of urine and sometimes ear wax

Treat: With early diagnosis, a diet with minimal levels of leucine, isoleucine, and valine (milk, meat, eggs) will prevent neurological damage. Some patients respond to high doses of thiamine (a cofactor of BCKDC)

Ind: Part of universal neonatal screening, particularly prevalent in children of Amish, Mennonite, and Jewish descent

4 Tumor Markers

Gen: Molecules that are produced in tumor cells, which can be used for the identification of specific tumors as well as prognosis, assessment, and monitoring

Classified as tumor-specific antigens (TSA), present only on tumor cells and tumor-associated antigens (TAA), present on some tumor cells and also some normal cells

Normal levels usually do not entirely rule out tumor/recurrence

Ind: Used to detect or monitor malignancy
- Before the first treatment (surgery, chemo-, hormone- or radiotherapy)
- After surgery or after the start of therapy
  - First control usually 5-10 days after therapy (according to the type of the corresponding tumor marker)
  - Every 3 months during the first 2 years
  - Every 6 months in the 3-5 years
  - Prior to each new therapy
- In case of suspected recurrence or metastasis
- When renewed staging

4.1 Clinically Relevant Tumor Markers

CEA: **Carcinoembryonic antigen**

Norm: <5.0 µg/L

↑: <10 µg/L   Mild (cirrhosis; inflammation or adenocarcinoma)
   >10 µg/L   Suspected malignant process
   >20 µg/L   Almost certainly a malignant process

Interpretation:
- Carcinomas: colon, stomach, pancreas, breast cancers, as well as medullary thyroid and bronchial carcinomas
- Colon-CA: correlates with tumor mass and spread
- Excellent marker with particularly high values for hematologic metastases: bone, liver, lungs
- Benign (values usually <10 µg/L): Liver disease (hepatitis, alcohol, cirrhosis), pancreatitis, GI inflammation, pulmonary inflammation or smoking
- Combined with other tumor markers to increase sensitivity

Pathophysiology:
- Glycoprotein shed from the surface of malignant cells
- Expression particularly in GI tract (especially colon mucosa) and pancreas. In addition, vaginal epithelium

Pancreatic cyst fluid: Useful for distinguishing (with CA19-9, amylase) mucinous from non-mucinous (pseudo, serous), and/or likely malignant (adenocarcinoma)

<5 ng/mL likely serous cystadenoma, pseudocyst, cystic neuroendocrine tumor, mets

>200 ng/mL highly suspicious for mucinous cysts, the greater the CEA, the more likely malignant

Peritoneal fluid: Useful for distinguishing benign from malignant (~7% of all ascites; peritoneal carcinomatosis-53%, massive liver mets causing portal hypertension-13%, peritoneal carcinomatosis plus massive liver metastasis-13%, hepatocellular carcinoma plus cirrhosis-7%, and chylous ascites due to lymphoma-7%).

>6.0 ng/mL is suspicious for malignancy (sensitivity 48%, specificity 99%), especially in tumors known to increase CEA (lung, breast, ovarian, gastrointestinal, colorectal)

<6.0 ng/mL may be seen in lymphoma, mesothelioma, leukemia, melanoma, hepatocellular

Pleural fluid: Useful for distinguishing benign (CHF, pneumonia, PE, cirrhosis) from malignant. Nonsmoking, healthy adults should have low levels.

>3.5 ng/mL suspicious for malignancy (sensitivity 52%, specificity 95%), especially in tumors known to increase CEA (lung, breast, ovarian, gastrointestinal, colorectal)

<3.5 ng/mL seen in normal patients, also seen in mesothelioma, lymphoma, leukemia, melanoma

CSF: Detecting meningeal carcinomatosis (60% of patients) or brain metastasis from carcinoma. Normal <0.6 ng/mL

NSE: **Neuron-specific enolase**

AKA non-specific enolase

Norm: <12.5 µg/L

↑:   <25.0 µg/L Mild (hemolysis, cerebral ischemia).
>25.0 µg/L Lung Ca, neuroblastoma, (APUDoma and large cell ca ~10%)

Interpretation:
- Carcinomas: Lung, neuroblastoma (Sensitivity 85% for cut-off of 25 µg/L), APUDoma (Sensitivity 35% for cut-off of 25 µg/L), leukemia
- Benign: hemolysis, cerebral ischemia/disease, benign lung disease (5% >12 µg/L), uremia

Pathophysiology:
- One of the 11 enzymes of glycolysis, catalyzes 2-phosphoglycerate to phosphoenolpyruvate
- In the neurons, enolase is the Gamma-subunits, also in nerve cells and neuroendocrine cells of the intestine, lung, and endocrine organs, such as thyroid, pancreas, pituitary

CYFRA 21-1: **Cytokeratin-19 fragments**

Norm: <3.3 ng/mL

↑: >3.3 ng/mL
High normal/mild elevations may be lung disease (pneumonia), GI (Crohn's/UC), gyn disease/cancer, GU disease/cancer
High elevation: Non-small cell lung carcinoma
>10 ng/mL: Cancer, (benign only in extremely rare cases <1%)

Interpretation:
- CA: non-small cell lung ca (particularly squamous); not organ specific, all solid tumors may have increase
- Benign: GI disorders, renal insufficiency
- No dependence on gender, age, pregnancy

Pathophysiology:
- Insoluble cytokeratin as part of cell support structure
- In contrast, the fragments are serum soluble
- Two specific monoclonal antibodies (Ks 19.1 and BM 19.2)
Pleura fluid: If significantly higher than the serum (>20.9 ng/mL): sensitivity 71% and specificity 82% for malignancy

SCC-Ag: **Squamous cell carcinoma (AKA TA-4)**

Norm: <2 g/L

↑:
<10 g/L Mild elevation: cirrhosis, pancreatitis, lung disease
>10 g/L Highly suspicious for malignancy

Interpretation:
- Carcinoma: squamous of the cervix, lung, esophagus, anus, HEENT
  - Cervix (sensitivity 83%, specificity 95%)
  - Lungs (sensitivity 25%-75%, specificity 95%)
  - HEENT (sensitivity 35%, specificity 95%)
- Benign: Cirrhosis, pancreatitis, renal insufficiency, pulmonary disease, benign skin diseases (psoriasis, eczema)

Pathophysiology:
- SCC: glycoprotein with molecular weight of 42 kD, carbohydrate content 0.6%
- A subfraction of TA-4-antigen, the neutral form remains inside normal tissue, the acidic forms are released during SCC or epithelial damage

Note: In specimen preparation and processing, contamination with skin and saliva must be avoided (false positives). Smoking has no effect

CA. 15-3: **Carbohydrate–Antigen 15-3**

Norm: <30 U/mL

↑:
<50 U/mL Mild elevation: may be benign
>50 U/mL Highly suspicious for malignancy

Interpretation:
- Carcinoma: **Breast**; only increased in the advanced stage: Lung, prostate, liver, ovary, cervix, endometrium
- Benign: benign breast disease/tumor (rarely >40 U/mL; fibroadenoma <50 U/mL), ovarian cysts, PID, liver disease, sarcoid, lupus, TB, lactation and pregnancy

Pathophysiology:
- Circulating epitope of a protein produced by MUC1 gene. Mucinous-Glycoprotein (300 kD)
- Related to CA27.29 (AKA BR27.29, more sensitive and specific)

CA. 19-9: **Carbohydrate–antigen 19-9**
("gastrointestinal cancer antigen")

Norm: <50 U/mL
<100 U/mL Mild elevation - usually benign
>100 U/mL Suspicious for malignancy (rarely, may be benign up to 500 U/mL)

Interpretation:
- Carcinoma: **pancreas**, stomach, biliary, colorectal
- Benign: cirrhosis, chronic hepatitis, acute and chronic pancreatitis, biliary tract disease (PSC); cholestasis
- **Neither sensitive or specific enough for screening**

Pathophysiology:
Modified Lewis blood group antigen. **Rare patients Lewis-negative (3%-5%), do not express CA19-9**

Pancreatic cyst fluid: Useful in assessment of pancreatic cysts (with CEA, amylase); <37 U/mL more consistent with serous cystadenoma or pseudocyst (Sensitivity 19%, Specificity 98%)

Peritoneal fluid: Useful for distinguishing benign from malignant (~7% of all ascites; peritoneal carcinomatosis-53%, massive liver mets causing portal hypertension-13%, peritoneal carcinomatosis plus massive liver metastasis-13%, hepatocellular carcinoma plus cirrhosis-7%, and chylous ascites due to lymphoma-7%)
>32 U/mL is suspicious of malignancy. (sensitivity 44%, specificity 93%)
Normal levels may be seen in mesothelioma, leukemia/lymphoma, melanoma

Pleural fluid: Useful for determining benign (CHF, pneumonia, PE, cirrhosis) from malignant
>20 U/mL is suspicious for malignancy (sensitivity 35%, specificity 95%), significantly higher in CA 19-9-secreting malignancies (pancreas, cholangio, colorectal, stomach, bile duct, lung, ovarian).
Normal levels may be seen in leukemia/lymphoma, mesothelioma, melanoma

CA 72-4: Carbohydrate-antigen 72-4

Norm: <6.7 U/mL
↑: >6.7 U/mL

Interpretation:
- Carcinoma: stomach, ovarian, non-small cell lung, pancreas, esophagus
- Compared to other markers (CEA, CA.19-9) strikingly high diagnostic specificity vs. benign diseases

- Increased levels are rarely found in benign or inflammatory processes, but may be seen in cirrhosis, pancreatitis, pneumonia, obstructive lung diseases

Pathophysiology:
A mucin-like circulating tumor-associated glycoprotein

CA 125: **Carbohydrate-antigen 125**

Norm: <35 U/mL

↑: >35 U/mL
Higher values, more likely benign. Even low elevations suspicious when monitoring for recurrence

Interpretation:
- Carcinoma: **ovarian**, endometrial, pancreas, cholangio, stomach, lung, cervical, liver, uterine, breast; increases proportional to stage
- Benign: peritoneal irritation, pleural effusion, ovarian cysts, PID, cirrhosis, pancreatitis, cholelithiasis, hepatitis, pregnancy, endometriosis

Pathophysiology:
A glycoprotein (MUC16) normally expressed in ovary, fallopian tube, peritoneum, pleura, pericardium, colon, kidney, stomach

PSA: **Prostate specific antigen**

Norm: Varies with age

<2.0 µg/L	<40 years
<2.5 µg/L	40-49 years
<3.5 µg/L	50-59 years
<4.5 µg/L	60-69 years
<6.5 µg/L	70-79 years

↑:

<10 µg/L	BPH (malignancy in 20%-30% of cases)
>10 µg/L	Suspicious for malignancy (or acute inflammation)
>20 µg/L	Highly suspicious for malignancy

Interpretation:
- **Prostate cancer**
- Benign: Benign prostatic hyperplasia **(BPH), prostatitis,** prostate infarct
- Increases after **digital rectal examination (DRE), biopsy,** prostate massage, normalization within 3 d-6 wk
- **An increase of >0.8 µg/L/year or by 70% within a year has sensitivity of 90% and specificity of 90%-100%**
- Values >0.2 ng/mL are considered evidence of biochemical recurrence of cancer in men after prostatectomy

fPSA/tPSA ratio:
Free PSA (fPSA) and total PSA (tPSA): PSA has different isoforms:10%-30% free PSA circulating unbound in the serum, 70%-90% forms a complex with alpha-1-antichymotrypsin. Patients with prostate cancer have a lower free PSA compared with patients with BPH. This may aid in the differentiation of carcinoma vs hyperplasia. This improves early detection as well as reduces unnecessary biopsies. Ratio <0.10: increased probability of prostate cancer
Ratio >0.25: increased probability of BPH

Pathophysiology:
A glycoprotein produced in the prostate gland, the urethral lining, and the bulbourethral gland. Usually PSA concentration in the serum is low, unless disruption of the prostate. PSA is largely organ-specific, but not tumor specific
The American cancer society recommends annual DRE and serum PSA beginning at age 50 years. Younger for those in high-risk groups (African Americans or men with a first-degree relative diagnosed at a younger age)

AFP: | **Alpha-Fetoprotein**

Norm:

<6 U/mL	>1 year
>100,000 ng/mL	Neonates (100 ng/mL by 150 days)
<500 U/mL	Mild elevation: hepatitis
>1200 U/mL	Practically diagnostic of malignancy

Interpretation:
- Carcinoma: **Hepatocellular**, hepatoblastoma, non-seminomatous germ cell tumors (embryonal, yolk sac - see HCG below) of **testis/ovary**, stomach, cholangio, pancreas, lung, breast, advanced colorectal (other tumors usually show liver mets); the majority of values are less than 500 KIU/L, in only 4% values >500 KIU/L.
- Benign: cirrhosis, hepatitis, **pregnancy**

Pathophysiology:
A glycoprotein that migrates with alpha-1-proteins on SPEP. Produced in GI tract, liver, and yolk sac of the fetus

HCG: **Human chorionic gonadotrophin**

Total-HCG
<5 U/L men, women (premenopausal, not pregnant)
<10 U/L women (postmenopausal)
Beta-HCG
Norm: <0.2 U/L
↑: >25 IU/L   Pregnancy, as early as 1 wk post-conception

Interpretation
- CA: germ cell tumors of testes/ovary
  - Embryonal carcinomas: most AFP- and HCG-positive
  - Pure seminoma: always AFP-negative, and only rarely HCG-positive
  - Choriocarcinoma: Always HCG-positive, and AFP-negative
  - Yolk sac tumor: Always AFP-positive, HCG-negative
  - Differentiated Teratoma: always HCG- /AFP-negative
  - Mixed tumor: depends on composition
- Also pancreas, GI, hepatocellular, lung, breast, kidney
- Benign: pregnancy: normal, ectopic, molar (higher levels than expected)
- False-elevations may be seen in patients with human antianimal or heterophilic antibodies

Pathophysiology:
A glycoprotein with two non-covalently associated subunits, alpha and beta, related to TSH, LH and FSH. Produced during pregnancy by the placental syncytiotrophoblasts, helps maintain the corpus luteum

4.2   Sensitivities for (Selected) Solid Tumors

Lung tumors

- Small cell:
  NSE (54%), CYFRA 21-1 (16%-55%), NSE and CYFRA 21-1 (62%)
- Non-small cell:
  CYFRA 21-1 (49%), CEA (29%), SCC (17%)
- Squamous cell:
  CYFRA 21-1 (60%), SCC (31%), CEA (18%)
- Adenocarcinoma:
  CYFRA 21-1 (42%), CEA (40%), CYFRA 21-1 + CEA (55%).

Breast

CA15-3: Specificity 95% when >28 U/mL
- Primary Diagnosis: Sensitivity 20% to 30%
  - Node-negative cases: Sensitivity 16% (>25 U/mL)
  - Node-positive cases: Sensitivity 54% (>25 U/mL)
- Recurrent: Sensitivity 30%; distant mets: Sensitivity 50%-90%
CEA: Sensitivity between 27%-75%, depending on the stage of the disease
CA15-3 + CEA:
- Primary diagnosis: Sensitivity 30%-60%
- Recurrent: Sensitivity 56%; distant mets: Sensitivity 60%-80%

Colorectal

CEA: Increases according to stage
I (0%-20%), II (40%-60%), III (60%-80%), IV (80%-85%)

Pancreas

CA 19-9: Sensitivity 70%-95%, specificity of 72%-90%
CEA: Sensitivity 35%-50%

Stomach

CA 72-4 (40%-46%), CA 19-9 (30%-34%), CEA (20%-24%)
- Primary diagnosis (sensitivities at specificity of 95%)
CA 72-4 (69%), CEA (54%), CA 19-9 (48%)
- Distant mets (sensitivities at specificity of 95%)
CA 72-4 + CEA (68%-72%),
CA 72-4 + CA 19-9 (64%),
CEA + CA 19-9 (64%),
CA 72-4 + CEA + CA 19-9 (74%)
- Tumor-Marker -combinations (sensitivities at specificity of 95%)

Hepatocellular

AFP: Sensitivity 60%-95%, specificity 75%

Ovarian

CA-125: >35 U/L sensitivity 82%-96%; >65 U/mL sensitivity 74%-78%
- Staging sensitivities >65 U/mL:
  I: 66%, II: 74%, III: 94%, IV: 100%
- Histology sensitivities
  - Serous: >65 U/mL (sensitivity 81%-98%)
  - Endometrioid: >35 U/mL (sensitivity 60%-75%)
  - Undifferentiated: >35 U/mL (sensitivity 57%-88%)
  - Mucinous: >35 U/mL (sensitivity 45%-67%); >65 U/mL (sensitivity 9%-69%)

Prostate

PSA: >10 µg/L (sensitivity 68%, specificity 90%)
PSA-increase Rate: increase of >0.8 µg/L/year or >70% within a year (sensitivity 90%, specificity 90%-100%)

PSA (µg/L)	Positive predictive value %	Negative predictive value %
<2.5	10	90
<10	25	70
>10	50-60	50

Cervix

SCC: >2.5 µg/L sensitivity 59%
  - Primary squamous: sensitivity 45%-83%
  - Recurrent squamous: Sensitivity 66%-84%
  - Adenosquamous: sensitivity 56%; adeno: sensitivity 0%-23%
CEA: Sensitivity 32% >3 µg/L

Bladder: (muscle invasive)

CYFRA 21-1: Sensitivity 52%-56%, specificity 95%
  - Stage I: 4-16%, II: 33%, III: 36%, IV: 73%
TPA: Sensitivity 40%, specificity 95%

Pleural effusion

Malignant:
- **CEA:** Sensitivity 52%, specificity 95% >3.5 ng/mL
- **CYFRA 21-1:** Sensitivity 62%, specificity 95%, >65 µg/L
- **CA 15-3:** Sensitivity 48%, specificity 97% >25 U/mL

Adenocarcinoma:
- ↑CEA and CYFRA 21-1 in effusion
- In pleural effusion, CEA is the best to differentiate mesothelioma (normal) and other malignant tumors (increased)
  > 2.3 µg/L: sensitivity 83%, specificity 95%

Pleural mesothelioma:
CYFRA 21-1-concentration in mesothelioma pleural effusion associated with histological type. Higher concentrations found in epithelioid vs sarcomatoid and biphasic

- **General:**
  - ↑CYFRA 21-1, normal CEA in effusion
  - Serum: CYFRA 21-1 and CEA are normal
- **Epithelioid:**
  - ↑↑ CYFRA 21-1, normal CEA in effusion
  - Serum: CYFRA 21-1 and CEA are normal

Ascites

Malignant:
- **CEA:**
  - >2.2 µg/L: sensitivity 83%, specificity 83%, PPV 75%, NPV 89%
  - >2.5 µg/L: sensitivity 45%, specificity 100%
  - >3.0 µg/L: sensitivity 51%, specificity 100%
- **CA 19-9:** >30 KIU/L: sensitivity 52%, specificity 100%, PPV 100%, NPV 50%
- **AFP:** Values >30 KIU/L: sensitivity 52%, specificity 100%

Clinically relevant tumor markers and their weighting in different tumors:

	CEA	CA 19-9	CA 72-4		
Stomach	▨ 2nd	■ 1st	■ 1st		
Pancreas	▨ 2nd	■ 1st			
Biliary tract	▨ 2nd	■ 1st			
Colon	■ 1st	▨ 2nd			

	CEA	CA 125	CA 15-3	CA 72-4	SCC
Breast	▨ 2nd		■ 1st		
Ovary		■ 1st		▨ 2nd	
Cervix	□ opt				■ 1st
Endometrium		▨ 2nd			

	AFP	HCG
Liver (HCC)	■ 1st	
Germ cell ⇒ Chorion	■ 1st	■ 1st

	PSA	CYFRA 21-1
Prostate	■ 1st	
Bladder		■ 1st

	CYFRA 21-1	NSE	CEA
Lung, small cell	▨ 2nd	■ 1st	
Lung, non-small cell	■ 1st		▨ 2nd

	CEA	SCC
HNO	□ opt	□ opt
Esophagus	□ opt	□ opt

	CEA	Calcitonin	HTG
Thyroid gland	□ opt		■ 1st
C-Cell		■ 1st	

■ Marker 1st choice
▨ Marker 2nd choice or marker first choice with certain restrictions
□ Optional Marker or marker 1st or 2nd choice with certain restrictions

AFP	Alpha-1-fetoprotein	**HCG**	Human chorionic gonadotropin
CA 15-3	Carbohydrate antigen 15-3	**HTG**	Human thyroglobulin
CA 19-9	Carbohydrate antigen 19-9	**NSE**	Neuron-specific enolase
CA 72-4	Carbohydrate antigen 72-4	**PSA**	Prostate-specific antigen
CA 125	Carbohydrate antigen 125	**SCC**	Squamous-cell-carcinoma antigen
CEA	Carcinoembryonic antigen		
CYFRA 21-1	Cytokeratin-fragment 19		

5   Lipids

Cholesterol, triglycerides (TG), and phospholipids are the main lipids in the body. Since lipids are insoluble in water they are transported as lipoproteins with a hydrophilic surface.

Total cholesterol is not in itself sufficient for the detection and differentiation of disorders of lipid metabolism and transport. However, routine determination of all lipid parameters is too complex and expensive. Therefore, the work up of hyperlipoproteinemia is performed in a step-wise fashion.

Step I:	Basic screening should be performed on every patient, in particular those with other cardiovascular risk factors; the majority of the lipid metabolism disorders can be determined by: • **Total cholesterol** • **Triglycerides**
Step II:	When there is increased total cholesterol, the following is recommended: • Control of the elevated values (diet, meds) • Determination of **HDL and LDL** (for convenience, sometimes these are obtained originally, especially if high levels are expected in Step 1) • Possibly exclusion of secondary lipid metabolism disorders (depending on levels, age risk factors, etc)
Step III:	Further studies depend on the question: • Lipoprotein electrophoresis • Lp(a) • Apo-lipoproteins (A-I, A-II, B, possibly C-II, C-III, E) • Apo-E-polymorphism • LDL receptors • Lipoprotein lipase and hepatic triglyceride lipase in heparinized plasma • Fractionation of the lipoproteins and determination of cholesterol and triglycerides in the individual groups

5.1   Cholesterol

Func: A sterol (modified steroid) consisting of 4 rings, a hydrocarbon side chain, and a hydroxyl group. It is an essential **component of cell membranes and subcellular compartments** (eg, mitochondria), and is **precursor of steroid hormones and bile acids**

Ind: Evaluate coronary risk (along with triglycerides), monitor hypercholesterolemia and therapy
Preventative health care (starting at 20 years, then every 5 years)

Path: Circulating cholesterol is 60%-75% endogenous synthesis and 25%-40% dietary intake; 70% is esterified. Dietary cholesterol esters are hydrolyzed in the duodenum, absorbed in the jejunum, esterified in the enterocytes to chylomicrons, and delivered into the blood where 90% are excreted in the bile as bile acids and sterols. The remaining 10% is excreted in the feces through enterohepatic recirculation
High cholesterol is **one of the risk factors of early atherosclerosis.** The amount of risk is partially dependent on total cholesterol, LDL, and the ratio of **LDL to HDL**

HDL: High Density Lipoprotein cholesterol; "good" cholesterol, the smallest lipoprotein with the highest protein to lipid ratio (>50%), has a protective effect and functions as **anti-atherogenic**, carries cholesterol from body back to liver. Determined by precipitating VLDL and LDL from the serum; the HDL remains and can be measured enzymatically. Increased with increased physical activity (exercise). Values <5 mg/dL occur in **Tangier disease**, in association with cholestatic liver disease, and in association with diminished hepatocyte function
Tangier disease: Autosomal recessive disorder with low cholesterol, nl - ↑ TG, and absent HDL and apo A-1

LDL: Low Density Lipoprotein cholesterol: "bad" cholesterol, **contributes significantly to atherosclerotic plaques.** May be isolated by ultracentrifugation, the difference between total cholesterol and the cholesterol in the supernatant after precipitation. However, usually determined mathematically from the total cholesterol (TC), triglycerides (TG) and the HDL using the **Friedewald formula**:

$$LDL = TC - HDL - TG/5$$

Note: This may only be applied to **fasting serum** without chylomicrons and the when **triglycerides <400 mg/dL**

Prod: Predominantly in the liver, but also skin, intestine, (60%-75%); or dietary intake (25%-40%)

Food sources: Cholesterol is only found in animal products
- Particularly high cholesterol: meat (especially organ meats), animal fats, egg yolks, shellfish and crustaceans
- The amount ingested is variable but always less than that formed by endogenous synthesis

Norm: **Total cholesterol:**

<200 mg/dL	Desirable
200-239 mg/dL	Borderline high
≥240 mg/dL	High

HDL:

≤40 mg/dL	Low
41-60 mg/dL	Normal (Borderline low in children)
>60 mg/dL	High (Normal in children)

LDL:

≤100 mg/dL	Optimal (<70 - h/o heart disease and/or diabetes)
101-129 mg/dL	Near optimal
130- 159 mg/dL	Borderline high
≥160 mg/dL	High

LDL-HDL ratio:

≤3.5	Optimal
3.6-5	Borderline high
>5	High

↑ Hypothyroidism, cholestasis, nephrotic syndrome, diabetes mellitus, hypercholesterolemia, familial combined hyperlipidemia (excess production of apolipoprotein B-100), thiazide diuretics, OCPs
Primary hypercholesterolemias are inherited and secondary hypercholesterolemias are acquired and represent the most common form; often associated with elevated triglycerides; and may be higher with high HDL

↓ High metabolic states (malignancies, multiple traumas, surgery, chronic infections), hyperthyroidism, malnutrition, malabsorption syndrome, hepatic insufficiency

Note: Fasting is not required for total cholesterol, but is preferable. Fasting is required for a full lipid panel, especially if HDL is used to calculate LDL (since triglycerides are used in the calculation)

5.2 Triglycerides

Func: Triglycerides are neutral fats that consist of **glycerol and three fatty acids.** If the fatty acid chains consist solely of single bonds that means they are "saturated" with the maximum hydrogen ions. If there is one double bond there is one less hydrogen ion (monounsaturated) and 2+ double bonds equals polyunsaturated. Liver synthesizes triglycerides into VLDL which functions as a transport system for lipids in the blood. The more triglycerides that are released in the peripheral tissues via **lipoprotein lipase** (LPL), the more the density increases: VLDL to IDL ("Intermediate Density Lipoprotein") to LDL (Low Density Lipoprotein). Triglycerides themselves have a comparatively **low atherogenic effect,** but when specifically combined with an elevated LDL that leads to high risk for atherosclerotic cardiovascular disease

Ind: Estimation of coronary risk (with TC, LDL, HDL), hypertriglyceridemia, monitoring therapy.
Preventative health care: **starting at 20 years,** then every 5 years if no abnormality

Prod: Primarily absorbed from the diet in the small intestine as chylomicrons and then transported to the liver

Norm: Serum triglyceride level is heavily dependent on the dietary habits; however, there is also a strong familial/genetic association
Adults:

<150 mg/dL	Normal
150-199 mg/dL	Borderline high
200-499 mg/dL	High
≥500 mg/dL	Very high

Children:

<90 mg/dL	Normal
90-129 mg/dL	Borderline high
≥130 mg/dL	High

↑ Diabetes mellitus, obesity, hypothyroidism, liver disease, nephrotic syndrome, pregnancy, steroids, OCPs/estrogen therapy, spironolactone, cortisol disorders, excessive alcohol consumption
Very high levels (>1,000 mg/dL) can trigger **acute pancreatitis**

↓ Malnutrition, severe anemia, hyperthyroidism, burns, exudative enteropathy, Fredrickson Type A-B-Lipoproteinemia, vitamin C, fibrates, heparin therapy

Mat: Serum (**12 h fasting**), prolonged occlusion of the veins can lead to falsely high values

5.3   Fredrickson Classification

Classification of Familial Hyperlipoproteinemias

Lipid disorders may be classified by the lipoprotein profile or the serum concentration of cholesterol and TG. However, they do correlate well as VLDL and chylomicrons are largely TG and LDL is largely cholesterol. Early onset atherosclerosis is the most common and most well-known consequence of hyperlipidemia, seen when LDL or IDL are too high (increased cholesterol). High TG by itself represents a low risk for atherosclerosis. Eruptive xanthomas are seen with elevated VLDL or chylomicrons (TG), and peri-orbital xanthelasma may be seen with high LDL. Pancreatitis is associated with high levels of TG (>1000 mg/dL).

Type	Lipoproteins increased	Disorders	TC	TG	Age	Additional features
I	Chylomicrons	Lipoprotein lipase deficiency	↑	↑↑↑	<10 y	Pancreatitis Xanthomas
IIa	LDL	Hypercholesterolemia	↑↑↑	↑	<30 y	Early atherosclerosis Xanthomas (tendon)
IIb	LDL and VLDL	Apolipoprotein E def	↑↑↑	↑↑↑	<30 y	Early atherosclerosis Xanthomas
III	IDL	Dysbetalipoproteinemia	↑↑↑	↑↑↑	Often adult	Xanthomas (Palm/sole)
IV	VLDL	Combined hyperlipidemia	↑	↑	>50 y	Early atherosclerosis Xanthomas
V	VLDL and chylomicrons	Hypertriglyceridemia	↑	↑↑↑	Adult	Pancreatitis Xanthomas

Special features:
Familial apolipoprotein C-II deficiency may look like I or V
Familial combined hyperlipidemia may look like II
Familial hypertriglyceridemia may look like IV
Low atherosclerosis risk: Type I and V

5.4   Refrigerated Standing Plasma Test

Initial evaluation of dyslipidemia involving increased TG. Not routinely performed, largely replaced with other methods (eg, electrophoresis). Fasting serum is placed in 4°C refrigerator for several hours. The chylomicrons with 85%-90% triglycerides forms a creamy layer over the serum

- Clear serum indicates lower triglyceride levels
- Cloudy serum indicates increased VLDL (triglycerides)
- A creamy ring at the top indicates large quantities of chylomicrons; the presence of chylomicrons may be seen with clear serum (type I) or with cloudy serum (type V)

5.5   Lipoprotein Electrophoresis

Performed similarly to SPEP, but stained with fat stain (Oil red O, sudan black). The protein content of the lipoproteins determines the speed, the alpha-lipoprotein migrates the fastest, chylomicrons the slowest. More accurate than the standing plasma test

	TG	Cholesterol	Phospholipids	Protein
Chylomicrons	~90%	5%	4%	2%
Pre-beta-Lipoproteins (VLDL)	50%	20%	20%	10%
Beta-lipoproteins (LDL)	10%	45%	25%	20%
Alpha-lipoproteins (HDL)	5%	15%	30%	50%

5.6   The Main Lipoproteins

	Chylomicrons	VLDL	LDL	HDL
Main lipid	Triglyceride (Exogenous)	Triglyceride (Endogenous)	Cholesterol	Cholesterol
Density	0.95	1.0	1.05	1.10

(cont.)	Chylomicrons	VLDL	LDL	HDL
Apoprotein	B-48, A-1, C, E	B-100, C, F	B-100	A-1, C, E, Lecithin cholesterol acyl transferase (LACT)
Origin	Intestines	Intestines, liver	Intravascular: final product of VLDL degradation	Liver, intestine, intravascularly; final product of chylomicron and VLDL degradation
Function	Transport of dietary lipids to liver	Transport of triglycerides to peripheral cells	Transport of cholesterol to peripheral cells	Return of cholesterol from peripheral cells to liver
Half-life	30 min	Hours	Days	Days
Electro-phoresis	Point of origin	Pre-beta	Beta-lipoprotein	Alpha-lipoprotein
Transport	Intestine to liver	Liver to periphery	Liver to periphery	Periphery to liver

5.7   Lipoprotein(a) [Lp(a)]

Func:
- A LDL particle that also has an apolipoprotein (a) covalently linked to apolipoprotein B-100. Has 34 different isoforms and is structurally similar to plasminogen
- Independent risk factor for coronary heart disease and stroke. Serum concentration related to genetic factors, diet and meds have little impact, therefore not routinely performed on health individuals
- Clinical importance especially with other risk factors (increased LDL, family history, smoking, obesity, diabetes, low HDL, etc)
- The relative risk for CHD with increased Lp(a) and increased LDL is ~3x higher than without Lp(a) increase

Ind: To provide additional information on coronary heart disease (CHD) risk

Norm: <30 mg/dL

↑   Increased risk for MI and stroke

Met: Immunochemical measurement of Apo(a)

6　Carbohydrate

6.1　Diabetes Mellitus

A disease of impaired glucose metabolism. Long-term treatment centers around controlling the blood sugar levels to prevent hyperglycemia and ketoacidosis. Chronic complications include atherosclerosis/cardiovascular disease, nephropathy, peripheral neuropathy, and retinopathy

Classification:

Type 1 – Primary insulin-dependent diabetes:
- **Beta-cell defect, which leads to an absolute deficiency**
- Mostly immune-mediated (Autoimmune disease - Ab against pancreatic beta cells)
- Often triggered by viral infections
- HLA-associated (DR3 and/or DR4 in >90% of patients)
- The cause for 10% of all diabetes cases are preventable

Type 2 – Primarily non-insulin dependent diabetes:
- Can be due to **relative deficiency** due to a secretory defect or due to **insulin resistance**
- Type 2a: Normal weight, approximately 10% of cases
- Type 2b: Obesity, 80% of cases

Others:
- Diseases of the exocrine pancreas (pancreatitis, cystic fibrosis, hemochromatosis)
- Endocrinopathies (Cushing's syndrome, acromegaly, pheochromocytoma)
- Chemically induced (glucocorticoids, neuroleptics, alpha interferon, pentamidine)
- Genetic defects in insulin action
- Other genetic syndromes, with which diabetes can be associated
- Infections
- Rare forms of autoimmune mediated

Gestational diabetes (during pregnancy):
- Usually resolves after pregnancy, but may remain
- Patient at high risk for recurrence with future pregnancies

Impaired glucose tolerance:
- Should not be regarded as an independent disease, but as a phase of disturbed glucose metabolism
- Represents an early stage of diabetes

Diabetic ketoacidosis:
- Occurs in insulin-dependent diabetes, type 1 more common than type 2
- Often has inciting event: failure to take insulin, infection, trauma
- Marked hyperglycemia, ketosis, anion gap acidosis; plus hyponatremia, clinical hyperkalemia with overall hypokalemia, neutrophilia, hyperamylasemia, hyperlipasemia, pre-renal azotemia
- Early signs/symptoms: Nausea, cramping, polyuria, polydipsia,
- Late signs/symptoms: Hyperventilation (Kussmaul respiration), altered mental status, coma, death

Note: **Must administer K^+ along with insulin** to avoid marked hypokalemia as insulin causes increased cellular uptake of glucose, H^+, and K^+

6.2   Diagnosis of Diabetes

- **Fasting plasma glucose:**
  - Normal: 70–100 mg/dL
  - **Impaired glucose tolerance: 101–125 mg/dL**
  - **Diabetes: ≥126 mg/dL**
- **Random plasma glucose:**
  - **>200 mg/dL** (with clinical symptoms)
- **Confirmations** (especially if marginal alterations, glycosuria):
  - Daily blood glucose checks
  - Oral glucose tolerance test: 75 g oral glucose intake, 2 h plasma glucose check, >200 mg/dL = positive

6.3   Glucose in the Blood

- **Normal fasting plasma: 70–100 mg/dL**
- **Random plasma: 70–140 mg/dL**

Note: NaF tube is preferred: If blood is left in non-separated tube glycolysis will reduce glucose by 5–10 mg/dL/h

6.4   Hyperglycemia

Elevated blood glucose:
Diabetes mellitus, Graves' disease, acromegaly, acute myocardial infarction, adrenal hyperfunction, pheochromocytoma, anesthesia, shock, carbon monoxide poisoning, CNS disorders (meningitis, trauma, tumors)

Fasting plasma glucose:
Diabetes: ≥126 mg/dL
Glucose Impairment: ≥101 mg/dL

Hyperglycemia hyperosmolar nonketotic coma:
- Occurs in non-insulin-dependent diabetes, type 2; rarely type 1
- Less common than DKA, but more fatal
- Patients have extreme hyperglycemia (>600 mg/dL), hyperosmolarity, and normal pH, ketones, and HCO_3, along with altered mental status and dehydration (increased BUN:creatinine ratio)

6.5   Hypoglycemia

Blood glucose below the normal range:
- Usually caused by overdose of insulin and/or oral anti-diabetic medications (sulfonylurea)
- Critical limit: 45 mg/dL

Symptoms:
- Expression of adrenergic counter-regulation: cold sweat, trembling, hunger, palpitations, pallor
- Neurologically: abnormal coordination, hallucinations, ataxia, altered consciousness - may lead to hypoglycemic shock, sometimes agitation and anger

Causes:
- Excessive physical labor/exercise
- Malnutrition, fasting, or malabsorption syndrome
- Congenital metabolic disorders
- Severe hepatic dysfunction (such as cirrhosis, hepatitis - can't clear insulin or convert glycogen)
- Alcohol consumption when blood glucose concentrations are low (on empty stomach) leads to a further reduction of glycemia

Note: NaF tube is preferred: If blood is left in non-separated tube glycolysis will reduce glucose by 5-10 mg/dL/h

6.6 Mellituria

- Generic term for sugar in the urine, more specific terms: glycosuria, fructosuria, lactosuria, pentosuria
- Most common is glycosuria, a symptom of diabetes

6.7 Glycosuria

Excretion of glucose in the urine:
- **Hyperglycemic glycosuria:** results from elevated plasma glucose above the renal threshold (generally between 150-180 mg/dL)
- **Normoglycemic glycosuria:** results from reduced renal threshold: Pregnancy, toxic and metabolic tubular injury

Important: if present, need to rule out diabetes via blood sugar testing or oral glucose tolerance test

Main indication: Diabetes screening test

Norm:
Random: <15 mg/dL
24 h: <30 mg

6.8 Oral Glucose Tolerance Test (OGGT)

Administration of oral glucose and observation of the serum glucose levels

In healthy individuals, values decrease rapidly to within normal range due to insulin secretion

In delayed or missing insulin secretion the return to baseline is slower.
Ind: Latent diabetes mellitus, renal diabetes, gestational diabetes; to stimulate and analyze endogenous insulin secretion

Prep:
- 3 days normal carbohydrate rich diet (at least 150-200 g/day) and normal physical activity
- Preferably 12 h fasting, before beginning the test (best in the morning between 8-9 am)

Test:
- Draw specimen for fasting blood glucose
- Administer **75 g of glucose** orally in 300 mL of water
  - May alternatively administer via IV
- Draw blood glucose at 60 min, 120 min, if necessary, after 180 min

Diabetes mellitus	Venous plasma	≥200 mg/dL
	Venous whole blood	≥180 mg/dL
	Capillary whole blood	≥200 mg/dL
Glucose intolerance	Venous plasma	140-199 mg/dL
	Venous whole blood	120-179 mg/dL
	Capillary whole blood	140-155 mg/dL

6.9   Ketone Bodies

(Beta-hydroxybutyrate (BHB), acetoacetate acid, acetone)

Func: Generated from metabolism of amino acids, carbohydrates, and fatty acids
More common in **Type 1 diabetes**, but can rarely occur in Type 2
BHB is most common (~75%), followed by acetoacetate (20%), and acetone (5%)
BHB/acetoacetate ratio between 3-7:1 in severe ketosis

Ind: **Differential diagnosis of metabolic acidosis;** particularly ketoacidemia, diabetic coma and non-ketotic hyperosmolar coma

Prod: Increased production during times of hypoglycemia (fasting, starvation, metabolic disorders [diabetes, glycogen storage diseases], malnutrition [frequent vomiting, alcoholism])

Norm: Plasma BHB after overnight (12 h) fast: 0.21-2.81 mg/dL
Urine ketones after overnight (12 h) fast: <50 mg/L

↑ Fasting, starvation, diabetic/alcoholic/pancreatic ketoacidosis, lactic acidosis (sepsis, intoxication, hypoxemia, malignancy), hereditary metabolic disorders, extreme physical exertion, uremia

Mat: Urine, serum

Met: **Serum (quantitative determination of beta-hydroxybutyrate):**
  • Serum is de-proteinized to prevent acetate decarboxylation to acetone
  • Conversion to acetoacetate by beta-hydroxybutyrate-dehydrogenase (beta-HBDH) is measured

Urine (qualitative detection of acetoacetate and acetone):
- 5 drops of Na-Nitroprusside solution and 1 mL 20% NaOH is added to 2 mL urine
  - Will turn blue/violet in the presence of acetoacetate or acetone
- Test strip method: Same concept, but performed by dipping a test strip into urine sample

Note: **Nitroprusside does not react with BHB.** Urine method will not identify elevated BHB (the most abundant ketone)

6.10 Hemoglobin A1c (HbA1c)

Func:
- Hemoglobin with a non-enzymatically attached hexose molecule; a retrospective measure of carbohydrate metabolism over the past **2-3 months**
- **Fasting is not necessary** (largely independent of circadian rhythms, dietary, and other short-term fluctuations in serum glucose concentrations)
- Occurs over the lifespan of the RBC and is dependent on the blood sugar levels
- Minimal variability among patients

Nomenclature:
HbA0 - Unglycosylated HbA group
HbA1 - Glycosylated hemoglobin A (glycosylation of the N-terminal amino acid (valine) of partly degraded hemoglobin with various carbohydrates)
- HbA1a - glycosylated beta chains of HbA1:
  - HbA1a1 - glycosylation with fructose-1,6-diphosphate
  - HbA1a2 - glycosylation with glucose-6-phosphate
- HbA1b - HbA1 with unknown reactant
- HbA1c - ~80% of HbA1, glycosylation with D-glucose
  - L-HbA1c - labile aldose form
  - S-HbA1c - stable ketose form

Ind: **Diagnosis or monitoring long-term glycemic control** in diabetics; not useful for daily monitoring

Prod: Glycosylation of proteins is a constant process; occurs over the lifespan of the RBC and is dependent on the blood sugar levels

Norm: 4%-6%

Evaluation of a glucose control:	**Borderline:** 6.1%-6.5% **Diabetes:** >6.5%
Therapeutic goals:	Adults: <7.0% Teens: <7.5% Children: <8.0% Toddlers: 7.5%-8.5% Therapeutic goals may need to be adjusted in patients with significant complications, comorbid conditions, and/or cardiovascular disease
↑	Poor blood glucose control Satisfactory control: <7.0% Moderate control: 7.1-7.5% Poor control: >7.5%
Mat:	Serum/plasma, blood
Met:	High performance liquid chromatography (HPLC - most common), electrophoresis, affinity chromatography, immunoassay
Note:	• As HbA1c is a long-term reflection of blood glucose levels, a patient who recently achieved good control will still have high HbA1c levels for several weeks; and conversely, a patient who has started to have poor control will still have low levels • Falsely low levels may be seen in hemolytic anemia • Falsely high levels may be seen in polycythemia or post-splenectomy • Patients with rare homozygous disorders (HbCC, HbSS, HbEE, HbSC) will not have Hb A, hence HbA1c is not measurable - may use **fructosamine** • Some rarer Hb variants will interfere with testing (HbD, HbE, HbFukuoka, HbPhili, HbRaleigh). More common variants (HbF, HbC, HbS)

6.11   Fructosamine

Func: Glycated serum proteins with a shorter half-life than HbA1c (20 days); a retrospective measure of carbohydrate metabolism over the past **2-3 weeks**

Ind: **Monitoring intermediate-length glucose control** in diabetes; to monitor insulin therapy

Prod: Albumin is preferred (80% of glycated proteins); non-enzymatic addition of glucose to the NH_2 group that occurs over the lifespan of the protein and is dependent on the blood sugar levels

Norm: 200-285 µmol/L

↑   Poor blood glucose control
Satisfactory control: <317 µmol/L
Moderate control: 317-345 µmol/L
Poor control: >345 µmol/L

Mat: Serum

Met: Fructosamine test (photometric determination of reduced ketoamine)

Note: As the fructosamine test is a photometric test, any color generating compound may interfere (vitamin C, bilirubinemia). Newer, more specific tests are available
Reference ranges vary by patient's age, gender, and laboratory methods. In general, a 60 mg/dL increase in blood sugar yields an ~2% rise in HbA1c and ~120 µmol/L rise in fructosamine. Some use the calculation below to relate fructosamine with HbA1c yielding the following results:
Fructosamine = (HbA1c =1.61) x 58.8

Fructosamine	HbA1c
200 µmol/L	5.0%
258 µmol/L	6.0%
288 µmol/L	6.5%
317 µmol/L	7.0%
346 µmol/L	7.5%
375 µmol/L	8.0%
435 µmol/L	9.0%
494 µmol/L	10.0%

6.12 Insulin

Func:
- Protein hormone that regulates glucose uptake and utilization, protein synthesis and triglyceride metabolism; blood levels parallel blood glucose levels (ie, directly proportional)
- Type 1 diabetes is due to insulin deficiency (islet cells destruction), type 2 diabetes is due to insulin resistance
- Whipple triad: classic findings in insulinomas; hypoglycemia <45 mg/dL with typical symptoms that is relieved with glucose ingestion; Insulin:Glucose ratio often >180

Ind: Monitoring diabetes, monitoring insulin therapy, suspected insulinoma

Prod: Pancreatic islet/beta cells; released in response to hyperglycemia

Norm: 2.5-25 µIU/mL

↑ Insulinoma (elevated even during hypoglycemia), early type 2 diabetes

↓ Type 1 diabetes (progressive decline with ongoing destruction), late type 2 diabetes

Mat: Serum

Met: Immunoassay

Note: Cross-reactivity with exogenous recombinant human insulin
Test interference with anti-insulin antibodies and heterophile antimouse antibodies

6.13 C-peptide (Connecting Peptide)

Func:
- 31 amino acid midportion of proinsulin that may be involved in endothelial function and bone and renal circulation; mainly used to **measure insulin secretion** (longer half-life than insulin: ~30 min vs. 5-10 min)
- Insulin: Stimulates cellular glucose uptake and suppresses glycogenolysis, gluconeogenesis, and ketogenesis
- Discordant c-peptide/insulin molar ratio (nl<1) indicates either exogenous insulin (therapeutic, factitious) or anti-insulin autoantibody (bound insulin has longer half-life), molar ratio >1
- Maintained normal molar ratio (<1) in insulinoma and sulfonylurea

Ind: Diagnostic work-up of hypoglycemia (insulinoma, factitious insulin administration), early insulin deficiency (suspected prediabetes type 1), monitoring insulin levels in diabetics or post pancreatic/islet cell transplant

Prod: Pancreatic beta cells, **C-peptide and insulin arise from the proinsulin in equal quantities;** excreted by the kidneys

Norm: 1.0-4.0 µg/L

↑ Insulin producing tumor, renal failure, sulfonylurea toxicity, secondary insulin elevation (obesity, glucose intolerance, early type 2 diabetes), insulin-antagonist hypersecretion (Cushing's, acromegaly)

↓ Pancreatic failure/decreased insulin secretion (type 1 diabetes, long-standing type 2 diabetes)

Mat: Serum, fasting (at least 8 h after last high-dose biotin administration)

Met: Immunoassay (cross-reactivity with proinsulin)

Note
- **C-peptide suppression test** - C-peptide levels are measured after exogenous insulin induced hypoglycemia (<60 mg/dL) → **insulinoma - lack of suppression**
- **Falsely low levels may be seen with specimen hemolysis** or with marked elevations (>180 µg/L - hook effect)
- Test interference with heterophile antimouse antibodies, or antibodies to ruthenium or streptavidin

6.14 Lactate

Func:
- A **metabolic product of anaerobic glycolysis**, increased during oxygen deprivation states (inhibition of aerobic glycolysis); the normal lactate/pyruvate ratio is 10-20:1; cardiac muscle can get 60% of its energy from lactate; the liver and kidneys are less dependent on lactate for the gluconeogenesis; during oxygen deprivation, the liver meets the energy requirements by the anaerobic glycolysis
- **Lactic acidosis** is a sign of deteriorated cellular oxidative processes and is characterized by hyperpnea, muscle weakness, fatigue, altered mental status, coma, and death
- McArdle disease: Autosomal recessive glycogen storage disease type V; glycogen phosphorylase deficiency leading to defective glycogenolysis in muscle cells characterized by myoglobinuria, fatigue, muscle cramps, stiffness, and weakness

Ind:	Diagnosis and monitoring lactic acidosis, detection of tissue hypoxia (septic shock, poisoning); metabolic acidosis; suspected McArdle-syndrome, diagnosis of cerebral and meningeal disorders (in CSF)
Prod:	Muscles; red blood cells, brain, adrenal medulla; metabolized by liver
Norm:	**Blood:** 0.5 to 2.2 mmol/L **CSF:** 1.2 -2.1 mmol/L
↑	• **Blood:** Hyperlactatemia without acidosis: physical activity, carbohydrate infusion, elevated insulin, hyperventilation compensation, postoperative. Hyperlactatemia with acidosis: clinically subdivision into lactic acidosis with or without impaired tissue perfusion; heart failure, shock/circulatory failure, hypovolemia, diabetes, congenital metabolic disorders, toxins (ethanol, methanol, salicylates) • **CSF:** Bacterial meningitis, ischemia, epileptic seizure
↓	McArdle's disease - reduced lactate formation; function test: muscle ischemia test
Mat:	Blood - NaF tube, from vein; CSF
Met:	Enzymatically
Note	**Falsely high levels may be seen with prolonged tourniquet use.** Some methods do no measure D-lactate (uncommon cause of lactic acidosis)

6.15 Glucagon

Func:	• 29 amino acid peptide hormone that stimulates **glycogenolysis and gluconeogenesis. Functions opposite of insulin, ie, glucagon raises blood glucose levels** in order to maintain a sufficient supply of glucose to the brain • Hyperglucagonemia leads to hyperglycemia and can be seen in diabetes/ketoacidosis • Glucagonoma syndrome: rash (necrolytic migratory erythema, stomatitis, glossitis), weight loss, diabetes, and diarrhea
Ind:	Diagnosis and post-surgical monitoring of glucagonomas; limited utility in diagnostic work-up of hypo- or hyperglycemic episodes

Prod: Pancreatic alpha cells (and hypothalamus); cleaved from a larger precursor peptide; secretion stimulated by hypoglycemia as well as amino acids, fatty acids, catecholamines, and the sympathetic nervous system; secretion is inhibited by normal/elevated glucose and somatostatin

Norm: <80 pg/mL
Levels are inversely related to blood glucose and **much higher in neonates**

↑ Glucagonoma, neuroendocrine tumors (carcinoids), rarely hepatocellular carcinoma

6.16 Glucagon Test

Func: Measurement of catecholamines and insulin after glucagon administration

Ind: Determination of residual insulin secretion in newly diagnosed type 1 diabetes, suspected insulinoma, suspected pheochromocytoma

Mat: • Blood
• At least 12 h without alcohol, coffee, tea, or nicotine; 24 h without drugs that stimulate catecholamine release

Met: • For suspected pheochromocytoma: Determine baseline catecholamines and blood pressure
For newly diagnosed patients with type 1 diabetes: Determine baseline insulin
• 1 mg IV glucagon
• Re-determine the appropriate parameters after 5, 10, and 15 min
Increase in catecholamines to >3x baseline and increase in blood pressure >20 mmHg: suspicious for pheochromocytoma
Increase in insulin to >135 mIU/L: suspicious for insulinoma (only 50% sensitive)

Note • May cause nausea and vomiting, particularly at doses >1 mg and rapid injection
• Hypersensitivity reactions are possible
• Relative contraindication: blood pressure >170/110 mmHg: risk of hypertensive crisis

6.17 Congenital Disorders

Inborn errors of catabolism and anabolism of any of the 3 main monosaccharides: fructose, galactose, and glucose

6.17.1 Fructosuria

- Autosomal recessive disorders that render patient unable to metabolize fructose
- Hepatic fructokinase mutation is most common; catalyzes the first step in fructose metabolism; deficiency leads to asymptomatic fructosuria
- Hereditary fructose intolerance is due to deficiency of hepatic, renal and intestinal fructose-1,6-diphosphate aldolase that leads to poor feeding, failure to thrive, liver and kidney failure, and death; patients asymptomatic unless they consume fructose or sucrose
- Hepatic fructose-1,6-diphosphatase deficiency leads to impaired gluconeogenesis, hypoglycemia, and marked metabolic acidosis; growth and development are normal with proper recognition and nutritional support

6.17.2 Galactosemia

- Inability to metabolize galactose
- Most common monogenic carbohydrate metabolic disorder caused by mutation in galactose-1-phosphate uridyltransferase
- Discovered in neonates after feeding (especially breast milk - lactose); leads to failure to thrive, liver failure, cataracts, developmental delay, mental retardation, and infertility
- Milder form seen with galactokinase deficiency - uridine diphosphate galactose-4-epimerase which breaks down galactose byproduct; associated with cataracts, but not other signs/symptoms; can be limited to RBCs
- Galactose can also be slightly increased in severe liver disease (decreased metabolism)

6.17.3 Other urinary saccharides

- Usually clinically irrelevant
- Elimination of fructoses and pentoses (xylose, arabinose) typically after fruit consumption
- Lactose: Occasionally in late pregnancy

6.17.4 Lactose intolerance

- Most common carbohydrate metabolic disorder (up to 90% have autosomal dominant mutation that allows lactase production after infancy - especially in areas of the world with high milk ingestion rates)
- Causes issues with lactose absorption leading to nausea, bloating, gas, and diarrhea after dairy consumption
- In adolescents can get regression of lactase activity
- Congenital lactase deficiency
- Transient lactose intolerance (in premature infants)
- Testing. Lactose challenge test

6.17.5 Glycogen storage disorders

- Group of mostly autosomal recessive congenital metabolic diseases with enzyme defects in which glycogen is insufficiently (or not at all) converted to glucose, or glucose metabolism
- Liver and skeletal muscle are commonly affected → hepatomegaly, hypoglycemia and muscle fatigue, weakness, cramping
- **Type I (Von Gierke's)** – glucose-6-phosphatase deficiency; hypoglycemia, hyperlipidemia, growth failure, lactic acidosis, hepatomegaly, but minimal muscle symptoms
- **Type II (Pompe's)** – acid alpha-glucosidase deficiency; hepatomegaly, muscle weakness → heart failure, death by 2 years
- **Type III (Cori's or Forbes')** – glycogen debranching enzyme deficiency; hypoglycemia, hyperlipidemia, hepatomegaly, and myopathy
- **Type IV (Andersen)** – glycogen branching enzyme deficiency; hepatomegaly, cirrhosis, failure to thrive, death by 5 years
- **Type V (McArdle's)** – muscle glycogen phosphorylase deficiency; muscle cramps, rhabdomyolysis, renal failure
- **Type VI (Hers')** – liver glycogen phosphorylase deficiency; hypoglycemia, hepatomegaly
- **Type VII (Tarui's)** – muscle phosphofructokinase deficiency; muscle cramps, growth retardation, hemolytic anemia
- **Type IX** – phosphorylase kinase deficiency; hypoglycemia, hyperlipidemia, hepatomegaly
- **Type XI** – glucose transporter defect; hypoglycemia, hepatomegaly
- **Type XII** – aldolase A deficiency; muscle cramps
- **Type XIII** – beta-enolase deficiency

6.18   Common Mono- and Disaccharides

Monosaccharides	Disaccharides
Glucose	Maltose, malt sugar: Glc-Glc
Galactose	Sucrose, cane sugar: Glc-Frc
Fructose	Lactose, milk-sugar: Glc-Gal

7 Enzymes

7.1 Alkaline Phosphatase

AKA Alk Phos, ALP

Func: A hydrolase enzyme responsible for dephosphorylation

Ind: Hepatobiliary disease, connective tissue disorders, certain bone disorders

Prod: ALP is ubiquitous in the body, but particularly concentrated in the **liver, bile ducts, bone, and kidney (ALPL)**, the intestines (ALPI), the placenta (ALPP), and white blood cells (LAP)

In healthy individuals, ALP in the serum comes from approximately **equal shares** from the **liver** and the **musculoskeletal system.** If the source is unclear, isoenzyme studies can be performed, as can heat stability testing (bone burns, liver lasts)

Norm: 40–140 IU/L

Varies with age and gender. High levels seen in children undergoing growth spurts and pregnant women

↑
- Liver: liver disease, biliary cirrhosis, hepatocellular carcinoma
- Intestinal: inflammatory bowel disease
- Bone: tumors/metastases, Paget's disease, osteomalacia/osteoporosis, other bone diseases, fractures
- Placenta: third trimester, seminomas

↓ Protein deficiency, severe anemia, hereditary ALP-deficiency, OCPs

7.2 Leukocyte Alkaline Phosphatase (LAP)

Func: A hydrolase enzyme responsible for dephosphorylation, specific to white blood cells

Prod: Mainly in neutrophils

↑ Reactive granulocytosis, lymphangitis, polycythemia vera (PV), essential thrombocytosis (ET), primary myelofibrosis (PM)

↓ Chronic myelogenous leukemia (CML), paroxysmal nocturnal hemoglobinuria (PNH) and acute myelogenous leukemia (AML)

7.3 Alpha-Amylase

Func: Digestive enzyme, breaks down carbohydrates into composite sugars. Salivary amylase (ptyalin) and pancreatic amylase cleave linear α (1,4) glycosidic links yielding dextrins and maltose; inactivated by stomach acid

Ind: Pancreatitis, unclear abdominal pain, parotid disease

Prod: Isoenzymes: **pancreatic and salivary** (S-also in tears, sweat, breast milk) The majority is secreted into GI tract, only a fraction enters the blood and is rapidly excreted into the urine

Norm: 30-140 IU/L Serum
25-400 IU/L Urine

↑
- **Pancreatitis** (>10x normal, easier to perform than Lipase, but less specific), tumors of the pancreas, ovary, or lung, ERCP, cholecystitis, severe gastroenteritis
- **Parotitis/Mumps** (3-5x normal), salivary gland trauma (eg, stones, intubation), renal insufficiency (decreased excretion)

↓ Genetic variant, decrease in pancreatic parenchyma (cancer, fibrosis/ chronic pancreatitis)

7.4 Cholinesterase (ChE)

Func: A family of serine proteases that hydrolyze the neurotransmitter acetylcholine into choline and acetic acid

Ind: Liver disease, pseudocholinesterase deficiency, prolonged apnea after surgery, pesticide poisoning

Prod: **Acetylcholinesterase** (AChE), AKA erythrocyte (RBC) cholinesterase, or acetylcholine acetylhydrolase, mainly found in CNS gray matter, **nerve synapses, neuromuscular junctions**, where it ends neurotransmission, or on **RBC membranes** where it is part of the Yt blood group antigens. Also in lung and spleen, but **not in the plasma**. Presence in amniotic fluid is evidence of birth defects (abdominal wall, neural tube).
Pseudocholinesterase (BChE or BuChE), AKA plasma cholinesterase, butyrylcholinesterase, or acylcholine acylhydrolase, found primarily in the liver, but also plasma, intestines, pancreas, spleen, and CNS white matter. Half-life 8-16 h. **Only BChE is of clinical importance for testing/ follow-up.**
The difference between the two is primarily their preferred substrates: the former - acetylcholine; the latter - butyrylcholine, aryl and alkyl esters. The function of the serum enzyme is unknown.

Norm: 8-18 U/mL

↑ Enteropathy, diabetes mellitus, steatosis, hyperlipoproteinemia, acute MI

↓
- Pseudocholinesterase deficiency (genetic mutation, manifests during surgery/dental procedures - response to neuromuscular blockers/anesthetic), **advanced liver disease** (acute toxic damage, or chronic hepatitis/cirrhosis, tumors), pesticide poisoning
- The decrease must be >75% before significant prolongation of neuromuscular blockade is seen
- Drugs to avoid: succinylcholine, mivacurium, pilocarpine, novacaine

Met: The Acholest paper test: a drop of the patient's plasma is applied to the substrate-impregnated test paper yielding a colorimetric reaction. The time is inversely proportional to the BChE activity
- <5 min - Above normal
- 5-20 min - Normal
- 20-30 min - Borderline low
- >30 min - Below normal

7.5   Creatinine Kinase (CK)

Func: AKA creatine phosphokinase (CPK). Muscle specific enzyme, skeletal >cardiac>smooth. Catalyzes the production of creatine and ATP from phosphocreatine (PCr) and ADP. This is a reversible reaction, therefore it serves as an energy reservoir (storage and production of ATP)

Ind: Major indication: **suspected myocardial infarction**

Prod: Isoenzymes: MM = skeletal muscle, MB = cardiac muscle, BB = CNS, smooth muscle. When healthy, practically only CK-MM in blood. Cells that consume ATP rapidly, especially muscle, but also brain, retina photoreceptors, inner ear hair cells, and spermatozoa

Norm: Varies greatly with sex and age. Reference levels not established for under 6 years

- 50-330 IU/L Men ≥18 years
- 40-175 IU/L Women ≥18 years
- 90-500 IU/L Boys 12-17 years
- 90-270 IU/L Girls 12-17 years
- 150-500 IU/L Boys 6-11 years
- 130-400 IU/L Girls 6-11years

↑ Myocardial infarction, myocarditis, muscular dystrophy, myositis, rhabdomyolysis (excessive exercise, antibiotics), acute renal failure

Met: A coupled enzyme reaction where NADPH formation is measured photometrically and is directly proportional to CK

7.6   Creatine Kinase of Cardiac Muscle (CK-MB)

Func: Muscle specific enzyme that catalyzes the production of creatine and ATP from phosphocreatine (PCr) and ADP

Ind: Acute myocardial infarction, but now often replaced by or used in conjunction with troponins (gold standard)

Prod: Cardiac muscle, but a small amount in skeletal muscle

Norm: <6.7 ng/mL (Men)
<3.8 ng/mL (Women)

↑
- Myocardial infarction: Increases in 4-8 h, max. 12-24 h, nl after 3-4 days
  Note: 10% will have no CK-increase
- Severe unstable angina, polymyositis, rhabdomyolysis, crush injuries, CO poisoning, pulmonary embolism, muscular dystrophy
  Note: CK-MB rarely >30% of total, values >50% of total CK probably represent unusual Beta-subunit synthesis

Met: "Sandwich" electrochemiluminescence immunoassay using 2 CK-MB antibodies (one labeled)

7.7   Macro-CK

A variant of CK, which may migrate between MM and BB on the gel, falsely increasing CK-MB
Two major types:
- **Type 1: Enzyme-antibody complex**, Usually CK-BB with IgG>IgA, rarely IgM, CK-BB without can be very debilitating, usually in women >70 years
- **Type 2: Non-immunoglobulin bound oligomer from mitochondrial CK (CK-MI)**, increased in paraneoplastic syndrome and cirrhosis

Ind: Discordant CK-increases:
- Persistent enzyme activity without a dynamic curve
- CK-MB >25% of total-CK

7.8   Gamma Glutamyl Transferase (GGT)

Func: Participation in amino acid transport into the cells

Ind:
- Currently the most sensitive indicator to diagnose and monitor liver disease, screening/monitoring occult/chronic alcoholism
- Rises earlier and persists longer than other enzymes (AST, ALT, etc)
- Helpful to determine if increased alk phos is from musculoskeletal/ growth spurt, pregnancy (GGT normal)

Prod: Primarily liver, kidney, pancreas

Norm:
9-50 U/L	Men >18 years
7-28 U/L	Boys 1-17 years
6-38 U/L	Women>1 years

↑ Acute and chronic hepatitis (2-5x), cirrhosis, steatosis, liver tumors/ metastases (>10x), cholestasis, drugs (eg, OCPs, anticonvulsants, steroids, thiazides), pancreatitis, pancreatic tumors, MI (~50%)

Met: Enzyme colorimetric method measured at 405 nm

7.9   Glucose-6-Phosphate-Dehydrogenase (G6PD)

Func: Intraerythrocyte reduction of glutathione

Ind: Unclear etiology in chronic Coombs-negative nonspherocytic hemolytic anemia

Path: Decreased formation of NADPH due to deficient reduction of glutathione, older erythrocytes accelerated reduction, Increased RBC Heinz bodies (oxidized, denatured hemoglobin)

Epi: The **most common enzyme deficiency in hemolytic anemia. X-linked recessive**, >300 mutations, variably symptomatic (chronic hemolysis), most commonly asymptomatic with acute hemolytic episodes triggered by drugs (eg, sulfonamides, anti-malarials), infection, or **fava beans**. High frequency in patients of **Southeast Asian/ Mediterranean** descent, and abnormal variants in African Americans may lead to normal levels even with hemolysis

Norm: 8-14 U/g Hb

↓ G6PD deficiency, 0-20% of normal

Met: Spectrophotometric measurement of the enzyme activity (NADPH production)

7.10 Pyruvate Kinase (PK)

Func: Catalyzes the last step of anaerobic glycolysis

$$PEP + ADP \leftrightarrow pyruvate + ATP$$

Ind: Unclear etiology in chronic hemolytic anemia despite thorough initial work-up

Path: **Faulty anaerobic glycolysis**
→ **ATP depletion**
  → Increased rigidity of RBCs, cells shrink
    → **Accelerated degradation of RBCs** in spleen

Epi: Second most common RBC enzyme defect (after G6PD deficiency); high frequency in patients of central/northern European and north American descent

Norm: >50% Asymptomatic
Most with severe hemolytic anemia have enzyme activity <30%

↓ Autosomal recessive inherited enzyme deficiency
- Homozygous: variable symptoms of mild, compensated, hemolytic anemia to severe hemolysis with severe anemia, hepatosplenomegaly, macrocytosis, poikilocytosis, relatively few reticulocytes
- Heterozygous PK: asymptomatic, enzyme activity is 50% of normal

Met: Spectrophotometric measurement of enzyme activities in hemolysate; no exact correlation between enzyme activity and severity of anemia: enzyme activity alone unsuitable for diagnosis

7.11 Transaminases

7.11.1 Aspartate aminotransaminase (AST)

AKA glutamic oxaloacetic transaminase (GOT)

Func: A pyridoxal phosphate dependent enzyme that catalyzes the reversible transfer of an amino group between Asp and Glu; necessary for amino acid metabolism, glutamate then deaminated to form ammonium, then excreted as urea; and amino acid biosynthesis, citric acid cycle

L-Aspartate (Asp) + α-ketoglutarate ↔ Oxaloacetate + L-glutamate (Glu)

Ind: **Liver disease**, heart disease (MI: only AST↑, not ALT)

Prod: Liver, heart, skeletal muscle, kidney, brain, pancreas, lung, WBCs, RBCs
Two isoenzymes: 80% mitochondrial (liver), 20% cytoplasm (RBCs, heart)

Norm: < 48 U/L   Men
< 43 U/L   Women
< 55 U/L   Children

↑ ↑↑↑ **Liver disease** (hepatitis, cirrhosis, steatosis, mets), **heart attack** (increase 4-8 h, max 16-48 h, nl 3-6 days), carbon tetrachloride poisoning
↑ Skeletal muscle injury (muscular dystrophy, myositis, trauma), pancreatitis

7.11.2 Alanine aminotransaminase (ALT)

AKA glutamate pyruvate transaminase (GPT)

Func: A pyridoxal phosphate dependent enzyme that catalyzes the reversible transfer of an amino group between alanine and α-ketoglutarate

Glutamate + Pyruvate ↔ α-ketoglutarate + alanine

Ind: **Liver disease** (persists longer than AST)

Prod: Mostly in the liver, fairly specific for liver disease.
Subcellular localization: 85% cytoplasm, mitochondria 15%

Norm: < 50 U/L   Men
< 40 U/L   Women
< 25 U/L   Children

↑ Liver disease associated with **hepatocyte destruction** (hepatitis, cirrhosis, steatosis, mets)

7.12   AST/ALT Ratio

AKA De Ritis ratio

Values >1: Cirrhosis, liver mets, non-hepatic reasons (MI, trauma)
                Liver damage with necrosis

Values >2: **Alcoholic hepatitis, hepatocellular carcinoma**

Values <1: **Viral hepatitis**
                Liver damage of inflammatory nature

Note: Less useful when the liver enzymes are not elevated, or when
                multiple conditions co-exist

7.13   Glutamate Dehydrogenase (GLDH)

Func: A mitochondrial oxidoreductase enzyme that catalyses the reversible
           reaction between Glu and α-ketoglutarate, required for urea synthesis

$$\text{Glutamate} \leftrightarrow \alpha\text{-ketoglutarate} + NH_3$$

Ind: **Assessment of the severity (necrosis) and extent of acute liver
           damage**

Prod: Mainly in the liver, but also kidney and brain.

Norm: < 7 U/L   Men
           < 5 U/L   Women

↑   Liver disease with necrosis, obstructive jaundice, acute toxicity, acute
           ischemia (thrombosis)

7.14   (AST + ALT) – GLDH

A measure for the severity of liver damage at the cellular level
In general: <50 severe, >50 mild
>50: Acute viral hepatitis, alcoholic acute toxic hepatitis (GLDH mildly increased)
20–50: Acute flairs in chronic liver disease, cholestasis
<20: Obstructive biliary cirrhosis, liver mets, (GLDH moderately/markedly
increased)

7.15   Lactate Dehydrogenase (LDH)

Func: Catalyzes the reversible conversion of pyruvate (the final product of glycolysis) to lactate when O_2 is low, the reverse is the Cori cycle (liver). Increased lactate leads to negative feedback

Lactate + NAD^+ ↔ Pyruvate + NADH + H^+

Ind: Diagnosis/monitoring MI, PE, jaundice, anemia, organ damage, malignancy

Prod: All cells, especially heart, liver, skeletal muscle, kidney, lung, RBCs
Five isoenzymes: Two are cytochrome-c dependent, two are NAD(P) dependent. Each consisting of 4 polypeptides (H and M)

LDH 1 LDH 2	Cardiac muscle, RBCs, kidney	HHHH HHHM	H4 H3M
LDH 3	Lung, lymphocytes, platelets, endocrine glands	HHMM	H2M 2
LDH 4 LDH 5	Liver, skeletal muscle	HMMM MMMM	HM3 M4

Norm: 120-220 U/L   Adult
120-300 U/L   1-17 years
180-435 U/L   Infant
135-750 U/L   Neonate

Percentages
LDH 1 17%-31%
LDH 2 35%-48%
LDH 3 19%-29%
LDH 4 3.8%-9.4%
LDH 5 2.6%-10%

↑:   ↑↑↑ Megaloblastic anemia, pernicious anemia, Hodgkin's, malignancy (high turnover, esp. GI, lung), shock/hypoxia
↑ MI, myocarditis, pericarditis, PE (LDH3), pulmonary infarct, leukemia, hemolytic anemia, mononucleosis, muscle disorders (muscular dystrophy, myositis, trauma), liver disease (LDH5, not as high as AST, ALT), kidney disease (tubular necrosis, pyelonephritis)

Note: **RBCs have high LDH concentration → hemolysis of specimen will lead to false elevations**

7.16 Hydroxybutyrate Dehydrogenase (HBDH)

Func: Two isoenzymes of LDH (LDH 1 and LDH 2) also catalyze
2-hydroxybutyrate to oxobutyrate

Ind: MI (largely replaced by other cardiac markers, troponins, etc), hemolytic anemia

↑ MI (6-12 h, max 30-72 h, nl 10-20 d), hemolysis

7.17 LDH/AST Ratio

Helps decipher the cause of jaundice between prehepatic (hemolysis, dyserythropoiesis) and hepatic:
- LDH/AST <5 (37°C) Liver and biliary disorders
  (Exception: significant secondary liver involvement in anemia)
- LDH/AST >5 (37°C) Hemolytic disorders (>22 TTP>HELLP)
  (Exception: mononucleosis, some liver malignancies)

7.18 Lipase

Func: **Pancreatic enzyme that hydrolyzes glycerol esters of long-chain fatty acids** absorbed from food. Requires bile salts and cofactor-colipase for full activity

Ind: Suspected acute pancreatitis (acute upper abdomen), chronic recurrent pancreatitis, pancreatic injury

Prod: Pancreatic acinar cells

Norm: Lipase activity in the serum is low in healthy individuals, however, lipase levels rely on the reference ranges of the method used even more than most laboratory tests, in general:
10-70 U/L   Serum
< 4 U/L   Urine   Not excreted in urine like amylase

↑ **Acute pancreatitis (higher specificity [99%] and sensitivity than amylase)**
Acute: 3-6 h, max 20-30 h, nl 7-10 d; Obstructive chronic pancreatitis, acute flair in chronic pancreatitis, renal insufficiency (creatinine >3 mg/dL), drugs (cholinergics, opiates); very high values in cyst fluid are suggestive of pseudocyst

Met: Patients should be **fasting. Should not use collection tubes with glycerol lubricated stoppers or tubes containing citrate, oxalate, or EDTA.**

7.19 Acid Phosphatase (AP)

Func: Enzyme that removes phosphate groups during digestion. Maximum enzymatic activity at pH <7.0. Largely replaced with other tests

Ind: Evaluation of tumors and mets of the **bone/prostate; Gaucher disease**

Prod: Mainly in platelets, RBCs, reticuloendothelial system, bones, prostate. Stored in lysosomes and functions when fusion with endosomes occurs.
5 isoenzymes:
AP-1: RBCs
AP-2: Prostate (inhibition by tartrate)
AP-3: Platelets
AP-4: Monocytes
AP-5: Granulocytes, Gaucher cells, bone

↑ Bone disorders (Paget's disease, hyperparathyroidism, tumors/mets), Gaucher disease, prostate (cancer, prostatitis, DRE), thrombosis/embolism, hemolysis

Met: Best in the morning due to circadian values. Collection tubes should not contain heparin or oxalate (inhibit activity)

7.20 Leucine Aminopeptidases (LAP)

Func: Enzyme that hydrolyzes residues (preferentially leucine) from the N-terminus of proteins

Ind: Liver/biliary disease

Prod: Liver, biliary tree, pancreas, kidney, intestines, testes, breast, uterus

Norm: 1.0-3.3 U/mL

↑
- ↑↑↑ Intra- and extra-hepatic cholestasis, cirrhosis, liver toxicity damage, hepatocellular carcinoma
- ↑ Acute viral hepatitis, tumors in the tissues with high LAP-concentrations

7.21 Enzyme Localization

Mainly:
- Mitochondrial: AST (80%), ALT (15%), GLDH, AP
- Cytoplasmic: AST (20%), ALT (85%), LDH, CK
- Membranous: GGT

7.22 Laboratory Findings in Specific Diagnoses

- Acute viral hepatitis: ALT and AST, but ALT>AST; also: AP, GGT, GLDH
- Alcoholic liver disease: GGT, AST>>ALT
- Steatosis: ALT, ChE
- Chronic hepatitis: ALT, AST, ChE
- Liver tumors: AST, GLDH, GGT
- Hepatocellular necrosis: AST, ALT, GGT, GLDH
- Myocardial infarct: CK, CK-MB, cardiac troponin T and troponin I, myoglobin
- Biliary disease: AP, GGT
- Cholestasis: GGT, AP, LAP, bilirubin, GLDH, ALT, AST
- Pancreatitis: amylase, lipase

7.23 Half-Lives of Enzymes

Enzyme	Half-life	Enzyme	Half-life
AP	3–7 days	GLDH	16–18 h
Alpha–Amylase	9–18 h	GGT	3–4 h
CHE	10 days	GOT (AST)	12–14 h
CK	12 h	GPT (ALT)	50 h
CK-MM	20 h	LDH 1	4–5 days
CK-MB	10 h	LDH 5	10 h
CK-BB	3 h	Lipase	7–14 h

7.24 Cardiac Markers

Marker	Increases	Maximum	Normalization
Troponin T or I	3–8 h	24–48 h	7–14 days
Myoglobin	2–6 h	8–12 h	2 days
CK-MB	4–8 h	12–18 h	2–3 days
Total-CK	4–8 h	16–36 h	3–6 days
AST	4–8 h	16–48 h	3–6 days
LDH	6–12 h	24–60 h	7–14 days

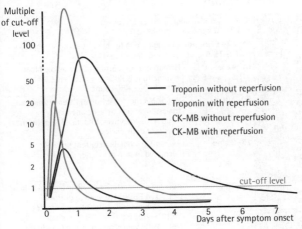

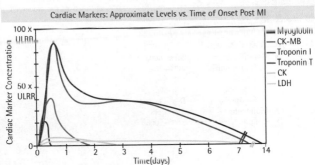

Cardiac Markers: Approximate Levels vs. Time of Onset Post MI

8   Hematology

Erythrocyte count	M: 4.3–5.6 x million/μL = 4.3–5.6 /pL F: 3.9–5.0 x million/μL = 3.9–5.0 /pL	
Hemoglobin (Hb)	M: 14–17.5 g/dL F: 12–15.5 g/dL	Hemoglobin in the blood, usually ~15 g/100 mL of blood; see also →124
Hematocrit (Hct)	M: 42%–50% W: 37%–45%	Hematocrit: proportion of the whole blood volume that is RBCs; see also →125 Hct = MCV x RBC count
Mean corpuscular volume (MCV)	80–100 fL	<80 = Microcytosis: Iron deficiency anemia, thalassemia, sideroblastic anemia >100 = Macrocytosis: Vitamin-B12 deficiency, folic acid deficiencies
Mean corpuscular hemoglobin (MCH)	27–33 pg	Average hemoglobin content per RBC; decreased in iron deficiency anemia
Mean corpuscular hemoglobin concentration (MCHC)	32–36 g/dL	Average concentration of Hb in a given volume of packed RBCs; measured in grams of hemoglobin per deciliter of erythrocytes MCHC = Hb/Hct Note: False values may occur in hereditary spherocytosis, sickle cell disease, and advanced hypochromic microcytic anemia

Reticulocytes: Immature RBCs; see also →123

Leukocytes: 4500–10000/μL = 4.5–10 x 10^9/L

- Granulocytes: 50%–80%
  - Neutrophils: 40%–70%
  - Bands: 0%–5%
  - Eosinophils: 0%–6%
  - Basophils: 0%–2%
- Monocytes: 1%–12%
- Lymphocytes: 20%–50%

Platelets:

Func: Essential in blood clot formation

Norm: $1.5–4.5 \times 10^5/\mu L$

Prod: Small fragments of megakaryocyte cytoplasm; median survival of 8–12 days; destruction in the spleen

↑   Thrombocytosis: inflammation, malignancy, postoperative, hemolysis, polycythemia, leukemia, splenectomy, chronic bleeding, infection

↓   Thrombocytopenia:
   • **Increased consumption:**
     Acute bleeding, infection, sepsis, DIC, certain medications, heparin-induced thrombocytopenia (type I and II), hypersplenism syndrome, autoantibody formation, hemolytic uremic syndrome (HUS, Gasser syndrome), thrombotic thrombocytopenic purpura (TTP, Moschowitz syndrome)
   • **Decreased production:**
     Cytostatic medications, aplasia, infiltration of the bone marrow (myelofibrosis), toxic medication, vitamin B12 deficiency, folic acid deficiency, iron deficiency; rarely, Fanconi syndrome, Wiskott-Aldrich syndrome

8.1   Erythrocyte Morphology

Anisocytosis	Variable size of RBCs; non-specific morphological feature of all anemias; seen even under normal conditions to small extent
Anulocytes	Extenuation of the ringed coloration of RBCs with a narrow band of hemoglobin in the periphery and a wider pale center, usually seen in high-grade iron deficiency
Basophilic stippling	Special form of polychromasia; corresponds to aggregation of RNA-containing ribosomes; may be accompanied by reticulocytosis; associated with specific anemias (hemolytic, sideroblastic), thalassemia, toxins (arsenic, lead), TTP
Cabot ring	Thread-like, loop- or figure 8-shaped, red colored, intra-erythrocytic inclusion; believed to be microtubule remnants of a mitotic spindle; indicative of RBC formation abnormality; found primarily after splenectomy, but also disorders of erythropoiesis, extramedullary hematopoiesis, severe anemia, and thalassemia

Codocyte	"Target cell, leptocyte" RBCs that look like a bull's eye with a red center with surrounding pallor and the usual peripheral ring; due to relative membrane excess (disproportional increase in membrane to volume); increased osmotic resistance (decreased osmotic fragility); occurs in iron deficiency, thalassemia, HbC, liver disease (decreased lecithin-cholesterol-acyltransferase activity)
Dacrocyte	"Tear drop cell", occur in myelophthisic anemia, especially in myelofibrosis (red cell membrane deformation due to marrow fibrosis 'squishing' the RBCs)
Drepanocyte: "Sickle cell"	Erythrocyte that contains hemoglobin HbS, is short-lived (<42 days – normal is 120 days), decreased elasticity, and under oxygen deprivation irreversibly deforms into sickle shape; typical of sickle cell anemia
Elliptocyte	"Ovalocyte", oval-shaped RBC with a difference between the two diameters of at least 2 µm; up to 10% is considered normal; seen in elliptocytosis (Dresbach's syndrome); predisposition to hemolytic anemia
Heinz body	"Heinz-Ehrlich body", precipitated denatured hemoglobin in the form of a spherical RBC inclusion; visualized using supravital stains (bromocresol green, crystal violet, methylene blue); occurs in toxic hemolytic anemia, splenectomy, hereditary Heinz body anemia (hemoglobin abnormality), and in neonates predisposed to oxidative damage by drugs
Howell Jolly body	DNA-containing nuclear remnant; occur after splenectomy, possibly with rapid red cell regeneration (eg, after hemolytic crisis) and in erythrocyte maturation disorders (pernicious anemia)
Normocyte	Regularly-sized, regularly biconcave disc-shaped RBC with normal hemoglobin content, central pallor ~1/3 the diameter, and diameter of 6.5-8.5 µm
Microcyte	Erythrocyte with normal shape, but reduced diameter (<6 µm), often also hypochromic
Macrocyte	Erythrocyte of normal shape, but increased diameter (>8.5 µm), often also hyperchromic
Macroovalo-cyte	Enlarged, slightly oval, hemoglobin-rich RBC with a diameter of 10-20 µm; almost exclusively seen in megaloblastic anemia caused by vitamin B12 and/or folic acid deficiency

Poikilocytosis	Varying cell shape; describes the presence of one or more of these malformed RBC types
Polychro-masia	Varying cell color; typically refers to a gray-blue staining of RBCs seen during increased RBC production (reticulocytosis); therefore usually associated with an elevated reticulocyte count and a slight macrocytosis. This "regenerative" blood is observed in hemolysis and after heavy bleeding, also lead poisoning or thalassemia
Reticulocyte	Immature RBC with slight grey discoloration and slightly increased size (leads to slight macrocytosis); see also →123
Rouleaux formation	Reversible erythrocyte aggregation in the form of coin-like money roll with obstruction of the blood flow, resolves upon dilution with saline; occurs in monoclonal gammopathy, burns, lipemia
Schistocyte	"Helmet cell" fragments of erythrocytes formed by mechanical shearing of intracapillary strained fibrin (thrombi) or mechanical device (eg, artificial heart valve); typically crescent-shaped with pointed ends; found in microangiopathic hemolytic anemia (HUS, TTP), DIC, burns, 'march' hemoglobinuria
Stomato-cytes	Erythrocyte with the shape of a stoma (mouth); occurs in alcoholism, liver disorders, or hereditarily; cells have increased passive permeability for Na^+ and K^+
Spherocytes	Erythrocytes with reduced diameter, loss of biconcave disc shape, and uniformly dense hemoglobin staining without central pallor; occurs in hereditary spherocytosis or hemolytic anemia; occasionally also in alcohol-induced hepatitis, splenectomy, hypertriglyceridemia, and Clostridium infection

8.2   Erythrocyte Sedimentation Rate (ESR)

Func: The rate at which RBCs sediment in 1 hour

Ind: **Screening test for inflammatory and neoplastic changes**

Norm Men <50 years: ≤15 mm
Men >50 years: ≤20 mm
Women <50 years: ≤20 mm
Women >50 years: ≤30 mm

↑ ↑↑: Infection, inflammation, leukemia, malignancy, necrosis, gammopathies, autoimmune diseases, nephrotic syndrome
↑: Anemia, pregnancy, postoperative

↓   Polyglobulinemia, polycythemia vera, sickle cell anemia

Mat: 2 mL citrated blood

Note:
- Less suitable than CRP to follow the course of acute illness, since ESR rises late and drops late
- The 2 h test has no additional value to the 1 h test, so it has been largely abandoned

8.3   Anemia

8.3.1   Disorders of erythropoiesis

Decreased number and/or hemoglobin content of RBCs; results in disorder of O_2 transport and deficient O_2-dependent functions. Often associated with increased bilirubin and secondary hemochromatosis

<14 g/dL	Men
<12 g/dL	Women

Stem cell defect	Reduction of erythropoiesis in the bone marrow (as opposed to erythroblast disorders with hyperplastic erythropoiesis in the bone marrow, see below); isolated disorder of erythropoiesis ("pure red cell aplasia") or of pluripotent stem cells: in combination with neutropenia and thrombocytopenia (panmyelophthisis)

Erythroblast defects	**Megaloblastic anemia:**
	• RBC development and maturation disorder, usually caused by vitamin B12 or folic acid deficiency
	• Increased incidence of megaloblasts in bone marrow and macrocytes in peripheral blood
	Iron deficiency anemia:
	• Most common form of anemia (80%), prevalence 5%-10%
	• Impaired formation of hemoglobin due to iron deficiency
	• Microcytic hypochromic erythrocytes
	• Causes:
	  – Acute or chronic blood loss (GI bleeding, heavy menses)
	  – Malnutrition, malabsorption
	  – Iron transport and recycling defect (sideroblastic anemia)
	  – Increased iron demand (growth, pregnancy, lactation, competitive sports)
	  – Iron distribution disorder (infection, inflammation, tumor)

| Erythro-blast defects (cont.) | **Aplastic anemia:**
Rare bone marrow failure disorder of all three cell lines (pancytopenia); associated with high mortality. In ~15% of cases the pancytopenia is preceded by a mono- or bicytopenia.
Etiology
• Idiopathic aplastic anemia (>70%), cause unknown
• Secondary aplastic anemia: toxic (in particular, benzene), medication, ionizing radiation, viral infections (parvo B19)
Myelodysplastic syndromes:
• Acquired clonal disorders of bone marrow stem cells with associated disturbance in maturation
• Leads to refractory anemia, thrombocytopenia, neutropenia, occasionally also lead to leukocytosis
• Mono-, bi-or tricytopenia with normal or increased bone marrow cellularity
Dyserythropoietic anemia:
Rare, familial refractory anemia with highly ineffective erythropoiesis (often abnormal multinucleated erythroblasts) and qualitative malfunction of the erythrocytes |
| Marked Displace-ment | **Myelophthisic anemia:**
Displacement of the hematopoietic bone marrow by tumor/neoplasia: leukemia/lymphoma, myelodysplasia, malignancy, myeloma, myelofibrosis, metastases of solid tumors
Erythropoietin deficiency:
AKA: Renal anemia
• Normochromic, normocytic, hypo-regenerative anemia
• Develops in chronic renal impairment due lack of erythropoietin (Epo) |

8.3.2   Blood loss

| Acute | Massive acute blood loss → risk of hypovolemic circulatory shock |
| Chronic | Chronic bleeding often leads to iron deficiency anemia. The most common causes are,
• GI tract: carcinomas, hemorrhoids, peptic ulcers, severe gastroesophageal reflux disease
• Genital: carcinomas, menorrhagia |

8.3.3 Increased red blood cell destruction

Often leads to jaundice
Jaundice:
AKA Icterus: yellowing of the skin, mucous membranes, sclera, and internal organs as a result of bilirubin deposition. Visible in the sclera from ~2 mg/dL and in the skin from ~3 mg/dL (depending on the base color of skin)

Corpuscular hemolytic anemia	
Membrane defects	Hereditary RBC membrane defects are caused by mutations in alpha (55%) and beta (30%) spectrin, ankyrin, protein band 3, protein 4.2, and glycophorin 3. Most are autosomal recessive and have variable symptomology
	Hereditary spherocytosis (HS):
	• Autosomal dominant synthesis defect of structural protein spectrin
	• Increased Na^+ and H_2O uptake into RBCs
	• Erythrocytes swell, take on a spherical shape and are destroyed prematurely in the spleen
	• Higher incidence in European descendants
	Hereditary elliptocytosis (HE):
	• Elliptocytes: Oval-shaped deformed RBCs (up to 10% is considered normal deviation)
	• Over 90% are asymptomatic; U.S. incidence believed to be ~0.05%; incidence increased in patients of African or Mediterranean descent (malarial resistance)
	Stomatocytic elliptocytosis (southeast Asian ovalocytosis):
	• Patients are of southeast Asian descent
	• Mild hemolytic anemia
	• Increased malarial resistance
	Hereditary pyropoikilocytosis (HPP):
	• Autosomal recessive variant typically in patients of African descent
	• Life-threatening hemolytic anemia with micropoikilocytosis (small and misshapen RBCs) that are markedly unstable at increased temperatures

Membrane defects (cont.)	Paroxysmal nocturnal hemoglobinuria: • Acquired erythrocyte-induced hemolytic anemia with increased hemolysis during sleep and hemoglobinuria (darkly colored morning urine) • Complement activation by surface structures of the erythrocyte, and subsequent hemolysis with reduction of acetylcholinesterase activity in the cell membrane
Enzyme defects	Glucose-6-phosphate dehydrogenase (G6PD) deficiency: • Reduction of intraerythrocytic reduced glutathione → hemolytic anemia with "oxidative stress" • Usually caused by medication (aspirin, antimalarials, sulfonamides, and certain antibiotics), but also illness, DKA, and sometimes foods (fava beans) • Heinz bodies within RBCs (oxidized, denatured Hb), "bite cells" (RBCs with Heinz body removed in spleen), elevated LDH, decreased haptoglobin, negative direct antiglobulin (Coombs') test, positive **fluorescent spot test** (measures NADPH by G6PD via fluorescent dye, false negatives in patients who are actively hemolysing) • X-linked recessive, most common human enzyme defect, especially in patients of African, middle eastern, or south Asian descent; different mutations lead to variable deficiency levels • Protection from plasmodium falciparum malaria • Most patients are asymptomatic; but may lead to neonatal jaundice +/- kernicterus, hemolytic crises, acute renal failure • Patients should be vaccinated to prevent infection-induced attacks; blood transfusions may be given in times of marked anemia; dialysis in renal failure, splenectomy may be performed in severe cases, folic acid and B12 levels should be watched and supplemented as needed Pyruvate kinase deficiency: • Inherited metabolic disorder characterized by faulty anaerobic glycolysis → lack of ATP • Autosomal recessive inheritance more common, but autosomal dominant variants exist; second most common enzyme deficiency hemolytic anemia (after G6PD); especially in patients of Amish descent

Enzyme defects (cont.)	• Atypical RBCs (echinocytes - "burr cells") with premature destruction in spleen • Different mutations lead to variable deficiencies, total lack of pyruvate kinase is fatal • Usually a- or mildly symptomatic, though may be present with neonatal jaundice +/- kernicterus, and severe cases have multiple hemolytic episodes; gallstones common • Treat with blood transfusions as needed, splenectomy may be performed in severe cases
Hemoglobin defects	**Thalassemia, see also →127** Autosomal recessive hereditary disorder of α or β hemoglobin with hypochromic, iron-refractory, hemolytic anemia **Sickle cell anemia, see also →129** • Autosomal recessive hereditary hemoglobinopathy caused by point mutation (Glu→Val in position 6 of beta hemoglobin chain) • RBCs can carry less oxygen, have a shorter life and take on a sickle shape in oxygen deficiency, resulting in the increased blood viscosity and thrombosis → infarction and organ damage! • In general, only homozygotes clinically manifest disease
Extracorpuscular hemolytic anemia	
Alloimmune hemolytic anemia	**Hemolytic disease of the newborn - erythroblastosis fetalis** • Formation of blood group-specific alloantibodies (Abs - IgG) by the mother against fetal RBCs • Abs cross placenta and cause fetal RBC destruction → reticulocytosis, anemia, hydrops fetalis (edema, heart failure, and death) • Hemolysis leads to jaundice +/- kernicterus • Occurs when there is maternal/fetal ABO or Rh mismatch and hemorrhage occurs (trauma, abortion, childbirth, placental rupture) causing exposure of the fetal RBCs to the mother's system, causing her to produce Ab • **RhD+ is the most common cause**, usually the second child, but may be seen in first child if the patient has been previously exposed to D antigen (blood transfusion); the reason why we give Anti-D IgG, "Rhogam," to all pregnant patients

Autoimmune hemolytic anemia (cont.)	• **Kell antigen** is also a common culprit, but any antigen present on the fetal RBCs that is not present on the mother's RBCs may cause disease
	• Mother will have positive indirect antiglobulin (Coombs') test
	• Child will have positive direct antiglobulin (Coombs') test; Note: may be negative after transfusion
	• Treat with intrauterine blood transfusions, early delivery; plasma exchange of the mother
	Anemia caused by autoantibodies against RBCs leading to premature destruction in the spleen → splenomegaly
	Primary: Idiopathic form (~50% of cases)
	Secondary: Underlying diseases, such as lymphoproliferative disorders (lymphoma, myeloma), paraneoplastic syndrome, autoimmune diseases (lupus, RA), infectious diseases (URI, syphilis, tuberculosis, viral, mycoplasma), drugs
	The resulting disease depends on the type of antibodies and their complement binding capacity
	Warm autoimmune hemolytic anemia (WAIHA, warm agglutinin disease):
	• Ab has maximal activity at body temperature (37°C)
	• Usually IgG, but may be IgA
	• Most common AIHA
	• Positive direct antiglobulin (Coombs') test
	• Treat with corticosteroids (first line), rituximab (anti-CD20), or immunoglobulins (expensive), splenectomy in severe cases
	Cold autoimmune hemolytic anemia (CAIHA, cold agglutinin disease):
	• Ab with maximal activity at low temperatures (28–31°C)
	• Usually IgM
	• In children, secondary forms are usually due to infection (EBV, HIV, mycoplasma, pneumonia)
	• Tell patient to avoid cold weather, treat underlying disorder, possibly rituximab in severe cases

Autoimmune hemolytic anemia (cont.)	**Paroxysmal cold hemoglobinuria (PCH, Donath–Landsteiner syndrome):** • Rare hemolytic anemia after cold exposure with resultant hemoglobinuria • Ab is polyclonal anti-P IgG • Usually after infection (viral - adenovirus, CMV, EBV, influenza, measles, rubella, varicella; bacterial - haemophilus, mycoplasma, syphilis) - Ab cross-reactivity between microorganism and P antigen • Very rarely after vaccination or idiopathic • Usually transient/self-limited; though chronic, usually mild, forms exist • May treat with transfusions or corticosteroids if necessary
Mechanical hemolytic anemia	RBCs are 'sheared' while passing through microscopic thrombi or passed valve → Leads to schistocytes (fragmented RBCs) on peripheral blood smear **Artificial heart valves** **Microangiopathic hemolytic anemia (MAHA)** associated with either: • **Hemolytic-uremic syndrome (HUS):** Hemolytic anemia, acute renal failure, and thrombocytopenia with ~8% mortality rate; predominately in children; usually following infection (esp. E. coli O157:H7 - Shiga-like toxin, also *Strep pneumoniae*); most recover fully, some with have chronic kidney disease. Systemic thrombotic microangiopathy: Vessel wall damage, leukocyte and platelet activation resulting in systemic inflammation and thrombosis with organ damage/failure and death Atypical HUS: Rare, genetic form resulting in chronic complement activation • **Thrombotic thrombocytopenic purpura (TTP):** Rare disorder leading to diffuse microthrombi formation causing organ damage/failure and ~90% fatality rate without plasma exchange and appropriate immunosuppression; due to Ab inhibition of ADAMTS13, an enzyme that cleaves von Willebrand factor (vWF) → increased platelet adhesion Also a rare genetic form: mutation causing dysfunctional ADAMTS13

Mechanical hemolytic anemia (cont.)	**Disseminated intravascular coagulation (DIC):** aka consumptive coagulopathy; abnormal systemic coagulation activation leading to diffuse microthrombi → platelet consumption → hemorrhage with a fatality ranging from 10-50% depending on cause; patients have organ damage from thrombi and life-threatening hemorrhage; **do not give platelets** - will just worsen thrombosis (unless immediate death from massive hemorrhage is imminent); can result from infection, malignancy, pregnancy complications, extensive tissue injury, and other rarer causes; patients will have prolonged PT, PTT, increased FSPs (D-dimer); may give FFP, but only effective treatment is to treat underlying cause **Severe burns:** Associated with hemolytic anemia frequently proportional to the severity and extent of burns; no clear pathophysiology; may be due to actual RBC damage by heat **March hemoglobinuria:** Name given to hemolysis due to repeated minor trauma seen in marathon running, hand drum playing, and marching; may lead to hemoglobinuria, but rarely leads to a symptomatic anemia
Red blood cell distribution defect	**Hypersplenism:** • Increased blood cell sequestration in the spleen with resultant splenomegaly • Anemia, granulocytopenia, thrombocytopenia or pancytopenia with a compensatory bone marrow hyperplasia

8.4   Diagnosis by Morphological Criteria

Microcytic anemia	Normocytic anemia	Macrocytic anemia
Spherocytic anemias, thalassemia, iron-deficiency; RBC number may be only mildly low, however, MCH and MCV significantly reduced	Red blood cells with normal cellular volume	Typically hyperchromic anemia with macrocytes, right shift of marrow without megaloblastic change occurs in liver disease (cirrhosis, hemochromatosis), also aplastic anemia (eg, benzene, radiation), or acute hemolysis

Hypochromic anemia	Normochromic anemia	Hyperchromic anemia
Reduced total hemoglobin content of the individual RBCs; color index <1.0 and MCH <27 pg. Most common is iron-deficiency; also sideroblastic anemia; possibly with abnormal hemoglobin structure	Normal color index (1.0) and normal MCH (28–32 pg) Most commonly acute bleeding, also aplastic anemia and most of the hemolytic anemias	Increased total hemoglobin in individual RBCs; color index >1.0 and MCH >32 pg; usually also with macrocytes Cell formation abnormal more often than Hb formation

Hypochromic, microcytic	Normochromic, normocytic			Hyperchromic, microcytic	
Ferritin	Reticulocytes			Vit. B_{12}/folic acid	
↓	N– ↓		↑	↓	N
Iron deficiency	- Thalassemia - Iron recycling defect - Hemoglobin-opathies - Sideroblastic anemia - Infection, chronic ESRD, malignancy (1/3 of cases, usually normochromic/normocytic)	- Infection, chronic inflammation, malignancy - Bone marrow disease (aplastic anemia, myelofibrosis, granulomatous process, leukemia, lymphoma, metastasis) - Chronic renal insufficiency (erythropoetin deficiencies) - Endocrine causes - Liver disease	- Bleeding - Hemolysis	- Vit.B12-deficiencies - Folic acid deficiencies	- Chronic liver disease - Kidney disease - Inflammatory disorders - Intoxication

8.5 Polycythemia

- Increased concentration of erythrocytes in the peripheral blood with elevated hematocrit, hemoglobin, and viscosity → possible thrombosis
- May lead to headaches, hepatosplenomegaly, HTN
- Treated by phlebotomy (removing red blood cells), or cytostatics (busulfan, hydroxyurea)
- Absolute: increased RBCs numbers in normal plasma volume (erythrocytosis)
  - Polycythemia vera: primary bone marrow myeloproliferative disorder often with Hct >55%; rarely transforms to leukemia; 95% have somatic JAK2 mutation (V617F)
  - Primary familial polycythemia: autosomal dominant mutation in the epo receptor
  - Chuvash polycythemia: autosomal recessive disorder of Chuvashian descendants with C5981 mutation of VHL gene
  - Secondary polycythemia: due to hypoxia (high-altitudes, heart disease, COPD, chronic sleep apnea)
    - Neoplasms (renal/von Hippel-Lindau), liver, adrenal (pheochromocytoma, adenoma)
    - Excessive transfusions or erythropoietin (epo)
    - Hb Chesapeake or Kempsey: greater O_2 affinity leads to more epo production
- Relative: increased concentration due to decreased plasma volume, usually due to dehydration or burns

8.6 Reticulocyte

Func: AKA proerythrocyte; immature RBC (1 day maturation); have mesh-like (reticular) network of ribosomal RNA (positive with supravital dyes - crystal violet, methylene blue), more glycolysis enzymes, and greater osmotic resistance

Ind: Measurement of effective erythropoiesis

Norm: 0.5%-2.0%

↑ Acute hypoxia, acute hemorrhage, hemolytic anemia, substitution therapy of iron deficiency anemia

↓   Iron/vitamin B12/folic acid deficiency, myelodysplastic syndrome, bone
           marrow suppression, renal anemia (decreased epo), iron utilization
           disorders (inflammation, tumors)

Mat: EDTA-blood

8.7   Osmotic Resistance

Opposite of osmotic fragility

Func: RBC susceptibility to rupture in hypotonic saline solution

Norm: • Incipient hemolysis in 0.44%-0.48% NaCl solution
           • Complete hemolysis in 0.30%-0.34% NaCl solution

↑   (Decreased fragility) pronounced microcytosis, especially in thalassemia,
           also sickle cell, iron deficiency

↓   (Increased fragility) spherocytosis, elliptocytosis

Mat: EDTA-blood

Note: Osmotic resistance is decreased after blood incubation of 24 h at 37°C

8.8   Hemoglobin

Func: Ferrous (Fe^{2+}) iron-containing, metalloprotein transporter of oxygen and
           carbon dioxide within RBCs and their precursors, as well as a buffer
           substance and antioxidant in various other tissues; ~1/3 of RBC content;
           O2 binding capacity of 1.34 mL/g; HbA1 (up to 97% of total Hb), HbA2
           (<3%) and fetal HbF (<1% in adults, except in some
           hemoglobinopathies), other rare variants
           Carbaminohemoglobin: Bound to CO_2 - blue color
           Carboxyhemoglobin: Bound to CO - cherry-red color
           Oxyhemoglobin: Bound to O_2 - 'blood'-red color

Ind: Anemia, polycythemia, disorders of water balance (dehydration,
           hyperhydration)

Norm: Men: 14.0 -17.5 g/dL; Women: 12.0 -15.5 g/dL

Note: Oxygen affinity decreased by ↓ pH (acidic), ↑ CO_2, and ↑ 2,3 BPG; conversely
           Oxygen affinity increased by ↑ pH (basic), ↓ CO_2, and ↓ 2,3 BPG

8.9 Hematocrit

Func: Proportion of whole blood volume that is RBCs

Ind: Anemia, polycythemia

Norm: • 42-50% (Men)
• 37-45 % (Women)

↑ Polycythemia, dehydration

↓ Anemia, hyperhydration

Mat: 1-2 mL of EDTA whole blood, or 50 µL capillary tube

Met: Automatic calculation of blood cell counters (Hct = MCV x RBC)
Centrifugation and read lower portion of the glass capillary as a percentage

Note: Falsely low levels may be seen in capillary centrifugation of microcytic, hemolytic samples

8.10 Methemoglobin

Func: Contains oxidized, **ferric (Fe^{3+}) iron** and is not suitable for oxygen transport (cannot bind O_2), has a dark bluish brown color; converted back to hemoglobin by NADH-dependent methemoglobin reductase

Ind: Suspicion of methemoglobinemia (congenital or from intoxication)

Norm: 0.2%-1.0%

↑ Congenital methemoglobinemia (NADH reductase or cytochrome B5 reductase deficiency)
 ■ Infants or pregnant women with nitrate toxicity → reduced NADH reductase activity
 • Toxins (aniline dyes, benzocaines, chlorates, chromates, nitrates/nitrites, sulfonamides) → lead to direct conversion of Hb to MetHb
 • HbH and HbM (resist reduction), G6PD deficiency (↓ NADPH) , or pyruvate kinase deficiency (↓ NADH)
 10%-20% - Mucous membrane discoloration
 20%-30% - Anxiety, dyspnea, headache
 30%-50% - Confusion, fatigue, palpitations, tachypnea
 50%-70% - Acidosis, arrhythmia, coma, seizures
 >70% - Death

Mat: Venous EDTA or heparinized blood

Note: Falsely high O_2 saturation on pulse oximetry
Treatment of cyanide poisoning involves converting Hb to MetHb (amyl nitrate) to bind the cyanide (cyanomethemoglobin)
Brown discoloration of dried blood partially due to formation of methemoglobin

8.11 Hemoglobin Electrophoresis

Func: Separation of Hb in order to quantify and/or identify variants

Ind: Suspected hemoglobinopathy (eg, HbS, HbC, HbE)

Mat: EDTA-blood

Type	Chains	Normal	Note
HbA1	α2β2	95%–97%	In high doses/chronic use
HbA2	α2δ2	1%–3%	↑ β-thalassemia
HbF	α2γ2	0.5%–2% (in adults, newborns) 50%–85%, by 6 months ≤10%	↑ β-thalassemia, persistent HbF, sickle cell anemia, megaloblastic anemia, rarely leukemias

8.12 Hemoglobin F (Fetal)

Func: α2γ2, O_2 transport in the fetus; binds O_2 with more affinity than hemoglobin A, allowing fetus to get oxygen from the mother (due to lack of interaction with 2,3-BPG)

- First produced at 10-12 weeks gestational age (before that embryonic hemoglobin)
- At birth HbF is replaced with adult Hb; present for ~first 6 months of life
- In certain blood disorders elevated HbF may persist: sickle cell disease, thalassemia
- γ on chr. 11

Ind: Suspected hereditary persistence of fetal hemoglobin (HPFH). Often seen on SPEPs in patients with sickle cells disease, thalassemias, or other blood disorders

Prod: Early fetal erythropoiesis is in the yolk sac; at 3-4 months gestational age (GA) - moves to spleen and liver; ~7 months GA moves to the bone marrow, where it remains throughout life (unless disease process occurs that cause extramedullary hematopoiesis

↑ Sickle cell disease, thalassemia, hereditary persistence of fetal hemoglobin, megaloblastic anemia, and rarely, leukemia

8.13   Thalassemia

Microcytic anemias (MCV ↓, MCH ↓): Synthesis disorders of Hb chains
- Autosomal recessive hemoglobin formation disorders due to decreased synthesis of structurally normal polypeptide hemoglobin chains resulting in hypochromic, iron refractory, hemolytic anemia
- Most common symptomatically is "classic" beta-thalassemia major with abnormal synthesis of β-chains and emergence of HbA2 ($\alpha_2\delta_2$) and HbF ($\alpha_2\gamma_2$)
- **Confers resistance to malaria**
- Can be seen in combination with other disorders: Sickle Cell, hemoglobin C, hemoglobin E, etc.

Beta-thalassemia major:
- AKA "classic" thalassemia, Cooley's anemia, Mediterranean anemia
- **Homozygous β-chain mutations**; 2 β-globin genes, 1 each on chr. 11
- β-chains are severely reduced or entirely absent → need for blood transfusions
- Marked overproduction of HbF, beginning insidiously often in early childhood and can rarely be lethal (due to increased O_2 affinity)
- In addition to a marked microcytic hemolytic anemia with resulting jaundice and hepatosplenomegaly, patients are at increased risk for infection and can get iron overload (from disease itself or multiple transfusions - iatrogenic; can be fatal), bone deformities (bone marrow expansion - most notable in the skull), and congestive heart failure and arrhythmias
- Increased prevalence of β-chain mutations in African Americans and patients of mediterranean descent

Beta-thalassemia minor:
- Heterozygous β-chain mutation
- β-chains are under-produced and degraded rapidly, usually with concurrent overproduction of HbA2 ($\alpha_2\delta_2$)
- Typically only a mild hemolytic anemia, with variably normal to low elevations in bilirubin, and moderate hepatosplenomegaly
- CBC w/smear: microcytic hypochromic, possibly with basophilic stippling, no peripheral erythroblasts
- Blast proliferation in the marrow; usually no gross skeletal changes
- Increased prevalence of β-chain mutations in African Americans and patients of Mediterranean descent (Greek, Italian)

Alpha-thalassemia:
- Insufficient production of the alpha chain.
- 4 α-globin genes, 2 each on chr 16 → **The greater the number of defective genes the less α-globin is produced** and the more severe the thalassemia
- 3 affected alleles leads to the formation of excess β- and γ-chains and the formation of tetramers: HbH (β_4) and HbBart's (γ_4)
- Homozygous alpha mutations (ie, all 4) usually leads to intrauterine death/congenital hydrops fetalis
- Increased prevalence in African Americans (-/α -/α) and Asian Americans (-/- α/α)

Alpha thalassemia chart		
# of defective alleles	Disease	Genotype
1	Silent carriers: 3 remaining alleles allow normal hemoglobin production Slightly ↓ MCV and MCH	-/α α/α
2	Alpha thalassemia trait: 2 remaining alleles allow nearly normal hemoglobin production Mild microcytic hypochromic anemia, non-responsive to iron α-thal-1: *cis* deletion, associated with Asian descent α-thal-2: *trans* deletion, associated with African descent	-/- α/α -/α -/α
3	Hemoglobin H disease: patients make HbH and HbBarts - both with increased O2 affinity microcytic hypochromic anemia with target cells, Heinz bodies and splenomegaly	-/- -/α
4	Incompatible with life. Death in utero or shortly after birth from hydrops fetalis HbBarts (γ_4)	-/- -/-

8.14 Sickle Cell Anemia (HbS)

- Hereditary hemoglobinopathy caused by point mutation on β-globin gene (Glu → Val at position 6)
- Homozygotes: HbSS - Sickle cell disease - symptomatic sickling of RBC's resulting in numerous complications:
  - Decreased O_2 carrying capabilities
  - Hemolytic crisis
  - Sickled cells form microthrombi → micro infarctions "vaso-occlusive crisis," joint pain, skin ulcers, organ damage/stroke, priapism
  - Sickled cells are removed from circulation by the spleen → hemolytic anemia, decreased RBC life-span, and autosplenectomy → increased infection with encapsulated organisms (eg, *Strep pneumoniae*, *haemophilus influenza*)
  - Aplastic anemia

- Avascular necrosis or osteomyelitis (Salmonella, Staph, gram negative bacilli from GI tract)
- Retinopathy, hemorrhage, or detachment
- Spontaneous abortions, IUGR, or pre-eclampsia
- Marked illness with malaria (as opposed to sickle cell trait)
- Heterozygotes: HbAS - Sickle cell trait - have minimal clinical manifestations
  - Confers resistance to malaria (as opposed to sickle cell disease)
- More common in patients of Mediterranean and African descent (~8% of African Americans are carriers)

8.15   Hemoglobin C (HbC)

Func:
- Autosomal recessive hemoglobinopathy resulting from glutamine to lysine substitution at 6th position of β-globin chain (E6K)
- Heterozygotes (HbAC): 30%-45% of total Hb is HbC, usually asymptomatic
- Homozygotes (HbC disease): >90% HbC; may be asymptomatic or may have splenomegaly and hemolytic anemia (typically mild) → jaundice, gallstones; may have joint pain; normal lifespan
- Peripheral blood smear (PBS) shows codocytes (target cells), microspherocytes, and HbC crystals
- Treatment usually not needed, may supplement with iron, B12, and folic acid to prevent anemia
- Common among African Americans (2%-3% in U.S.), also those of Mediterranean or Latin American descent
- Confers protection against malaria
- HbSC: will have target cells on PBS, but less sickling than HbSS → less acute vaso-occlusive events; Do have more retinopathy, ischemic bone necrosis, and priapism; 4%-5% of African Americans in the U.S.

8.16   Hemoglobin E

- Autosomal recessive hemoglobinopathy resulting from a single point mutation leading to a glutamine to lysine at the 26th position of β-globin chain (E26K)
- Heterozygotes (HbAE - trait): asymptomatic; may have decreased MCV and scattered codocytes (target cells)

- Homozygous (HbE - disease): mild splenomegaly and hemolytic anemia with codocytes on peripheral blood smear
- Most common among patients of Southeast Asian descent
- HbE/β-thalassemia: Moderate to severe anemia, hepatomegaly, bone injury, heart failure
- HbSE: mild hemolytic anemia, less vaso-occlusive crises

8.17 Porphyrins

Porphyrins are (mostly) naturally occurring organic compounds that form complexes with divalent and trivalent metal ions:
- Porphine - simplest porphyrin
- **Heme** - Iron containing porphyrin; some cytochromes and various enzymes such as catalase or peroxidase are hemoproteins

Porphyrinemia: Increased porphyrins in the blood
Porphyrinuria: Increased porphyrin (and precursor) excretion in the urine:
- Normal coproporphyrin excretion is 100 µg/day; uroporphyrin is excreted only in trace amounts
- Main indications are suspected hepatic porphyria, erythropoietic porphyria or lead poisoning.

Porphyrins are synthesized in the **citric acid cycle**:
- Heme synthesis begins and ends in the mitochondria with the middle portion of the cycle occurring in the cytoplasm

Porphyria:
Hereditary enzyme defect or acquired metabolic disorder with disturbed porphyrin synthesis affecting the hematopoietic system (bone marrow) and/or in the liver (erythropoietic, erythrohepatic, hepatic porphyria), with excessive precursor protein formation, organ deposits and excretion

Acute intermittent porphyria:
- Autosomal dominant metabolic disorder affecting heme production
- Due to decreased porphobilinogen deaminase activity (formally known as uroporphyrinogen I synthase) resulting in excessive porphobilinogen (PBG)
- Second most common porphyria (after porphyria cutanea tarda)
- Incidence probably underestimated due to long periods of latency

- Signs/symptoms: Dark red colored urine, PBG deposition in the liver, kidneys, ganglion and granule cells, abdominal cramps, constipation, liver dysfunction, polyneuritis, hypertension, cardiovascular disorders, and depression
- No skin findings
- Usually manifests after the puberty; episodes provoked by drugs or chemicals
- May be misdiagnosed with a psychiatric illness → psychiatric medications only worsen disease

Porphyria cutanea tarda:
- Autosomal dominant (~20%) or acquired (metabolic toxins, alcohol, barbiturates, hexachlorobenzene, iron overload/hemochromatosis) metabolic disorder affecting heme production
- Due to decreased uroporphyrinogen III decarboxylase activity resulting in excessive formation of δ-aminolevulinic acid and porphobilinogen
- Most common porphyria
- Signs/symptoms: Dark-red colored urine, mild photodermatosis with blistering and hyperpigmentation, onycholysis, hyalinosis cutis, hypertrichosis, hepatomegaly and cirrhosis, hypersideremia

Hepatoerythropoietic porphyria:
Homozygous form

Congenital erythropoietic porphyria (Günther syndrome):
- Autosomal recessive hereditary metabolic disorder affecting heme production
- Due to a defect in uroporphyrinogen III synthase
- Signs/symptoms: Dark-red colored urine, progressive photodermatitis with erythrodontia, protein deposition in skin, teeth and bones, abdominal pain, later mutilation of fingers, nose, ears, hemolytic anemia, and splenomegaly
- Symptoms often beginning in early childhood, but can present in adulthood
- Extremely rare, ~200 cases reported world-wide

Enzymes of the citric acid cycle and resulting porphyrias					
Porphyria	Enzyme affected	Substrate	Product	Chr	MOI
n/a	ALA synthase 1	Glycine, succinyl CoA	δ–ALA	3p	
X-linked sidero-blastic anemia	ALA synthase 2	Glycine, succinyl CoA	δ–ALA	X	
ALA dehydratase deficiency	ALA dehydratase	δ–ALA	PBG	9q	AR
Acute intermittent porphyria	PBG deaminase/ HMB synthase	PBG	HMB	11q	AD
Congenital erythropoietic porphyria	URO III synthase	HMB	URO III	10q	AR
Porphyria cutanea tarda	URO III decarboxylase	URO III	CPP III	1p	AD
Coproporphyria	CPP III oxidase	CPP III	PPP IX	3q	AD
Variegate porphyria	PPP oxidase	PPP IX	PP IX	1q	AD
Erythropoietic protoporphyria	Ferrochelatase	PP IX	Heme	18q	AD

ALA: Aminolevulinic acid, Chr: Chromosome, CPP: Coproporphyrinogen, HMB: Hydroxymethylbilane, MOI: Mode of inheritance, PBG: Porphobilinogen, PP: Protoporphyrin, PPP: Protoporphyrinogen, URO: Uroporphyrinogen, AD: Autosomal dominant, AR: Autosomal recessive

8.18   Complete Blood Count (CBC)

Func:

RBC count	4.5–5.9 million/μL (men)	4.6–5.0 million/μL (women)
Hb	14–17.5 g/dL (men)	12–15.5 g/dL (women)
Hematocrit	42%–50% (men)	37%–45% (women)
MCV	80–100 fl	
MCH	27–33 pg	
MCHC	32–36 g/dL	
WBC count	4.5–10 x 109/L	
Platelet count	1.5–4.5 x 10⁵/μl	

With differential white blood cell count:
- Evaluation of numbers and morphological changes of granulocytes and lymphocytes
- Percentages of WBC subtypes: either by conventional light microscopy (manual count) or automation
- Absolute numbers: by automation only
- Indication: suspected leukocytosis, leucopenia, infections, toxins, tumors and leukemia/lymphoma

Left shift:
- Increased percentage of precursor cells (A 'shift' to the left side of the maturation path)
- Often called when neutrophil precursors ('bands') >5%
- Seen in bacterial infections, toxins, metastatic tumors, leukemias, hemolysis
- "Reactive" picture: Increased band neutrophils and increased myelocytes -eg, acute bacterial infections
- "Pathological" picture: Increased band neutrophils, increased myelocytes and promyelocytes - eg, leukemia, such as in CML (chronic myelogenous leukemia)

Right shift:
- Relative increase of mature forms (ie, segmented neutrophils)
- Occurs in pernicious anemia, panmyelophthisis, etc.

Leukemic hiatus:
- A 'gap' in granulocyte maturation with numerous myeloblasts and mature segmented neutrophils, but few intermediate forms
- Often seen in acute leukemias

Leukocyte distribution:
Quantitative shifts can only be discovered in the event of significant deviation from normal
Qualitative changes, however, especially when significant atypia, are easier to identify and mark the importance of the blood smear evaluation

Normal distribution:
- Granulocyte: 50%-80%
  - Segmented neutrophils: 40%-70%
  - Band neutrophils: 0%-5%
  - Eosinophils: 0%-6%
  - Basophils: 0%-2%
- Lymphocytes: 20%-50%
- Monocytes: 1%-12%

8.19 Hematopoiesis

Erythropoiesis and **granulopoiesis** begin in the mesodermal blood islands of the embryonal yolk sac
- 3-4 months gestation: in mesenchymal cells of the fetal liver and spleen
- ~7th months gestation: begins in the mesenchyme of the fetal bone marrow
- After birth: exclusively in the bone marrow and the lymphoid organs (unless some abnormality)

Begins with pluripotent stem cells that make up the many generations of erythropoiesis, leukopoiesis and thrombopoiesis

Stem cells								
Bone marrow	Myelopoiesis/leukopoiesis						Erythro-poiesis	Thrombo-poiesis
	Mono-cytopoiesis	Granulopoiesis			Lymphocyto-poiesis			
		Myeloblast			Lymphoblast		Proerythro-blast ↓	Mega-karyoblast ↓
	Monoblast ↓ Promono-cyte ↓ Monocyte	Neutro-philic promyeloc yte ↓ Neutro-philic myelocyte ↓ Neutro-philic meta-myelocyte ↓ Neutrophilic band ↓ Seg-mented neutrophil	Eosino-philic promyeloc yte ↓ Eosino-philic myelocyte ↓ Eosino-philic metamye-locyte ↓ Eosino-philic band ↓ Eosinophil	Basophilic pro-myelo-cyte ↓ Basophilic myelocyte ↓ Basophilic metamyc-locyte ↓ Basophilic band ↓ Basophil	Pro-B cell ↓ Pre-B cell	Pro-T cell ↓	Basophilic normoblast ↓ Polychro-matic normoblast ↓ Orthochro-matic normoblast ↓ Reticulocyte	Promega-karyocyte ↓ Mega-karyocyte
Peripheral blood	Monocyte	Seg-mented neutrophil	Eosinophil	Basophil	B Cell	T Cell*	Reticulocyte ↓ Erythrocyte	Platelets
Tissue	Macro-phage/ histiocyte	Seg-mented neutrophil	Eosinophil	Basophil	B cell, plasma cell	T Cell		

Morphology and characteristics of the white blood cell (WBC)

Cell	Size	Nucleus			Cytoplasm	
		N/C Ratio	Nuclear shape	Chromatin	Color	Granules
Band neutrophil	12–16 µm	N<C	Bent rod shaped	Coarse, deeply colored	Inconspicuous, pale pink	Fine azurophilic fills much of the cytoplasm
Segmented neutrophil	12–15 µm	N<C	Segmented, 2–5 lobes	Coarse, deeply colored	Inconspicuous, pale pink	Fine azurophilic fills much of the cytoplasm
Eosinophil	12–16 µm	N<C	Segmented, usually bi-lobed, often partially obscured by granules	Coarse	Inconspicuous, pale pink	Chunky, purple to blue/black, filling cytoplasm
Basophil	12–16 µm	N≡C	Usually obscured by granules, segmented, usually bilobed	Coarse	Inconspicuous, pale violet	Chunky, purple to blue/black, filling cytoplasm
Monocyte	16–20 µm	N≡C	Usually kidney bean shaped, Emarginate	Clear, easy pale staining ("Cotton Candy")	Basophilic, pale blue-gray, often vacuoles	Unspecific. fine azurophilic
Lymphocyte	10–12 µm	N>C	Round	Dense deeply colored	Pale blue; cytoplasm usually narrow, crescent-shaped	Not usually seen unless activated
Plasma Cell	10–20 µm	N</≡C	Round, eccentrically located	Large dark clumps (clock-face/ spokes of a wheel)	Pale blue/violet with perinuclear hauff (clearing)	Not usually seen unless activated; Russell bodies → Mott cell
Blast	15–20 µm	N>C	Round or slightly oval possibly with slight indent	Delicate, loose, usually 1–5 nucleoli	Medium to deep blue, often with perinuclear lightening	No granules

Morphology and characteristics of neutrophils and precursors

Cell	Myelo-blast	Promyelo-cyte	Metamy-elocyte	Myelocyte	Band	Seg-mented neutrophil	Hyper seg-mented neutrophil
Avg size	18 μm	22 μm	20 μm	18 μm	15 μm	15 μm	15 μm
Nucleus	Round, loose chrom	Roundish, slightly marginate, mod. dense	Indented <50%, slightly marginate, mod. dense	Bean/kidney shaped, indented >50%, dense	C-or-S shaped, no segments, very dense	3–5 segments, extremely dense	>5 segments, extremely dense
Nucleoli	1–5	1–5	Ø	Ø	Ø	Ø	Ø
Cytoplasm	Baso-philic	Basophilic	Basophilic bis oxyphilic	Oxyphilic	Oxyphilic	Oxyphilic	Oxyphilic
Coarse granules	Ø	++	+ - ++	Ø	Ø	Ø	Ø
Fine mature-granules	Ø	Ø	Ø - +	++	++	++	++
Ability to divide	+	++	++	(+)	Ø	Ø	Ø
% of the WBC in blood	-	-	-	<2%	2%–5%	50%–70%	<2%
Right shift					+	+++	++
Slight left shift				+	+	+++	
Strong left shift			↑	↑	↑↑	↓↓	
Chron. myelosis	+	+	++	++	++	++	
Acute leukemia	+++	+		+	+	++	

Bone marrow differential

Granulocytopoiesis	Normal value (%)
Myeloblast	1–4
Promyelocytes	3–14
Neutrophilic myelocytes	6–18
Neutrophilic metamyelocytes	3–15

Granulocytopoiesis (cont.)	Normal value (%)
Neutrophilic bands	5-17
Segmented neutrophils	8-23
Eosinophils (including precursors)	0-9
Basophils (including precursors)	0-1
Monocytes	0-4
Lymphocytes	0-26
Plasma cells	0-3
Proerythroblasts	1-3
Normoblasts	7-34

Thrombopoiesis
Megakaryocytes: 0-5
Counts should be **500 cells**, 200 minimum
M:E ratio: Myeloid to erythroid ratio - Normal value: 2-4:1

8.20　Erythropoietin (EPO)

Func: Stimulates maturation and differentiation of RBCs and hemoglobin synthesis

Ind: DDx of anemia and polycythemia; suspected paraneoplastic syndrome

Prod: Kidney, stimulated by hypoxia, liver - minor production in adult, primary source in fetus

Norm: 4-25 U/L

↑
- Hypoxia (pulmonary, cardiovascular, anemia, bleeding, CO poisoning)
- Paraneoplastic syndrome
- 2 and 3 trimester of pregnancy (physiologic)

↓
- Chronic renal insufficiency
- Polycythemia vera

Mat: Serum, plasma

Met: ELISA, RIA

Note: Diurnal variations: Minimum shortly after waking, peak at night

8.21 Delta-Aminolevulinic Acid

Func: δ-ALA is a precursor in heme biosynthesis

Ind: Suspected porphyria; suspected lead poisoning

Norm:
- 1-15 µmol/L Blood
- 1-30 µmol/L Urine

↑ Acute intermittent porphyria, variegate porphyria, hereditary coproporphyria, lead poisoning

Mat: Whole blood, washed RBCs, urine

8.22 Bilirubin

Func: Degradation product of hemoglobin:
- Total bilirubin: Total amount of bilirubin (direct and indirect)
- Indirect/unconjugated bilirubin: Bilirubin that has not been processed by the liver; elevated in when the glucuronidation capacity of the liver is overwhelmed (liver disease, marked hemolysis)
- Direct/conjugated bilirubin: Partly albumin-bound, partly free; not normally present in the serum (<0.3 mg/dL)

Ind: Diagnosis and follow-up of jaundice

Prod:
- Formed by the breakdown of hemoglobin in the reticuloendothelial system in the spleen and in Kupffer cells of the liver.
- Conjugated in the microsomes of liver cells mainly with glucuronic acid
- Unconjugated bilirubin is lipid-soluble, but not water-soluble

Norm:	Total bilirubin	Indirect bilirubin	Direct bilirubin
Adults	≤1.0 mg/dL (≤17.1 µmol/L)	≤0.7 mg/dL (≤12 µmol/L)	≤0.3 mg/dL (≤5.1 µmol/L)
Neonate, premature	Birth ≤8 mg/dL 3-5 days ≤15 mg/dL (peak)	Increased	≤0.3 mg/dL
Neonate, term	Birth ≤6.0 mg/dl 3-5 days ≤12 mg/dL (peak)	Increased	≤0.3 mg/dL

↑   **Indirect**: Hemolytic anemia, neonatal jaundice, hemolytic disease of the newborn, Gilbert's syndrome
Direct: Liver disease: acute viral hepatitis, cirrhosis, steatosis, tumor, abscess, intra-and extra-hepatic cholestasis, Dubin-Johnson syndrome

Mat: Serum

Note: Bilirubin binds to the elastic fibers of the skin and conjunctiva and thus causes the yellowing.
- Scleral icterus: >2 mg/dL
- Jaundice visible in the skin: >3 mg/dL

The differentiation of direct from indirect bilirubin is easier when a total bilirubin is at least 2 mg/dL

Further investigations:
- Predominantly unconjugated hyperbilirubinemia
  - Hemolysis: Free Hb in the plasma, haptoglobin, reticulocytes, LDH
  - Rhabdomyolysis: Creatinine kinase
- Conjugated and unconjugated hyperbilirubinemia (proportions variable)
  - Liver damage: ALT, AST
  - Biliary tree: GGT, Alk Phos

Jaundice	Pathophysiology	Direct	Indirect	Total	Most common
Prehepatic	Over production → Glucuronidation capacity of the liver inadequate	↔	↑	↑	Hemolytic
Hepatic	Bilirubin conjugation defect	↑	↑	↑	Hepatitis
Posthepatic	Blockage of direct bilirubin excretion	↑	↔	↑	Cholestasis/tumor

8.23 Leukocytosis

- Increased number of leukocytes in peripheral blood
- May absolute granulocytosis, lymphocytosis, or monocytosis depending on etiology
- Reactive usually less elevated than leukemias, however, a distinction based solely on the number of leukocytes is not possible

Causes:
- Infectious diseases, local inflammation, leukemia
- Centrally induced: diencephalic disorders
- Physiologic: Pregnancy, infants/toddlers, after heavy physical labor (myogenic leukocytosis, motion leukocytosis), after eating (postprandial leukocytosis), drugs (corticosteroids, lithium)

8.24 Leukopenia/Leukocytopenia

- Reduced number of leukocytes in the peripheral blood
- Most common is granulocytopenia
- May see only slightly reduced total leukocyte count with absolute granulocytopenia if there is a relative increase of lymphocytes and monocytes

Causes:
- Massive consumption in bacterial infections, viral infections, increased splenic destruction
- Bone marrow damage/depression: (familial granulocytopenia, vitamin B12 deficiency, myelodysplasia), autoimmune diseases (SLE, reactive arthritis, Sjögren's syndrome, Felty's syndrome)
- Toxic drug-induced agranulocytosis: see with analgesics, antibiotics, anticonvulsants, antidepressants, antihistamines, antimalarials, anti-thyroid, antihypertensives, diuretics, allopurinol
  - Type I: Allergic reaction → immune complex type, dose-independent
  - Type II: Toxic injury of the precursor cells in the bone marrow, dose-dependent

8.25 Granulocytosis

Increased number of granulocytes in the peripheral blood
Causes:
Neutrophilia (eg, general infection/abscess), eosinophilia (eg, parasites, allergies), basophilia (very rare)

8.26 Agranulocytosis

- Severe reduction in granulocytes (marked granulocytopenia) due to disturbance of granulocytopoiesis with resultant severe secondary immune deficiency
- Highly decreased or absence of neutrophils (and usually eosinophils and basophils)
- Pronounced tendency for infection

Causes:
Allergic hypersensitivity reactions to medications (analgesics, antibiotics, sulfonamides, metal-containing preparations)

- As a result of inflammatory processes
- By paraproteins/immunoglobulins
- Bone marrow damage (drug induced, usually iatrogenic):
  - **Type I**: Rapidly occurring, dose-independent, due to immune complex formation (eg, acetaminophen)
  - **Type II**: Occurs gradually, dose-dependent, toxic bone marrow damage; first sign is general decline in condition and fever, later with mucosal ulceration, necrosis, regional lymphadenopathy, possibly enlargement of the spleen; peripheral blood may show relative lympho-and monocytosis

Cyclic agranulocytosis: 3-4 week leukopenic phases, favorable prognosis

- **Infantile hereditary agranulocytosis**: Autosomal-recessive familial agranulocytosis of infancy with hypoplastic bone marrow, inhibition of mature myelopoiesis, usually with absences of granulocytes and inflammatory skin conditions; poor prognosis

8.27 Neutrophilia

Increased numbers of neutrophils in the peripheral blood
Causes:
Acute and chronic infections (bacteria, fungi, protozoa); stress; acute disease (burns, intoxication, hemolysis, hemorrhage, acute cardiovascular disease); chronic diseases (autoimmune diseases, myeloproliferative syndrome, metastasis, hypercortisolism); drugs (glucocorticoids, contraceptives)

8.28 Neutropenia

- Reduced number of neutrophils in the peripheral blood → the extreme is agranulocytosis)
- Often not symptomatic until <1000/µL
- 500-1000/µL: increased risk of infection, particularly bacterial
- <500/µL: infection risk extremely high

Causes:
Infections, malignancy, medicines, bone marrow damage; other disorders: Lupus erythematosus, hypersplenism, cirrhosis, congenital neutropenia, cyclic neutropenia, megaloblastic anemia

8.29 Eosinophilia

Increased numbers of eosinophils in peripheral blood, bone marrow and/or tissues
Causes:
Allergies; parasitic infestations, collagen vascular diseases, chronic myeloid leukemia; after infections and intoxications; Hodgkin's disease; familial eosinophilia (usually asymptomatic)

8.30 Basophilia

Increased numbers of basophils in peripheral blood and/or bone marrow
Causes:
Rare finding, may be seen in chronic myeloid leukemia or pre-leukemia in myeloproliferative diseases

8.31   Monocytosis

Increased number of monocytes in the peripheral blood
Causes:
Tuberculosis, syphilis, subacute bacterial endocarditis, various chronic inflammatory diseases

8.32   Monocytopenia

Reduced number of monocytes in peripheral blood
Causes:
Absolute: hairy cell leukemia, aplastic anemia
Relative: Decrease in proportion of monocytes due to increase in another leukocyte (eg, neutrophilia)

8.33   Lymphocytosis

Increased number of lymphocytes in peripheral blood
Causes:
Lymphocytic response occures upon contact with an antigen, in particular during viral infections, and other infectious diseases: hepatitis, malaria, tuberculosis, syphilis, symptomatic phase of brucellosis; also in lymphatic leukemia
- Acute infectious lymphocytosis (Smith's syndrome): benign, febrile, disease probably caused by a lymphotropic virus (especially in infancy) with severe lymphocytosis, volatile catarrhal symptoms (cough, difficulty swallowing, conjunctivitis), possibly with morbilliform rash
- Relative: Increase in the proportion of lymphocytes due to decrease neutrophils (neutropenia with normal absolute lymphocyte count)

8.34   Lymphocytopenia

Reduced number of lymphocytes in the peripheral blood
Causes:
Acute-phase of infection; stress; hypercortisolism/Cushing's syndrome; drugs (glucocorticoids, cytostatics); congenital immunodeficiencies, familial lymphopenia with agammaglobulinemia (Swiss type)
Relative: Reduction in the proportion of lymphocytes due to increase in neutrophils (neutrophilia with normal absolute lymphocyte count)

8.35   Thrombocytosis/Thrombocythemia

- **Thrombocytosis:** Increase in number of platelets in peripheral blood, often reactive, due to hemorrhage, surgery, vigorous physical activity, inflammatory diseases, etc.
- **Thrombocythemia:** Severe, permanent increase in number of platelets in the peripheral blood, in particular, seen in myeloproliferative disorders (eg, polycythemia vera)

8.36   Thrombocytopenia

Decrease in number of platelets in the peripheral blood
Causes:
Due to shortened platelet survival time (platelet cytolysis, increased consumption, hypersplenism) or synthesis failure (bone marrow disease); acquired - most common; rarely congenital (Fanconi's anemia, Hegglin syndrome, Wiskott-Aldrich syndrome)

8.37   Infections

- Bacterial: more neutrophilia
- Viral: more lymphocytosis

8.38   Granulocyte Pathomorphology

- **Alder's anomaly:** Azurophilic granules in granulocytes, macrophages and lymphocytes; affected patients often suffer from Gargoylismus or dysostosis
- **Auer rods:** Azurophilic crystals in the cytoplasm of white blood cells (myeloblasts, promyelocytes, metamyelocytes), particularly in acute myeloid leukemia
- **Dohle-inclusion bodies:** Blue granulocyte inclusions seen in severe infections (eg, streptococci), burns, aplastic anemia and certain toxins
- **Pelger-Huet anomaly:** Lack of segmentation of the nucleus of granulocytes without clinical significance, autosomal-dominant inheritance
- **Pseudo-Pelger-Huet cells:** Similar morphology to Pelger-Huet anomaly cells; seen in infections, leukemia and bone tumors

- **Toxic granulation**: Amplification of neutrophil granules with coarse basophilic granules, often with cytoplasmic vacuolization and reduction of the peroxidase-positive granules, in severe infections, poisoning, burns and tumors
- **Hyper-segmentation**: More than 5 lobes; seen in megaloblastic anemia (vitamin B12 deficiency, folic acid deficiency)

8.39 Lymphocyte Pathomorphology

- **Toxic granulation**: Coarse basophilic granules, possibly with cytoplasmic vacuolization, in severe infections, poisoning, burns and tumors
- **'Smudge' cells**: During the blood smear technique, lymphocytes are prone to crushing and with certain diseases are particularly fragile and are visible as smudged, irregular patches without significant core structure; common finding in chronic lymphocytic leukemia (CLL).
- **Atypical nuclear forms**: Occurring mainly during viral illnesses, have kidney-shaped or atypical indented nucleus
- **Downey cells**: Occurring in infectious mononucleosis (EBV/CMV); atypical mononuclear, blood cell (polymorphic, lobed, rich with chromatin, often continuous nuclear border)

8.40 Leukemia

'White Blood'
Collective term for malignant transformation and maturation of white blood cells (leukocytes) with the appearance of immature, morphologically and biochemically distinguishable from the normal cell types, especially in blood and organs of hematopoiesis
The symptoms occur gradually through displacement of normal blood cells and infiltration of atypical cells in organs. Anemia, bleeding as a result of thrombocytopenia and infections due to immune deficiency are possible manifestations, as well as irritation, enlargements and reduction of function of affected organs
Lymphoid: Malignancy affects the lymphoid lineage
Myeloid: Malignancy affects the granulocyte/myeloid lineage

8.41 Acute Leukemia

Acute leukemia = immature cell leukemia

8.41.1 Acute lymphoblastic leukemia (ALL)

Func: Malignant; fatal without intensive therapy
- Decreased differentiation of leukocytes
- Anemia and thrombocytopenia, white blood cell count is often, but not always, increased (but sometimes the absolute WBC count is actually decreased and immature leukemic cells may be difficult to find on the peripheral blood smear)
- Bone marrow examination is essential
- Initially, the bone marrow is infiltrated by abnormal, immature cells, then hematogenous spread and infiltration of the organs (massive hepatomegaly is common)
- **Most common leukemia of infancy**
- Distinguishable by surface antigens into B, T and O-types
- Using combinations of cytotoxic drugs at fixed time schedules, there is often significant therapeutic successes; may resort to bone marrow transplantation; cranial irradiation and/or intracerebral chemotherapy usually performed when there is CNS infiltration

Ind: **FAB classification of ALL:**
L1 Infantile type: Small cells, regular nuclear shape, homogeneous chromatin, no nucleoli
L2 Adult type: Medium to large cells, irregular nuclear shape, heterogeneous chromatin, one or more nucleoli
L3 Burkitt type: Large cells, regular core shape, homogeneous chromatin, prominent nucleoli
Cytochemistry: all PAS (periodic acid-Schiff reaction) coarsely positive

Acute lymphocytic leukemia (ALL)				
Diagnosis	**% of ALL**	**Genetic abnormalities**	**Morphology**	**Clinical association**
B Lymphoblastic leukemia, not otherwise specified	75% of ALL cases occur in children 80-85% are precursor B cell type Precursor T cell type is more common in adults.	Lacking well categorized cytogenetic abnormalities	Varies: - Small cells with scanty cytoplasm and condensed chromatin - Large cells with blue to blue-grey cytoplasm	
B Lymphoblastic leukemia with recurrent genetic abnormalities		t(9;22)(q34;11.2);BCR-ABL1 (Ph+) t(v;11q23) MLL rearranged (MLL) t(12;21)(p13;q22); TEL-AML1 (ETV6-RUNX1) B-ALL with hyperdiploidy B-ALL with hypodiploidy t(5;14)(q31;q32);IL3-IGH t(1;19)(q23;p13.3); E2A-PBX1 (TCF3-PBX1)		Ph+, MLL, Hypodiploid portends to worse prognosis TEL-AML1, Hyperdiploid, portends a favorable prognosis with high cure rate
Lymphoblastic leukemia		Almost always show clonal rearrangements in T-cell receptor however, there is also simultaneous IGH gene rearrangements in 1/5 of cases		Typically presents with high WBC count and often a large mediastinal mass

8.41.2 Acute myeloid/myelogenous leukemia (AML)

- Second most common leukemia of infancy
- Distinction according to morphological criteria and surface antigens of atypical cells into myeloblastic, promyelocytic and myelomonocytic cells
- Worse response to chemo among all leukemias - often treated with bone marrow transplant
- **Auer rods (in myeloblasts and promyelocytes)**
- Hiatus leukemicus: no intermediate cells in the smear, the mature cells are from normal, non-leukemic granulocytopoiesis)
- Massive splenomegaly and enlarged lymph nodes may be seen
- Clinical: fatigue, weight loss, susceptibility to infections, bleeding tendency
- Special form: "Smoldering leukemia": slow-onset form of acute - mostly myeloid - leukemia

Acute myeloid leukemia (AML) with recurrent genetic abnormalities (chart based on 2008 WHO classification)				
Diagnosis	% of AML	Differentiation	Morphology	Clinical association
AML with t(8;21) (q22;q22);RUNX1 -RUNX1T1	5%	Neutrophil	-Abundant granular cytoplasm -Perinuclear clearing -Large orange granules	Initial bone marrow aspiration may show low number of blast cells (<20%), due to myeloid sarcoma infiltration
AML with inv(16) (p13.1q22) or t(16;16) (p13.1;q22); CBFB–MYH11	5%–8%	Myelo-monocytic	Immature eosinophilic granules	Myeloid sarcoma

Diagnosis (cont.)	% of AML	Differentiation	Morphology	Clinical association
Acute Promyelocytic Leukemia t(15;17) (q22;q12) PML-RARA	5%-8%	Myeloid	**Hypergranular:** -Bilobed nucleus -Large azurophilic granules -Bundles of Auer rods (faggot cells) **Microgranular:** -Bilobed nucleus -Submicroscopic granules -Bundles of Auer rods (faggot cells)	Associated with DIC Microgranular form associated with rapid doubling time
AML with t(9;11) (p22;q23); MLLT3-MLL	10% of pediatric AML, 2% of adult	Hematopoietic stem cell	-Monocytoid with large cytoplasm +/- basophilia -Azurophilic granules and vacuoles	May have DIC or myeloid sarcomas
AML with t(6;9) (p23;q34); DEK-NUP214	1%-2%	Hematopoietic stem cell	Non-specific, looks like all other AML except APML and Megakaryoblastic	Patients usually present with pancytopenia
AML with inv(3)(q21q26.2) or t(3;3) (q21;q26.2); RPN1-EVI1	1%-2%	Hematopoietic stem cell	-Hypogranular neutrophils with pseudo-Pelger-Heut anomaly -Giant hypogranular platelets common	Usually presents with normal or possibly increased platelet count
AML (Megakaryoblastic) with t(1;22) (p13;q13); RBM15-MKL1	<1%	Myeloid stem cell with predominant megakaryocytic differentiation	Atypical monolobated megakaryocytes with increased blasts	Restricted to infants and young children (<3 years of age)

Diagnosis (cont.)	% of AML	Differentiation	Morphology	Clinical association
AML with NPM1	2%–8% of peds, 27%–35% of adult	Hematopoietic stem cell	Strong association with monocytic and myelomonocytic leukemias	Often have extramedullary involvement Higher WBC and PLT counts compared to other AMLs
AML with CEBPA	15%–18%	Hematopoietic stem cell	No distinctive features (with or without maturation, less commonly myelomonocytic)	Higher hemoglobin levels than other compared to other AMLs

Acute myeloid leukemia with myelodysplasia-related changes

Diagnosis: >20% blood or marrow blasts

And any of:	And absence of both:
• Previous history of MDS • MDS related cytogenetic abnormality • Multilineage dysplasia	• Prior cytotoxic therapy • Recurrent cytogenetic abnormality described in AML with recurrent abnormalities

% of AML	Differentiation	Morphology	Clinical association
24%–35%	Hematopoietic stem cell	Multilineage dysplasia	Poor prognosis; less likely to achieve remission

Therapy related myeloid neoplasms

Therapy related AML and MDS and MPN occurring as late complications of cytotoxic or radiation therapy for a prior neoplastic disorder

10%–20%	Hematopoietic stem cell	Multilineage dysplasia, most commonly	Often will present 5-10 years after exposure to alkylating chemotherapy/ionization ration from treatment for solid or hematologic malignancy

Acute myeloid leukemia, not otherwise specified (NOS)

>20% myeloblasts in the peripheral blood or bone marrow

5% cases	Varied	Varied	Pt. usually present with bone marrow failure

Type	Name	MPO	Esterase
\multicolumn{4}{	l	}{FAB classification of AML (not routinely used anymore, included for completeness)}
M0	Morphologically and cytochemically not differentiable, only individual myeloid markers positive	–	–
M1	Myeloblast without maturation: rare granules, at least 3% myeloperoxidase positive	+	–
M2	Myeloblast with maturation: many azurophilic granules	++	–
M3	Promyelocytic leukemia: most numerous Auer rods	+++	–
M4	Myelomonocytic: as M2, but >20% promonocytes; M4eo: variant with abnormal eosinophilia	++	++
M5	Monocytic Leukemia M5a: Immature, undifferentiated form, mainly monoblasts; M5b: Mature form, predominantly promonocytes and monocytes	–	+++
M6	Erythroid Leukemia: Erythroblasts >50% in BM	–	–
M7	Megakaryoblastic leukemia	–	–

8.42 Chronic Leukemia

- Significantly increased white blood cell count (often >100,000)
- Characteristic peripheral smear

8.42.1 Chronic lymphocytic leukemia (CLL)

Func: A low grade lymphocytic malignancy, most common in the 6th-7th decade
- In addition to the general leukemic symptoms, also have generalized lymphadenopathy and hepatosplenomegaly
- Distinguishable by surface antigens into B cell-type (common) and T cell-type (rare, about 3%)
- In the blood: increasing relative and absolute lymphocytosis with gradually occurring anemia and thrombocytopenia (by leukemic displacement or autoimmune)

- Increase susceptibility to infection (decreased immunocompetent B- and T-cells)
- Characteristic 'soccer balls and smudge cells'

CLL prognostic factors:

Good prognostic indicator: IGHV gene rearrangement/somatic hypermutation

Adverse prognostic indicators:
- CD38 surface expression (>30% of cells)
- ZAP-70 cytoplasmic expression (>30% of cells)
- Elevated β2-microglobulin
- 17p (tp53) deletion/mutation (detection should move patient into the highest risk category within any clinical stage)
- 11q- Deletion
- Lymphocyte doubling time <12 months
- Possible factors: elevated serum thymidine kinase, abnormal serum free light-chains, increased interleukin-8, decreased micro RNA expression

Intermediate prognostic indicators (controversial):
- Trisomy 12
- 13q Deletion (most common chromosomal abnormality)

8.42.2 Chronic myeloid/myelogenous leukemia (CML)

- Most common between 3rd and 6th decades
- Philadelphia chromosome - t(9;22) (q34;q11) ABL;BCR
- Infiltration of the bone marrow with myeloid cells (mainly promyelocytes and myelocytes)
- Peripheral blood is massively flooded with cells of all maturation stages
- Blast crisis leads to displacement of the functional cell population (granulocyte deficiency - high infection risk)
- Frequently extreme splenomegaly (up to 5000 g), also hepatomegaly
- Variations: rare eosinophilic and the (controversial) basophilic
- History: insidious onset, treated with radiation therapy (especially splenic irradiation) and cytostatics, although there is a significant reduction in the high leukocyte count, there is still only a small increase in the mean survival and eventual evolvement into blast crisis; newer medications have recently been approved, or are in testing phases

Leukemia	ALL	AML	CLL	CML
Etiology (favorable factors)	Trisomy 21 Ionizing radiation, alkylating agents	Ionizing radiation, alkylating agents, benzene, Klinefelter, Patau	Familial predisposition, mostly men (2:1), trisomy 12	Ionizing radiation
Age	Children: 85% usually <4 y Adults: 15% usually >75 y	Adults: 80–90% Children: 10%–20%	Usually 60–70 y (90% >50 y)	Usually 20–60 y, average 45–50 y at diagnosis
Incidence	1/100000	<30 y: 1/100000 >80 y: 10/100000	3/100,000 M:F = 2:1	2/100000
Peripheral blood: WBC	Lymphoblasts, Hiatus leukemicus	Myeloblasts, Hiatus leukemicus	↑↑ Lymphocytes	↑↑↑ All levels of maturity, leukemic thrombi
Erythro.	↓↓ Anemia	↓↓ Anemia	~↓ Anemia	~↓ Anemia
Other		Auer rods (thin, rod-shaped cytoplasmic inclusions – granule formation defects)	Smudge cells and soccer balls, periportal hepatic infiltration	Philadelphia chromosome rearrangement t(9;22) ABL;BCR, ↓↓ leukocyte alkaline phosphatase, diffuse liver infiltration
Clinical and special, all: LN swelling	Leukemic meningitis	DIC (most common in the promyelocytic leukemia, 'M3'); Bleeding (GIT, pulm, cranial, retina)	Infections (Herpes zoster) often few symptoms, occasionally Mikulicz's Syndrome (parotid and lacrimal gland involvement)	Hepato-splenomegaly → abdominal pain

Leukemia (cont.)	ALL	AML	CLL	CML
Therapy	As early as possible and as aggressive as feasible Chemotherapy, possibly radiation, bone marrow transplantation if symptomatic	As early as possible and as aggressive as feasible Chemotherapy, possibly radiation, bone marrow transplantation if symptomatic	As early as necessary and as gently as possible Chemotherapy, possibly radiation, monoclonal antibodies (Alemtuzumab, Rituximab), bone marrow transplantation, symptomatic	As early as possible, as long as necessary Interferon-alpha, chemotherapy Imatinib (inhibitor tyrosine kinase) Bone marrow transplantation, symptomatic
Prognosis	Particularly good in childhood; total: 30% healing 70–80% remission rate, 5 year survival 80% 10 year survival 50%	60–80% remission undergoing chemotherapy, 5 year survival 30–60%	No prospect of permanent cure, mean survival: 6–8 years	Mean survival: 5 years, stages: 1 chronic stable 2 acceleration 3 terminal blast crisis

8.43 Myeloproliferative Syndromes (MPS)

Malignant transformation of pluripotent stem cells that leads to a clonal proliferation with accumulation of atypical and immature cells. Effects leukocytes, erythrocytes and megakaryocytes and depending on cell type most affected, allocated to individual subgroups

	Chronic myeloid leukemia	Idiopathic myelofibrosis	Polycythemia vera	Essential thrombo-cythemia
Peripheral blood				
Leukocytes	↑↑↑	↑↑ - ↓	N-↑	N-↑
Left shift	↑↑↑, basophils, eosinophils	↑↑ red cell precursors	N-↑	N-↑
Hb/RBCs	N	N - ↓	↑↑	N
Platelets	N - ↑↑ (50%)	N-↑	N - ↑↑ (60%)	↑↑↑
ALP-index	↓	N-↑	N-↑	N-↑
Bone marrow				
Granulopoiesis	↑↑↑	↑↑ - ↓	↑	N
Erythropoiesis	N - ↓	↑ - ↓	↑↑	N
Megakaryopo-iesis	N - ↑↑	↑ - ↓	↑	↑↑↑
Fibrosis	N - ↑	↑ - ↑↑↑	N-↑	N - ↑
Iron stores	↓	N - ↑	↓↓	N
ABL/BCR-Rearrangement	>95%	-	-	-
LDH	↑↑	↑↑	↑	N-↑
Vit. B$_{12}$	↑↑	N - ↓	↑	N
Splenomegaly	(↑)-↑↑	↑↑↑	N-↑	N-(↑)
Myeloid metaplasia	↑↑	↑↑↑	N-↑	N-↑
Special features	Philadelphia-Chromosome, Leucocyte alkaline phosphatase ↓	Xerophthalmia (Keratitis sicca, dry eyes)	Packed marrow	
In common	"Colorful picture" in the aspirate (Increase in WBCs, often with more eosinophils and basophils)			WBC diff. often inconspi-cuous

8.44 Myelodysplastic Syndromes (MDS)

- **Acquired clonal diseases** of the bone marrow stem-cell with defects of cell maturation, resulting in a refractory anemia, thrombocytopenia, neutropenia, and occasionally a leukocytosis
- **Disrupted metabolism** with **mono-, bi- or tricytopenia** with normal or increased cellularity of the bone marrow; patients often also have refractory macrocytic anemia (up to 90%) during the course of the disease
- Leading causes of death are infection, bleeding, and the development of thrombocytopenia or AML
- **Basic therapy:** Substitution of the blood cells (erythrocytes, platelets), and early treatment of infections
- **Treatment goal:** In the advanced stage reduction or elimination of blast population by chemotherapy and/or stem cell transplantations

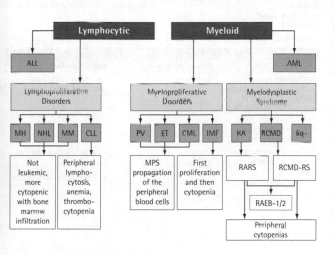

FAB classification

FAB subtype	Blasts in blood	Blasts in bone marrow	Other signs
Refractory anemia (RA)	≤1%	<5%	–
Refractory anemia with ringed sideroblasts (RARS)	≤1%	<5%	Ringed sideroblasts >15% in the BM
Refractory anemia with excess blasts (RAEB)	<5%	5%–20%	–
Chronic myelomonocytic leukemia (CMML)	<5%	5%–20%	Peripheral monocytes >10³/μL
RAEB in transformation* (RAEB-T)	≥5%	21%–30%	Variable Auer rods

* RAEB-T: diagnosis can be made by detection of Auer rods even at a low blast count

WHO classification

Disorder	Peripheral blood	Bone marrow
Refractory cytopenia with unilineage dysplasia (RCUD), Refractory anemia (RA), Refractory neutropenia (RN), Refractory thrombocytopenia (RT)	No or few blasts (< 1%)	Unilineage dysplasia (≥10% of cells)
		<5% Blasts
		<15% ringed sideroblasts
Refractory anemia with ringed sideroblasts (RARS)	Anemia	Dysplasia only of RBCs
	No blasts	<5% Blasts
		≥15% ringed sideroblasts

Disorder (cont.)	Peripheral blood	Bone marrow
Refractory cytopenia with multilineage dysplasia (RCMD)	Bi- or pancytopenia	Dysplasia present in ≥10% of 2 or more cell myeloid cell lines
	No or few blasts < 1%	No Auer-rods
	No Auer-rods	<5% blasts in KM
	Monocytes <1000/μL	<15% ringed sideroblasts
Refractory anemia with excess blasts-1 (RAEB-1)	Cytopenia	Uni- or multilineage dysplasia
	<5% Blasts	5%–9% blasts
	No Auer-rods	No Auer-rods
	Monocytes <1000/μL	
Refractory anemia with excess blasts-2 (RAEB-2)	Cytopenia	Uni- or multilineage dysplasia
	5%–19% Blasts	10%–19% Blasts
	Auer-rods ±	Auer-rods ±
	Monocytes <1000/μL	−
MDS unclassified (MDS-U)	Cytopenia	Dysplasia in <10% of cells in ≥1 series of cells With typical MDS Cytogenetics
MDS with del [5q] ("5q-syndrome")	Anemia	Megakaryocytes count normal or increased, with hypolobulated nuclei
	Platelets normal to increased	No Auer-rods
	No or few blasts (<1%)	<5% blasts
		cytogenetics: isolated del (5q)
Acute leukemia	≥20% blasts	≥20% blasts

8.45 Plasma Cell Disorders

8.45.1 Plasma cell myeloma

Multiple myeloma, symtomatic myeloma:

- A malignant disorder of plasma cells caused by proliferation of a single clone
- Frequent invasion of adjacent bone resulting in bone pain and fractures
- Plasma cells may infiltrate multiple organs and produce a variety of symptoms
- Monoclonal (M) protein overproduction can lead to renal failure (light chains - Bence Jones protein) or hyperviscosity of peripheral blood

Clinical and laboratory signs (approximate percent):
- Hb <12 g/dL (72%)
- Bone lesions/fractures (80%)
- Renal failure (20%)
- Hypercalcemia (10%)
- M-spike on serum protein electrophoresis, SPEP (80%)
- M-spike on serum protein immunofixation, SPIF (>90%)
- IgG (50%)
- IgA (20%)
- Light chain only (15%)

Diagnostic criteria: (All 3 required)
- Clonal plasma cells >10% on bone marrow biopsy or in any quantity in a biopsy from other tissues (plasmacytoma)
- Monoclonal protein in either serum and/or urine
  (Note: rare cases of non-secretory myeloma)
- End-organ damage related to the plasma cell disorder: **Related organ or tissue impairment (ROTI)**; commonly referred to as "**CRAB**":
  - Hyper**C**alcemia
  - **R**enal insufficiency due to myeloma
  - **A**nemia (hemoglobin <10 g/dL)
  - **B**one lesions (lytic or osteoporosis with pathologic fractures)

Good prognostic indicators:
- Cyclin D1 overexpression
- Low serum β2-microglobulin
- 5q amplification
- Translocation (11;14) or (6;14)
- Hyperdiploidy
- CXCR4
- Normal serum free kappa/lambda light chair ratio
- IgG subtype

Adverse prognostic indicators:
- Chromosome 13 deletion
- Chromosome 17p deletion
- High serum β2-microglobulin
- Hypoploidy/aneuploidy
- Translocation (4;14) or (14;16)
- BTK expression
- Increased N-cadherin (>6 ng/mL)
- Low serum prohepcidin
- Near tetraploidy
- IgA and IgD subtypes
- ISS and TGFβR2 hypermethylation

8.45.2 Monoclonal gammopathy of undetermined significance (MGUS)

Func: A premalignant disorder of plasma cells that have not met criteria for myeloma

Diagnostic criteria: (All 3 required)
- Serum monoclonal protein <30 g/L
- <10% clonal plasma cells on bone marrow biopsy
- No myeloma ROTI

8.45.3 Asymptomatic "smoldering" myeloma

Considered an 'early,' 'inactive,' or 'precursor' form of myeloma, almost always becomes full myeloma without proper treatment
Diagnostic criteria: (#1 and/or #2, #3 required)
- Serum paraprotein >30 g/L
- >10% clonal plasma cells on bone marrow biopsy
- No myeloma ROTI

8.45.4 Solitary plasmacytoma

A mass lesion of clonal plasma cells without any other signs or symptoms
Diagnostic criteria: (All 4 required)
- Biopsy-proven clonal plasma cell lesion of bone or soft tissue
- Normal bone marrow biopsy
- Normal skeletal work-up (only the solitary lesion)
- No ROTI

8.45.5 Waldenström's macroglobulinemia

Disorder of B cells leading to increased IgM and blood hyperviscosity; Sometimes considered an indolent lymphocytic lymphoma
Diagnostic criteria: (All 3 required)
- IgM monoclonal gammopathy
- >10% lymphoplasmacytic infiltration on bone marrow biopsy
- Other lymphoproliferative disorders excluded

8.45.6 Systemic amyloidosis

Systemic amyloid deposition due to overproduction of light chains
Diagnostic criteria: (All 4 required)
- The presence of amyloid-related systemic syndrome (renal, liver, heart, GI tract, nervous system, etc)
- Biopsy confirmed amyloid deposition of any tissue (Congo Red)
- Proof that the amyloid is light-chain based (immunohistochemistry, sequencing)
- Evidence of a monoclonal plasma cell proliferation making the light chain (not present in ~5% of patients, diagnosis made with caution)

8.45.7 POEMS syndrome

Rare plasma cell proliferative disorder; progressive and often fatal without treatment, more common in middle aged men

Diagnostic criteria: (All 3 required)
- Monoclonal plasma cell disorder
- Peripheral neuropathy
- At least one of: **O**rganomegaly, **E**ndocrinopathy, **E**dema, **S**kin lesions (hyperpigmentation, hypertrichosis, hemangiomas), papilledema, sclerotic bone lesions (>98%)

9 Hemostasis

Hemostasis	Fibrinolysis
Activation of endogenous and exogenous cascade	Activation of endogenous and exogenous cascade
Formation of thrombin	Formation of plasmin
Formation of fibrin (build the clot)	Cleavage of fibrin (break the clot)

9.1 Primary Hemostasis

Step I	**Vascular hemostasis:** • Reflex constriction of vessels by mechanical stimulation or insult at the injury site, particularly within the arteries and arterioles • Release of vasoconstrictor substances such as serotonin, kinins, prostaglandins → causing additional vasoconstriction. → slowed blood flow → allows for platelet aggregation
Step II	**Platelet aggregation:** • Platelets adhere to exposed collagen fibers caused by the injury of the vascular endothelium. Adhesion requires the presence of the Von Willebrand factor (bridging) • Upon adhesion to subendothelial structures, platelets are stimulated to activation and subsequent secretion • Activated phospholipids on the platelet membrane flip outward (flip-flop mechanism) to form a net-like matrix vital to the coagulation process • Platelet shape changes with protrusion of pseudopodia and secretion of platelet storage granules containing thromboxane A2, ADP, PAF, and serotonin into the surrounding medium which further propagates clot formation • This self-propagating systems leads to further activation of platelet-plasmatic coagulation cascade

9.2   Secondary Hemostasis

Plasmatic coagulation:
- Process carried out by the plasma coagulation factors
- Proceeds in 3 phases with distinction between endogenous and exogenous cascade systems according to whether the operations of activation is led by tissue thrombokinase (linked activated thrombokinase), from injured tissue (extrinsic), or by platelet thrombokinase (intrinsic) released by activated platelets

Phase 1	Intrinsic: Platelet thrombokinase (from platelet factor 3 = partial thromboplastin) causes the activation of a cascade of coagulation factors XII, XI, IX. Factor IX is activated by factor VIII phospholipids and factor X **Duration of cascade:** minutes (only if the extrinsic pathway is not activated)	Extrinsic: Tissue thrombokinase (Coagulation factor III) leads to the activation of Factor VII, in the presence of Factor X phospholipids **Duration of cascade:** seconds (Performance of this system is limited by the factor VII, which is rapidly consumed)
Phase 2	Activation of thrombin from prothrombin by activated factors X and V, phospholipids, and calcium ions	
Phase 3	Thrombin activates fibrinogen, and causes the formation of fibrin monomers In addition, thrombin also activates factor XIII, which is responsible for polymerization of fibrin. The result is a solid clot and coverage of injury defect with subsequent retraction	

9.3   Global Coagulation Tests

Evaluation of the coagulation system as a whole, based on relatively nonspecific (functional) screening tests which include:
- Bleeding time
- Thrombelastogram

9.4 Phase Specific Coagulation Tests

Evaluation of a disturbance to the endogenous, exogenous, or common pathway of coagulation which include:
• Quick test (inversed PT/INR→ decreased when PT is prolonged)
• Partial thromboplastin time (PTT or aPTT)
• Thrombin time (TT) and prothrombin time (PT)
→ Higher sensitivity than the global tests; Caveat: Detection of individual factors deficiencies is possible but only for significantly decreased values (<30%-50% of the normal, not sensitive!)

9.5 Factor Specific Tests

Quantitative and qualitative assessment of individual clotting factors, indicated for suspected congenital or acquired deficiency or defect of one or more coagulation factors

9.6 Stages of Blood Loss

Stage 1: All tests normal, only intravascular volume loss with hypotension (immediate)
Stage 2: Hemoglobin and hematocrit ↓ (after 4-6 h)
Stage 3: Reactive reticulocytosis with increased reticulocyte count → decreased MCH (after 2-3 days)

9.7 Bleeding Time

Def: Test for detecting disorders of primary hemostasis
Incision is made in the skin and time needed for the bleeding to stop on its own is measured
→ Nonspecific test that detects only pronounced defects in coagulation
→ Normal bleeding time does not exclude platelet function disorders

Ind: Detection of primary hemostasis disorders:
• Nonspecific assessment of platelet function, especially in (borderline) thrombocytopenia
• Screening test in suspected hemorrhagic disease, especially platelet disorder and von Willebrand syndrome

Norm: ≤6 min subaqueous bleeding time (method according to Marx)
2-7 min (method according to Ivy)
3-9 min (method according to Simplate)

↑
- Von Willebrand syndrome
- Platelet disorder/dysfunction
- Congenital conditions: Glanzmann's disease, Bernard-Soulier syndrome, storage pool disease, Wiskott-Aldrich syndrome, etc.
- Underlying diseases: severe uremia, severe cirrhosis, hyperviscosity syndrome, high concentrations monoclonal immunoglobulins
- Medications: platelet aggregation inhibitors (abciximab, aspirin/NSAIDS, clopidogrel, ticlopidine), prostacyclins, higher molecular weight dextrans, antibiotics
- Thrombocytopenia (when platelet count is less than 100,000, prolongation of bleeding time correlates with decreasing platelet count)
- Vascular defects/increased vascular fragility (=> Rumpel-Leede test)
- Decreased hematocrit (<30% may prolong bleeding time)

Note: Potential sources of error are based on different penetration depth, skin perfusion (temperature, shock), skin thickness, drainage problems (ear clips, blood pressure cuffs, sleeves)

Caution: Must be aware if patient is taking drugs containing acetylsalicylic acid (aspirin) or platelet aggregation inhibitors → may lead to excessive bleeding

9.8   Coagulation Activation as a Result of Vascular Injury

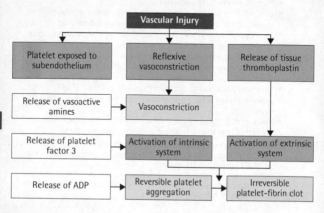

9.9   Clotting Factors

Factor	Name	Vit K dependent	% Activity for NL function	Half-life (hours)
I	Fibrinogen	N	30	150
II	Prothrombin	Y	30	80
III	Tissue factor, thromboplastin	N	N/A	<1
IV	Calcium ions	N	N/A	N/A
V	Proaccelerin	N	40	24
VI	Accelerin (Va)	N	20	N/A
VII	Proconvertin	Y	40	6
VIII	Antihemophilic factor A	N	30	12

Factor (cont.)	Name	Vit K dependent	% Activity for NL function	Half-life (hours)
IX	Antihemophilic factor B, Christmas-Factor	Y	30	24
X	Stuart-Prower factor	Y	30	60
XI	Rosenthal factor	N	20	80
XII	Hagemann factor	N	<5	70
XIII	Fibrin-stabilizing factor	N	<5	150
XIV	Fletcher factor	N	<5	35
XV	Fitzgerald factor	N	<5	150
vWF	von-Willebrand factor	N	30	15

9.10 Coagulation Inhibitors

Abbreviation	Name	Function
AT	Antithrombin	Inhibits factors IIa, IXa, Xa, XIa, XIIa
PC	Protein C	Inhibits factors Va and VIIIa
PS	Protein S	Cofactor of protein C

9.11 Coagulation Cascade

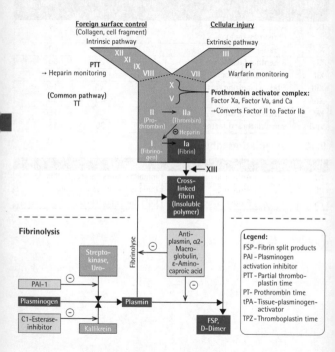

9.12   Prothrombin Time (PT)

Func: Evaluation of factor VII (extrinsic system) and the Factors X, V, II, I (common pathway; more sensitive than PTT). Tissue factor and thromboplastin added to citrated plasma with excess calcium and the time to clot formation is measured in seconds

Ind:
- Evaluation of hemorrhagic disease
- Vitamin K deficiency
- Monitoring of treatment with vitamin K antagonist (Coumadin/warfarin)
- Assessment of the synthetic function of the liver in severe parenchymal liver disease (eg, cirrhosis)
- Preoperative screening for coagulopathy

Prod: Liver

Norm: Times vary by lab based on what reagents are used
~8-14 sec
70%-120%

↑ >120%: usually artificial due to traumatic blood draw or exposure to cold

↓
- Vitamin K deficiency (vitamin K antagonists, malnutrition/diet, intestinal malabsorption, cirrhosis/liver disease)
- Consumption (blood loss coagulopathy, fibrinolysis)
- Hereditary deficiency
- Fibrinogen deficiency, dysfibrinogenemia
- Hemophilia

Mat: Citrated plasma

70%-120%	Normal range, does not exclude mild factor deficiencies
50%-70%	With normal PTT implies still normal hemostasis, possibly due to limited synthetic capacity of the liver
30%-50%	Suggestive of hemorrhagic diathesis, low risk and unlikely to bleed
15%-30%	Therapeutic range warfarin (VKA) therapy
5%-10%	Severe hemorrhagic diathesis, high risk with tendency to spontaneous bleeding
</= 4%	Risk of life-threatening bleeding, administer FFP immediately

International normalized ratio (INR):

Func: Only useful for monitoring oral anticoagulant therapy. Enables standardization of Prothrombin Time (PT). Variations among thromboplastins result in differing sensitivity to warfarin and can give different PTs for the same amount of anticoagulation. Requires the International Sensitivity Index (ISI)

$$INR = (Patient\ PT/NPT)^{ISI}$$

* The advantage of the INR is the improved comparability of results

Note: In the presence of lupus anticoagulant, hirudin, or argatroban the INR may overestimate the amount of anticoagulation. In this case a chromogenic factor X assay may be used

INR 0.8-1.2	Normal range, no anticoagulation
INR 2.0-3.0	Low dose anticoagulation (therapeutic)
INR 3.0-4.5	High-dose anticoagulation (supratherapeutic)

9.13 Activated Partial Thromboplastin Time (aPTT)

Func: Screening test to detect defects of the intrinsic system (Factors XV, XIV, XII, XI, IX, VIII) and the common final pathway (X, V, II, I)
- Activation of coagulation with partial thromboplastins which are missing tissue factor and thus require a longer period of time compared to complete thromboplastins
- To improve activation the Activated PTT (aPTT) is determined by adding contact activators of FXII (eg, silica, kaolin, celite or ellagic acid added) and excess calcium
- For determination of the aPTT, the factors of the contact phase activation are recorded (prekallikrein and high molecular weight kininogen)

Ind: Evaluation of hemorrhagic disease:
- Monitoring unfractionated heparin treatment*
- Monitoring of the substitution therapy in hemophilia A and B
- Preoperative screening for coagulopathy

Norm: Coagulometric (28-40 sec); Chromogenic Method (90-120 sec)

↑ Single factor deficiency (generally <30%; intrinsic or common, PT more sensitive in latter), coagulopathy, heparin, lupus anticoagulant (not fixed with mixing study), anti-FVIII (not fixed with mixing study), hemophilia A and B

↓ Indicates potential risk for hypercoagulability

Met: **Coagulometric** - Measurement of the clotting time following the addition of thromboplastin/ surfactant substances

Chromogenic - Activation of plasma and measuring the absorbance with sulfatide

* **Activated clotting time (ACT):** May be used to monitor higher-dose heparin treatment (when aPTT is immeasurable; >150 sec). Quick test performed on whole blood using a tube that contains intrinisic pathway activator. Norm: 70-180 s, heparin: >400 sec. Less precise than aPTT due to contributing factors (platelets, hematocrit, etc). FXa assay is favorable to ACT if time permits, used to monitor low molecular weight heparin or higher-dose heparin where aPTT is unreliable

Possible causes of prolongetd PTT		
Etiology	**PT**	**Additional work-up**
Anti-FVIII Ab	nl	Anti-FVIII assay
Common pathway deficiencies (FX, V, II)	Prolonged	Specific factor assays
DIC	Prolonged	Fibrin split products
Intrinsic pathway deficiencies (FXII, XI, IX, VIII, pre-kallikrein, HMWK)	NL	Specific factor assays
Heparin	Usually normal (PTT>PT)	Heparin neutralization
Hirudin	Prolonged	History
Liver disease/cirrhosis	Prolonged (PT>PTT)	History, liver function tests
Lupus anticoagulant	Prolonged (PT>PTT)	Lupus anticoagulant assay
Vit. K deficiency/Warfarin	Prolonged (PT>PTT)	FII, VII, IX, X assays

Possible sources of error in anticoagulation monitoring	
PTT inappropriately shortened (Underestimate)	**PTT inappropriately prolonged (Overestimate)**
• Acute phase reactions • ATIII deficiency (Renal disease) • Increased FVIII • Pregnancy	• Antiphospholipids • DIC • Factor deficiencies • Liver disease
Work-up	**Work-up**
ATIII levels, FVIII levels; HcG levels	Fibrin split products; Lupus anticoagulant

9.14   Thrombin Time (TT)

Func: Conversion of fibrinogen to fibrin by addition of thrombin to the patient's plasma

Ind:
- Suspected disturbance in fibrin polymerization/stabilization
- Suspected fibrinogen deficiency or dysfibrinogenemia (both TT and RT prolonged)
- Hyperfibrinolysis (rapid destruction of fibrin polymers)
- Thrombolytic therapy monitoring (eg, TPA/alteplase, streptokinase)

Norm: 17–24 sec

↑ **Heparin therapy**, disruption of fibrin (fibrinolysis), fibrinogen deficiency, dysfibrinogenemia, amyloidosis

9.15   Reptilase Time (RT)

Func: AKA hemocoagulase, a proteolytic enzyme derived from the venom the American Lance Viper snake; when reptilase is added to plasma it results in the conversion of fibrinogen to fibrin by cleaving fibrinopeptide A

Ind:
- Prolonged TT with suspected hyperfibrinolysis
- Consumptive coagulopathy (X and Y fragments of fibrin degradation products cause)

Norm: 12–21 sec

↑ Hypofibrinogenemia, dysfibrinogenemia, hyperfibrinolysis, amyloidosis

Note: **Unaffected by heparin**

Distinguishing dysfibrinogenemia from hypofibrogenemia is typically done with mixing studies: the former will only partially correct, the latter should completely correct

9.16   Recalcification Time

Func: Addition of calcium back into citrated blood, time to clot is measured. Largely replaced with other tests. General test that identifies the presence of coagulation abnormality, which requires further clarification

Norm: 80–120 sec

9.17 Fibrinogen

Func: Factor I; soluble plasma glycoprotein, converted to fibrin by thrombin

Ind: Hemorrhagic disease, dysfibrinogenemia, monitoring fibrinolysis

Prod: Liver

Norm: 200–400 mg/dL   Half-life 3–5 days

↑ Acute-phase reactant: Infections, non-infectious inflammation, postoperative, neoplasms (esp. pancreas, lung), large burns, nephrotic syndrome, cirrhosis, pregnancy/hormone therapy; diabetic ketoacidosis, cholestasis

↓ Abnormal or decreased synthesis: Acquired - liver failure and loss of synthetic function, poisoning (amatoxin, etc.), asparaginase therapy, physiologically in newborns, Hereditary - dys-, hypo- or afibrinogenemia (very rare)
Increased consumption: Coagulation with / without fibrinolysis, fibrinolytic therapy, severe blood loss, treatment with asparaginase

Mat: Citrated plasma

Note: Kinetic fibrinogen assays may be falsely low in patients with dysfibrinogenemias, markedly elevated FSPs (eg, thrombolytic therapy or DIC), or Ab to bovine thrombin. In these cases end-point determinations via nephelometric assays are better

9.18 Fibrin Split Products (FSPs)

D-Dimer is a type of FSP formed only by plasmin-mediated fibrin degradation: Indicates fibrin has been formed and then degraded

Func: Cleavage of fibrinogen to fibrin by plasmin; using monoclonal antibody for differentiated detection of fibrinogen splitting products (FSP), fibrin degradation products (FDP), and fibrin splitting products (D-dimers)

Ind:
- Fibrinogen split products: Hyperfibrinolysis (abnormal bleeding, DDx between intravascular coagulation and hyperfibrinolysis, retrograde assessment of fibrinolytic therapy (rarely used)
- D-Dimer: Intravascular activation of coagulation with secondary fibrinolysis (DVT, PE, DIC)

Norm: <250 ng/mL   D-Dimer units
             <0.5 µg/mL   Fibrinogen units
             A normal D-Dimer has a very high negative predictive value to rule out in vivo thrombosis (~95%; DVT, PE)

↑   Intravascular fibrinolysis, intravascular coagulation with subsequent fibrinolysis, fibrinolytic therapy, thromboembolism, thrombosis, wound healing, liver disease, pregnancy, malignancy, meds (furosemide, ADH analogues, nicotinic acid derivatives)

Note: In confirmed DVT → D-dimer antigen concentration can suggest:
             Normal range or below the respective critical value → likely incomplete vascular occlusion (about 95% probability, assuming normal fibrinolytic activity)
             D-Dimer determination of a suspected DVT is always a diagnosis of exclusion and additional testing should be utilized to rule out other etiologies; imaging and physical examination of extremities is usually required for confirmation

Mat: Citrated blood

Met: Latex agglutination assay: Patient's plasma mixed with anti-FSP/anti-D-dimer covered latex beads → agglutination = positive. Serial dilutions can be done to provide a titer
             ELISA assays may be done for quantitative measurements

9.19   Hyperfibrinolysis

Def: Elevated fibrinolysis (clot degradation) due to increased activation of plasminogen to plasmin which can result in bleeding when excessive
             Platelet count: normal
             Fibrinogen: reduced
             Fibrin: detectable

9.20 Platelet Function Tests (PFTs)

AKA Platelet aggregometry, thromboelastogram (TEG - similar method)

Func: A qualitative functional test of platelet activity, endogenous coagulation function and fibrinolysis
  • Blood in a cuvette is stirred continuously and monitored for aggregation by light transmission (resistance in TEG). (Normally no spontaneous aggregation)
  • Platelet aggregation agonists are added (ADP, epi, arachidonate, collagen, ristocetin)
  • The results are transferred onto a linear curve recording time on the y-axis and transmittance on x-axis (resistance in TEG)
  • **TEG:**
    - The period of time to start of clot formation is referred to as reaction time (r)
    - The time to reach the threshold amplitude is referred to as thrombus formation time (k)
    - The third measurement is the maximum amplitude (MA) given in mm. After reaching the MA, the curve narrows normally due to initiation of fibrinolysis

Ind: Suspected coagulopathy with hemorrhagic diathesis and normal tests (PT, INR, aPTT, TT, platelet count, fibrinogen, bleeding time); monitoring hemophilia therapy

Norm: >60% aggregation to agonists. Biphasic curve with low-dose ADP and epi: primary and secondary aggregation (latter from degranulation). Monophasic curve (primary only) with high-dose ADP, collagen 9 after short lag, and ristocetin (> 1.2 mg/mL)

  TEG: Reaction time (r): 10-16 min
  Thrombus formation time (k): 4-6 min
  Maximum amplitude (MA): 47-60 mm

  Abnormal response:
  • **ASA/NSAIDS:** Most common, patients must not have ingested for 7 days. Will show decreased aggregation with arachidonate
  • **Bernard-Soulier:** Response to everything but ristocetin
  • **Glanzmann thrombasthenia:** Decreased GpIIb/IIIa; poor response to all agents except ristocetin
  • **Myeloproliferative disorders:** Poor response to epi
  • **Storage pool defects:** Absent secondary phase with epi and ADP

Mat: 5 mL of platelet rich plasma (slow-centrifuged whole blood); kept at room temp to avoid platelet activation and immediately processed

9.21 Antithrombin (AT)

AKA Antithrombin III

Func:	• Most effective inhibitor of activated coagulation proteases; physiological coagulation inhibitor (AT deficiency with coagulation activation → high risk of thrombosis)
	• Binds heparin (The basis for the detection of AT by affinity chromatography)
	• Potentiated by heparin (Heparin is ineffective in the absence of AT)
Ind:	Consumptive coagulopathy, thrombophilia screening, lack of PTT extension under high-dose heparin, liver disease, nephrotic syndrome, asparaginase monitoring
Prod:	Liver, vascular endothelial cells
Norm:	10-15 IU/L
	>60% Activity adults
	>40% Activity neonates-6 months
↑	Cholestasis, treatment with warfarin
↓	DIC, heparin, OCPs, liver disease/cirrhosis (loss of synthesis/function), nephrotic syndrome, asparaginase therapy, hereditary alpha-1-AT deficiency
Mat:	5 mL of citrated plasma, immediately processed or immediately centrifuged and frozen
Met:	**Functional:** More clinically useful; usually measured spectrophotometrically based on inhibition of thrombin and Xa - uninhibited thrombin or Xa will activate a chromogen and is inversely proportional to AT
	Antigenic: If functional is abnormal may be performed to distinguish between type I and type II deficiency

9.22 Protein C

Func:	• Vitamin K-dependent factor that serves as a natural inhibitor of factors V and VIII
	• Activated by thrombomodulin-bound thrombin and Ca^{2+}; accelerated by protein S
	• Causes activation of fibrinolysis by neutralization of plasminogen activator inhibitor-1 (PAI-1)

Ind: Thrombophilia, DIC, liver disease, purpura fulminans in newborns.
Prior to initiation of vitamin K antagonists: **Skin necrosis**

Prod: Liver

Norm: 2-6 mg/L
70%-140%   Activity
Neonates have naturally low levels

↓   Hereditary protein C deficiency
- Heterozygous protein C deficiency: Protein C activity: 20%-70%
  - Type I: reduced concentration and activity of protein C
  - Type II: normal concentration, decreased activity of protein C
- Homozygous protein C deficiency: protein C activity: <1%
- Acquired protein C deficiency - including Vitamin K deficiency,
  parenchymal liver disease, DIC

Mat: Citrated plasma, patient must be off anticoagulants for 1 wk (1 month
post-thrombosis)

9.23   Protein S

Func:
- Vitamin K-dependent cofactor of activated protein C
- 40% Free protein → detectable in the blood in active form
- 60% Bound protein to C4b-binding protein (and biologically inactive)
- Congenital deficiency can lead to thromboembolic complications in
  early childhood → Consider Protein C and S deficiency in a young
  child with thromboembolic event

Ind: Thrombophilia, liver disease

Prod: Liver

Norm: 17-35 mg/L
70%-150%   Activity (free protein)

↓
- Hereditary Protein S deficiency syndromes include:
  - Reduced synthesis of Protein S (quantitative deficiency)
  - Adequate synthesis but deficient function (qualitative deficiency)
- Acquired protein S deficiency included Vitamin K deficiency,
  parenchymal liver disease

Mat: Citrated plasma

9.24 Activated Protein C-Resistant/Factor V Leiden

Def: A common hereditary mutation leading to "resistance" to activated Protein C inhibition resulting in hypercoagulability
- Cause in >90% of cases: mutation in the factor V gene (~5% of all Europeans, high incidence)
  - Single amino acid change from Arginine to Glutamine at position 506
  - Active form of coagulation factor V (FVa) is cleaved abnormally making it resistant to inhibition by Protein C
- Risks:
  - Heterozygous: 5-10-fold increased risk of thrombosis
  - Homozygous: 50-100-fold increased risk of thrombosis

Ind: Thrombophilia (esp. in unexplained/recurrent thromboembolism in patients <45 years)

Norm: >2.3 ([APTT+APC]/[APTT-APC])
Neonates show natural protein C resistance due to low endogenous levels

↓ APC Ratio 1.5-2.3 → heterozygote Factor V mutation
APC Ratio <1.5 → likely homozygote Factor V mutation

Mat: Citrated plasma

Met:
- Screened for with mixing studies (patients plasma diluted with FV-deficient reagent, then PTT measure with and without added protein C, deficient people will not correct). Affected by the presence of a lupus anticoagulant
- Molecular PCR is the gold standard method of detection and differentiation between hetero- and homozygous mutation carriers; molecular-based identification can be particularly useful in heterozygotes that may have a questionable or asymptomatic clinical picture

9.25 Spontaneous Clot Lysis Time

Func: 1 mL of whole blood is allowed to spontaneously clot in a small tube with or without thrombin additive, then observed for spontaneous clot lysis at 37°C. Not routinely performed

Norm: ~24 h

↓ Hyperfibrinolysis

Met: 1 mL non-citrated whole blood

9.26 Euglobulin Lysis Time (ELT)

Func: Measures overall fibrinolytic capacity

Norm: 5-24 h

↓ Hyperfibrinolysis

Met: Citrated platelet-poor plasma is mixed with acid in a glass test tube. The acidification causes precipitation of clotting factors (euglobulin fraction - fibrinogen, fVIII, PAI-1, tPA, plasminogen, α2-antiplasmin). The euglobulin fraction is then added to a borate solution and clotting is activated via CaCl. The clot is then observed for lysis either by eye (older method) or spectrophotometrically

9.27 Plasmin

Func: Cleaves fibrin and fibrinogen to fibrin split products. Fibrin (-ogen) split products in turn inhibit fibrin polymerization. Generated from plasminogen via plasminogen activators (ie, tissue plasminogen activator [tPA], urokinase-type plasminogen activator [uPA])

Ind: Thrombophilia, monitor fibrinolytic reserves in thrombosis, monitoring fibrinolytic therapy, suspected hyperfibrinolysis, ligneous conjunctivitis (association w/homozygous plasminogen deficiency)

Prod: Derived from plasminogen via rearrangement of arginine-lysine binding site
Plasminogen is a glycoprotein synthesized in the liver, half-life ~2 days

Norm: 0.2 g/L Plasminogen
>75% Activity

↑ Plasminogen is an acute-phase reactant; also, paraneoplastic syndrome (prostate, lung, bladder), diabetes, pregnancy/estrogen therapy/OCPs

↓   Acquired: Fibrinolytic therapy, coagulopathy, cirrhosis
Inherited: Rare autosomal recessive; increased risk of thromboembolic disease and ligneous conjunctivitis (homozygous)

Mat: Citrated plasma

9.28   Platelet Disorders

Bernard-Soulier syndrome:

- AKA hemorrhagiparous thrombocytic dystrophy. Autosomal recessive coagulopathy due to decreased GPIb (receptor for vWF) leading to thrombocytopenia and giant platelets
- PFTs normal to all agonists (ADP, thrombin, epi, etc.) but abnormal with ristocetin (similar to vWD)

Symptoms: Easy bruising, heavy menses, epistaxis, prolonged bleeding times, mucosal bleeding

Glanzmann thrombasthenia:

- Autosomal recessive hemorrhagic disease with significantly prolonged bleeding times due to platelet defect: GPIIb/IIIa deficiency leads to lack of PLA1 antigen
- PFTs abnormal to all agonists (ADP, thrombin, epi, etc.) but ristocetin (ristocetin normal)
- Poor induction of clot retraction despite normal platelet counts
  - Type I with reduced ATP levels
  - Type II with normal ATP levels

Symptoms: Skin and mucous membrane bleeding, prolonged bleeding time, no enlargement of the spleen

Platelet Storage Disorders:

Dense granules: Store ADP, ATP, serotonin, histamine, and Ca^{2+}, required for second wave of platelet aggregation

Chediak-Higashi and Hemansky-Pudlak syndrome:
Platelet counts normal, but absence of dense granules
Symptoms: Epistaxis beginning in childhood, prolonged bleeding, oculocutaneous albinism. C-H has granulocyte and platelet inclusion granules whereas H-P has macrophage inclusions

Wiskott–Aldrich syndrome:
- X-linked recessive disorder characterized by the triad of eczema, immunodeficiency and thrombocytopenia
- Platelets are small; low IgM, elevated IgA, IgE, variable IgG),

Symptoms: Petechiae, bruising, epistaxis, bloody diarrhea, eczema, recurrent bacterial infections, +/- splenomegaly, autoimmune disorders, and malignancy (mainly leukemia/lymphoma)

Alpha granules: IGF1, PDGF, TGFβ, PF4 (heparin binding), thrombopondin, fibronectin, vWF. Express P-selectin and CD63

Grey platelet syndrome:
- Autosomal recessive disorder (chr 3p) characterized by the absence of alpha granules leading to pale platelets on Wright stain. Proteins normally contained within granules released into the bone marrow leading to myelofibrosis
- Aggregation is abnormal to all agonists except ADP

Symptoms: Thrombocytopenia, prolonged bleeding, myelofibrosis

Acquired: Most common platelet disorders

ASA/NSAIDS: Inhibit cyclooxygenase 1 (COX-1), an enzyme involved in thromboxane A2 (TXA2) production; TXA2 stimulate dense granule release from platelets causing second wave aggregation; ASA inhibition lasts for the life of the platelet, ~10 days (acetylates the enzyme)

Circulatory bypass machines: Thrombocytopenia and dysfunction resulting from decreased α and dense granules

Clopidogrel and Ticlopidine: Inhibit platelet aggregation via ADP-mediate activation

GPIIb/IIIa inhibitors: Abciximab (ReoPro), Eptifibatide (Integrilin), Tirofiban (Aggrastat); prescribed to prevent thrombosis; effects similar to Glanzmann (Impaired aggregation to all agonists except ristocetin)

Myeloproliferative disorders (MPD): Thrombosis and bleeding associated with clonal defects in megakaryocytes; may be seen even with normal platelet counts; esp. polycythemia vera (PV) and essential thrombocythemia (ET)

Paraproteinemia: Common cause of dysfunction, esp. in classes that can form multimers (IgA, IgM), though most commonly seen IgG due to prevalence; defect proportional to concentration

Uremia: Mild defects of bleeding time and platelet aggregation; improved with dialysis, DDAVP, and estrogen

Platelet disorders			
Defective phase	Mediators involved	Inherited diseases	Acquired defects
Adhesion	GPIb and vWF	Bernard-Soulier von Willebrand disease	Paraproteinemia
Degranulation	Agonists/granules	Platelet release defect Storage pool disease	Aspirin
Aggregation	Fibrinogen and GPIIb/IIIa	Glanzmann	Dysfibrinogenemia

Common clinical manifestations in bleeding disorders		
	Coagulation disorders	Platelet disorders
Deep hematomas	Common	Rare
Delayed bleeding	Common	Rare
Hemarthroses	Common	Rare
Mucosal bleeding	Rare	Common
Petechiae	Rare	Common
Gender	Male	Female

9.29 Heparin

Natural

Func:
- Inhibits platelet aggregation and promotes fibrinolysis and fat clearance
- Binds to and activates antithrombin (AT) (>1000x activity increase) which then deactivates thrombin and other factors (especially factor Xa, but also XIIa, Xia, IXa, and Ia)

Prod: Basophils and mast cells

Therapeutic

Func: A fast-acting anticoagulant for prevention and treatment of thrombosis and embolism. Comes in 2 forms: unfractionated (half-life ~1-2 h) and low-molecular-weight (half-life 6-8 h). Heparin binds to endothelial cells and is engulfed by macrophages, decreasing binding to AT

Prod: Previously derived from mucosa of pig or cow, but now often synthetic

Note: Serious side-effects include heparin-induced thrombocytopenia (HIT - rare, see below), elevation of serum aminotransferase levels (~80%), and hyperkalemia (~8% - due to heparin-induced aldosterone suppression) Rarely alopecia and osteoporosis occur with chronic use
Antidote: Protamine sulfate and toluidine

9.30 Anti-Xa Activity

Func:
- Used to monitor unfractionated (UFH) or low molecular weight heparin (LMWH)
- Coagulation factor Xa is a target of several anticoagulants
- Used as a surrogate marker of the heparin concentration in the blood

Heparin:
- Inhibits multiple coagulation factor, especially factor Xa
- UFH: unfractionated, high molecular weight heparin, anti-IIa and anti-Xa activity, monitored by aPTT
- LMWH: fractionated, low molecular weight heparin, predominantly anti-Xa (ratio of anti-IIa: anti-Xa = 1:2-4)
  - If necessary, monitor by Anti-Xa activity

Danaparoid:
- A heparinoid, that predominantly inhibits factor Xa
- Anticoagulation of patients with heparin-induced thrombocytopenia type II (HIT II-unable to receive heparin)
  - If necessary, monitor by Anti-Xa activity

Ind: Monitoring Anti-Xa activity during LMWH, Danaparoid or specific anti-Xa inhibitors is recommended in the following situations:
- Severe renal or hepatic insufficiency
- Extremely high (>150 kg) or low body weight (<40 kg)
- Pregnancy
- Newborns or young children(<12 years)

LMWH has shown better bioavailability and longer half-life compared to UFH in weight-adjusted adult dosing, thus monitoring anti-Xa activity is typically not indicated in a clinically stable patient

Norm: <0.1 IU/mL

Mat: Citrated plasma collected 4 h after subcutaneous administration (maximum level) or after at least 12 h during time-independent intravenous therapy (IV drip)

Sample stability ~**1 h**: rapid transport and processing

Interpretation:

- Prophylactic administration of a low molecular weight heparin after 4 h → 0.2-0.4 IU/mL
- Therapeutic maintenance (steady-state) doses → 0.6-0.8 IU/mL

Anti-Xa activity >1.0 IU/mL significantly increased → risk of bleeding

- aPTT prolongation during therapy → signs of overdose/supra-therapeutic
- Lower anti-Xa activity than expected: Antithrombin deficiency (Heparin acts primarily via antithrombin; If AT deficiency → decreased heparin effect → lower Anti-Xa)
- Platelet factor 4 (PF4):- Released from degranulating platelets (dense granules), binds to heparin making it ineffective; seen in prolonged storage of blood samples at room temperature (processing in <1 h is necessary)

9.31 Coumarins (Warfarin)

Func: Esters of coumaric acid, a glycoside found in many plants (sweet clover, Tonka nut) existing as an α-pyrone derivative. Building block in many applications: fluorescent indicator, anticoagulants (coumarin derivatives), antibiotics (eg, coumermycin, novobiocin), and pesticide/rodenticide (how it was first discovered)

Most important use of coumarins is as inhibitors of coagulation:

- Vitamin K esterase antagonists
- Inhibition of liver synthesis of Vitamin K-dependent coagulation factors II, VII, IX, X

Antidote: Vitamin K

9.32 Specific Coagulation Factor Deficiencies

- Hemophilia A: Factor VIII
- Hemophilia B: Factor IX
- Other factor deficiencies very rare
- Vitamin K deficiency: Factors II, VII, IX, X
- Liver disease/cirrhosis: Factors I, II, V, VII, IX, X (esp VII - lowest half-life)
- Synthesis of all factors → LIVER (except factor VIII - capillary endothelium)
- Intestinal malabsorption leading to vitamin K deficiency (II, VII, IX, X)
- PT detects the factors VII, X, V, II, I

Factor assays typically performed when screening test (PT, PTT, TT) abnormal and there is full correction when mixed 1:1 with normal plasma (factor inhibitor will not correct completely)

Specific factor assays usually performed via mixing studies (mixing with plasma with a known factor deficiency and looking for correction of PT (II, V, VII, X) or PTT (VIII, IX, XI, XII) or both (I, II, V, X); often followed by serial dilutions. An inhibitor is likely if dilutions result in serial increase of activity

Chromogenic/antigenic assays available for FII, VII, VIII, IX, X)

Except FVIII, all factors are low in neonates <6 months

Mat: Citrated plasma tested or frozen within 2 h

Factor V deficiency:
Autosomal recessive, chr 1; PT and PTT prolonged, TT normal, bleeding time may be prolonged; most common is Factor V Leiden (see above)

Factor VII deficiency:
Rare autosomal recessive disorder associated with severe bleeding; chr 13; no association between FVII levels and bleeding severity; PT prolonged, PTT, TT and bleeding time normal; vitamin K dependent; activated by Tissue Factor III; a complete lack of FVII is incompatible with life; mutation homozygotes have levels of 1%-2% and may have severe bleeding; acquired deficiencies from liver disease, warfarin or vitamin K deficiency

Factor X deficiency:
Rare autosomal recessive; chr 13; synthesized in liver and vitamin K dependent; activated by FVIIa or FIXa-VIIIa complex, and Russell viper venom; Xa converts prothrombin to thrombin; PT, PTT, and DRVVT are prolonged; TT and bleeding time are normal; **Amyloidosis** is the only cause of acquired isolated FX deficiency; Acquired deficiency in association with other factor deficiencies seen in liver disease, warfarin and vitamin K deficiency

Factor XI deficiency:
Autosomal recessive; chr 4, "**Hemophilia C**"; found mainly in Ashkenazi Jews (5%-10%); very low levels may still be clinically normal

Factor XII deficiency:
Rare autosomal recessive condition that essentially never leads to bleeding diathesis despite prolonged pTT

Factor XIII deficiency:
Rare autosomal recessive, 2 subunits, chr 6 and 1; cross-links fibrin clot; PT, PTT, and TT normal; homozygotes have mild delayed bleeding: umbilical stump bleeding, frequent miscarriages, hypertrophic scars; gene polymorphism (Val34Leu) may help prevent DVT and may lead to increased risk of intracranial hemorrhage; acquired deficiencies seen with liver disease, DIC, or inflammatory disease (IBD, HSP)

Combined deficiencies:
FV and VIII: most common, believed to be caused by gene mutation, chr 18, leading to decreased ERGIC-53 which is important for intracellular transport
FII, VII, IX, X, protein C and S: second most common, vitamin K dependent factors, may be seen in newborns hence the vitamin K injection at birth, antibiotics that diminish the intestinal flora which produce vitamin K, malabsorption/malnutrition, and warfarin

Fibrinogen deficiency:
Afibrinogenemia and hypofibrinogenemia - autosomal recessive due to severely truncate proteins, dysfibrinogenemia - autosomal dominant due to missense mutations; 3 genes (α, β, γ), chr 4; most diseases in α locus; fibrinogen cleaved by thrombin to fibrin; binds to platelet GPIIb/IIIa to mediate aggregation

Afibrinogenemia: extremely prolonged PT and PTT and bleeding similar to moderate-severe hemophilia A

Hypofibrinogenemia: congenital or acquired (DIC, asparaginase, liver failure), bleeding occurs when <50 mg/dL. Umbilical cord hemorrhage is often the first sign in both a- and hypofibrinogenemia.

Dysfibrinogenemia: congenital or acquired (hepatobiliary diseases/cancer, renal carcinoma), asymptomatic ~50%, bleeding ~35%, thrombosis ~15%, associated with **frequent miscarriages**

9.33 Hemophilia

- Two main forms: Hemophilia A (Factor VIII) or B (Factor IX)
- Clinically indistinguishable, rare X-linked recessive hereditary coagulation defect with varying degrees of severity (variable penetrance) resulting in hemorrhagic diathesis including skin and mucosal bleeding, hemarthrosis (bleeding into joints), anemia, and thrombocytopenia
- 30% attributed to new mutation
- Simultaneous hemophilia A and B very rare

Hemophilia A (Factor VIII deficiency).
AKA Hemophilia vera, classic hemophilia, hemophilia I
- Hemophilia A is most common severe inherited hemophilia
- Early onset of symptoms, some manifest as newborns
- Almost exclusively young males
- Females are typically heterozygotes and are usually asymptomatic, but may rarely show mild hemophilia with localized tissue hemorrhage following mild blunt trauma and mild prolonged bleeding. Rarely show more severe hemophilia (homozygosity from carrier mother and affected father, very asymmetric lyonization of X chromosome, hemizygosity from Turner's syndrome). FVIII is a positive acute phase reactant: elevated in pregnancy

- FVIII <30% to prolong PTT; however platelet count, PT, and TT are usually normal
- Treatment:
  - Factor VIII substitution therapy - high molecular weight, remains intravascular; half-life ~12 h; may result in anti-FVIII Ab in ~20%
  - DDAVP (desmopressin) may be used in mild cases
  - Amicar (epsilon aminocaproic acid) - inhibitor of fibrinolysis that may be used in addition

Hemophilia B (Factor IX deficiency):
AKA Christmas disease, hemophilia II, German hemophilia
- Similar to Hemophilia A, but tends to be less severe
- Treatment: Factor IX substitution therapy - only 30% dose recovery; half-life ~8 h; may result in anti-FIX Ab

Residual factor activity	Severity of disease
30%-50% of normal	Subclinical (likely asymptomatic)
5%-30%	Mild hemophilia
1%-4%	Moderate hemophilia
<1% factor activity	Severe hemophilia

9.34   Factor-Inhibitor Induced Hemophilia

- Caused by the presence of inhibitors against factors VIII or IX resulting in coagulopathy
- Seen in hemophilia after repeated transfusions and/or factor substitution therapy
- Results from the formation of circulating antibodies to coagulation factors
- Clinical picture similar to hemophilia A (increased bleeding)

9.35 Von Willebrand Factor

Name	Abbreviation	Function
Factor VIII	FVIII	Procoagulant protein
Factor VIIIa	FVIIIa	Activated factor VIII
von Willebrand factor	vWF	Macromolecule of primary hemostasis
von Willebrand factor Antigen	vW: Ag	Antigenic determinant of vWF presence
Ristocetin cofactor activity	vWF: Rco	Biological activity of vWF
Factor VIII-to-vWF complex	FVIII–vWF complex	Circulating form of FVIII and vWF

Func:
- Most common inherited bleeding disorder (~1%); combined coagulation and platelet defect. Protects FVIII by binding to it and preventing premature proteolysis (AKA FVIIIR:Ag – FVIII related antigen)
- Allows bridge formation for platelet adhesion between activated platelets and subendothelium via GPIb
- Patients with blood type O have naturally low levels (~75%) - decreased risk of thrombosis and more severely affected by disorders

Ind: Hemorrhagic disease screening, monitoring therapy (**DDAVP** = 1-deamino 8 D-arginine-Vasopressin, vWF-containing factor VIII concentrate)

Prod: Vascular endothelium and megakaryocytes; stored in Weibel-Palade bodies in endothelium and α granules of megakaryocytes. Released as large multimers and degraded by proteases in the blood, most commonly to dimers

Norm: 50%–150%

↑ Increased with age, exercise, stress, and pregnancy

Mat: Citrated plasma
Note: Since vWF is a **positive acute phase reactant**, concentration fluctuates and repeated analysis is often required for diagnosis; collection is best early in the morning before physical exertion

Met: vWF concentration/vWF-antigen → immunodiffusion, ELISA
vWF activity/ristocetin cofactor

- Platelets are mixed with the antibiotic ristocetin and monitored for aggregation. The extent of platelet aggregation correlates with the ristocetin cofactor activity
- Ristocetin cofactor correlates to the presence of large multimers of vWF:
  - Decreased in vWF syndrome type 1, 2a, 2c
  - Not detectable in vWF syndrome type 3 (severe)
  - Elevated in vWF syndrome 2a and platelet-type (pseudo-vWD)

Syndromes: There are 4 vWD variations and 1 pseudo-vWD all based on the type of defect present

Type I: Most common; decreased synthesis of FVIII:C and vWF: normal structure and multimer pattern; (quantitative)
Clinical: Normal PT and platelet count, prolonged PTT and bleeding time, decreased FVIII and vWF activity; mucosal bleeding, nosebleeds, GI bleeding, menorrhagia, often hematoma
Symptoms of this particular type are not usually as severe as hemophilia → joint bleeding is rare

Type IIa: ~15% of cases; synthesis of a defective vWF, lack of large multimers (qualitative/functional)
Clinical: Normal PT, TT, and fibrinogen, prolonged PTT, FVIII and vWF may be normal or mildly decreased, ristocetin cofactor is decreased <50%
Moderately severe bleeding, increased compared to type I, but less than type III

Type IIb: Similar to type IIa, lack of large multimers (qualitative/functional); However, there is enhanced ristocetin-induced platelet aggregation (but not to cryoprecipitate exposure) and **marked thrombocytopenia and bleeding when given DDAVP: DO NOT give DDAVP!**
Clinical: Spontaneous binding of vWF to platelets due to mutation in GP1b, similar to platelet-type vWD, but in IIb there is selective binding of large multimers leading to increased clearance

Type IIM: Very rare disorder characterized by defective binding of vWF to GPIb, normal distribution of multimers (qualitative/functional)

Type IIN: Rare, autosomal dominant disorder caused by defective vWF that prevents binding to FVIII; normal multimer distribution and vWF levels, low FVIII (often confused with hemophilia A)

Type III: Severe, autosomal recessive disorder with essentially no vWF (quantitative)

Clinical: VWF:Ag and vWF.RC are greatly reduced or undetectable; FVIII:C also displays mild to severe reduction; severe bleeding tendency, significantly prolonged bleeding time, similar to hemophilia A including hemarthrosis and hematoma formation

Pseudo-/platelet-type vWD: Defect in GPIb leading to increased binding to vWF similar to IIb; however, in this disorder exposure to cryoprecipitate will lead to platelet aggregation

von Willebrand classification				
Type	FVIII	vWF: Ag	Ristocetin-induced aggregation	Multimer analysis
I	↓	↓-N1	-	Normal distribution, slightly decreased
IIa	N1-↓	N1-↓	↓↓	High molecular weight decreased
IIb	N1-↓	N1-↓	?	High molecular weight decreased
III	↓↓	↓↓	↓↓	All markedly decreased

9.36 Thrombocytopenias

General term for reduced platelet count. Differential depends on age of patient

Most common causes in neonates are infection induced bone marrow suppression (CMV, rubella, toxoplasmosis), NAIT, maternal ITP, and chromosomal abnormalities

In childhood the most common is ITP. Inherited causes should be considered if presentation within first year or if recurrent

In adults the most common causes are ITP, drugs (EtOH, antibiotics, anti-arrhythmics, heparin, thiazides), or hypersplenism (liver disease), but may also be seen in a variety of clinical settings including HIT, TTP, autoimmune disorders (lupus), infections (HIV, Hepatitis), lymphomas, antiphospholipid syndrome, and MDS

Note: It is important to review a peripheral smear to rule out satellitosis, clumping (may occur with EDTA), and large platelets which may be counted as RBCs by mechanical methods

Heparin induced thrombocytopenia (HIT):
A possible side-effect of heparin therapy. Only HIT type II is usually clinically relevant. Arterial thrombosis more common than venous, and bleeding diathesis is usually mild. Arterial thrombosis occurs in extremities (~10%), heart (MI ~4%), and CNS (stroke ~8%); venous thrombosis occurs in extremities (LE - DVT ~50%, UE ~10%), lungs (PE ~25%), and may lead to hemorrhagic adrenal necrosis

	HIT Type I	HIT Type II
Direct cause	Heparin effect	Specific antibody formation against heparin and platelet factor 4 (PF4)
Time to platelet reduction	1-4 days	5-20 days; -If re-exposed to heparin → platelets may drop immediately
Severity of thrombocytopenia	~100,000, not lower than 50% of baseline	30,000-50,000, lower than 50% of baseline
Incidence	5%-10%	Unfractionated heparin: <3% LMW Heparin: <0.5%
Thrombosis	None	About 30%-50% of cases experience clinical thromboembolic event, often subclinical thrombosis
Therapy	Continue heparin therapy	Discontinue heparin immediately; select and initiate an alternative anticoagulant (argatroban, danaparoid, lepirudin) Note: **Coumadin relatively contraindicated,** possible microvascular thrombosis; **platelet transfusion absolute contraindication**
Order blood counts	Before starting heparin therapy, and at least 2 times/week during heparin therapy	

Clinical diagnostic criteria for HIT	
Thrombocytopenia	Decreased platelet count more than 50% compared to highest value from day 5 of heparin therapy and in absence of other cause of thrombocytopenia (eg, major surgery, chemotherapy, sepsis, HELLP syndrome, thromboembolic event)
Thrombosis/ embolism	Evidence of thrombosis or embolism (in about 30% of cases this is seen before platelets significantly decrease)
Skin reaction	Necrosis and inflammation at heparin injection site
Systemic reaction	Acute anaphylactic reaction (<30 min following IV heparin bolus)

Laboratory investigation:

- Platelet count is a simple test for the early detection of HIT II
- HIT-antibody (Ab) only performed in clinical signs/symptoms
- Screening for HIT-Ab in asymptomatic patients without platelet decrease is not useful. Even if positive, there is not necessarily increased risk of complications (subclinical seroconversion)
- Clinically-significant HIT II with corresponding symptoms only manifests in a small proportion of patients with HIT-Ab, thus universal screening is not recommended
- The importance of laboratory detection of HIT-Ab is to confirm the clinical diagnosis
  - If there is clinical suspicion for HIT II, order HIT-Ab prior to subsequent doses of heparin. If positive, and with appropriate clinical picture, an alternative anticoagulant is needed with immediate discontinuation of heparin
  - HIT-Abs are only detectable for several weeks (usually undetectable by 3 months following final Heparin dose)
- The detection of antibodies to the heparin-PF4 complex
  - Does not indicate platelet activation
  - Therefore, confirmation by functional (qualitative) test is needed
- Rarely, there is a failure to detect HIT-Ab with immunological test
  - In cases of high clinical suspicion, but negative immunological tests → discontinuation of heparin with transition to alternative anticoagulant is recommended
  - Performing functional test and repeating immunological test may be helpful. The results can diverge in 10%-20% of cases. Combined testing increases sensitivity

- There is relatively high diagnostic sensitivity of the immunological and functional tests. However, the specificity of the functional test is significantly higher than the immunological test
- Overall, the results of laboratory tests must be assessed with the clinical situation and the pretest probability

Diagnostic confidence following test results	Immunological test	Function test	Platelet change after switching agent
Definite	Positive	Positive	Positive
Probably	Positive	Positive	Negative
	Positive	Negative	Positive
	Negative	Positive	Positive
Likely	Positive	Negative	Negative
	Negative	Positive	Negative
Excluded	Negative	Negative	Negative

Immunological test	Sensitivity	Specificity	Comments
Heparin–PF4 induced-antibody assay (HPIA)	91%–97%	74%–86%	ELISA, a high negative predictive value, low positive predictive value that was positive in 10%-50% of Heparin-exposed patients positive of which only a small proportion clinically manifest HIT → Test only when there is clinical suspicion of HIT II

Functional test	Sensitivity	Specificity	Comments
Serotonin release assay (SRA)	>95%	>95%	Radioimmunoassay - measurement of radioactively-marked serotonin release from test platelets after contact with patients serum
Heparin–induced platelet activation test (HIPA)	<80%	>90%	Measured of platelet activation by aggregation and sedimentation of test platelets after contact with patient's serum and heparin

Evaluation of platelet count during heparin therapy	
Clinical situation	**Frequency of platelet monitoring**
• At the start of heparin therapy with UFH/LMWH • If already started, immediately, or within 100 days	→ Before treatment (Baseline) → Repeat 24 h after the start of therapy
Anaphylactic reaction, thrombosis, acute inflammation, cardiorespiratory, neurological or other unusual symptoms (occuring acutely, <30 min after heparin administration)	→ Immediately
High HIT-II Risk (>1%) • Prophylactic administration of UFH after major surgical/orthopedic surgery • UFH at therapeutic doses	→ Repeat every 2nd day from day 4 to Day 14 (or the end of the Heparin) → Every 1-2 days from day 4 to day 14 (or end of heparin)
Moderate HIT-II Risk (0.1%-1.0%) • UFH to Internal Med/GYN patients • Prophylactic administration of LMWH after major surgical/orthopedic surgery • Post-surgical catheter flushing with UFH • One or more doses of UFH before converting to LMWH	→ At least every 2 days from day 4 to day 14 (or discontinuation of heparin)
Low HIT II Risk (<0.1%) • Prophylactic administration of LMWH in Internal Med/GYN patients • Catheter flushing with UFH, not post-surgery • Prophylactic administration of LMWH for small procedures	→ Before treatment; regular or repeat monitoring not necessary

Immune thrombocytopenic purpura (ITP):
Immune mediated thrombocytopenia; antigen target may be GPIb, GPIIb, GPIIIa, or GPV. Usually diagnosed clinically after other disorders are excluded, though may be confirmed with flow cytometry or ELISA (increased Ab on platelet surface)
Patients are otherwise healthy with only a markedly low platelet count (<30,000)
80% will respond to immunomodulatory medicine (methylprednisolone, IVIG; also best confirmation)
10% will be refractory to treatment
Splenectomy often performed for those refractory to treatment
2/3 have complete response
1/3 will relapse (treat with anti-CD20)
May also use other immunosuppressives (corticosteroids)

Neonatal alloimmune thrombocytopenia (NAIT/NATP):
Immune mediated thrombocytopenia due to anti-PLA1-Ab. 98% of population has PLA1 on their platelets. 80% of cases are due to PLA1 negative mother with PLA1 positive child. **~50% of first pregnancies** are affected, and all subsequent pregnancies. Neonates treated with **irradiated, washed maternal platelets**

Post-transfusion purpura (PTP):
Caused by anti-PLA1-Ab in a PLA1-negative patient given PLA1-positive platelets; Classically female patients ~7 days after transfusion, often with a history of prior transfusion or pregnancy. Patient's **own platelets are also destroyed**, leading to markedly low platelet counts. Usually recover with supportive treatment in several weeks

Thrombotic thrombocytopenic purpura (TTP):
Typically idiopathic disorder resulting in widespread microvascular thrombosis (esp. CNS, GI, kidney) leading to marked thrombocytopenia (<20,000; also **schistocytes** in the blood and **high LDH**); Patients usually fully recover with treatment (daily plasmapheresis + FFP) and rarely relapse. There is a **familial form** (chronic relapsing), as well as some association with **ticlopidine and pregnancy**
Classic Pentad: Thrombocytopenia, microangiopathic hemolytic anemia, neurologic symptoms, renal abnormalities, and fever
Abnormally large multimers of vWF found in circulation due to defective cleavage by protease **ADAMTS-13**
Platelet transfusion is contraindicated!

Hemolytic uremic syndrome (HUS):
Clinically overlaps with TTP (microvascular platelet thrombosis), but limited to the kidney, and occurs after infection with *S. dysenteriase* or *E. coli* O157:H7 due to exposure to Shiga toxin. Rare recurring form associated with complement pathway defect (factor H deficiency). Treatment consists of supportive care and antimicrobials (plasma exchange not helpful)

Other rare causes:

Alloimmune thrombocytopenia: Complication of multiple transfusions (classically seen during chemotherapy), due to anti-HLA-Ab against class I HLA (esp. A and B)

Congenital amegakaryocytic thrombocytopenia (CAMT): Autosomal recessive disorder that often presents in early life; due to a lack of megakaryocytes, hence a markedly low platelet count; mutation in MPL gene that encodes the thrombopoietin receptor; patients may develop full pancytopenia

May-Hegglin anomaly: Autosomal dominant disorder characterized by thrombocytopenia, giant platelets, and Dohle bodies (remnants of rough ER); MYH9 gene mutation, chr 22q; related to Fechtner, Epstein, and Sebastian syndromes, all autosomal dominant giant platelet disorders with mutations involving chr 22q, some also have Alport-like sensorineural hearing loss and kidney issues

Mediterranean macrothrombocytopenia: Considered a benign morphologic variant by some; a mild thrombocytopenia common to Southern Europe; caused by mutation on chr 17 leading to decreased vWF receptor (GPIb/Ix/V)

Quinidine-induced thrombocytopenia: Immune mediated disorder against GPIX

Thrombocytopenia with absent radii syndrome: Extremely rare disorder with unknown cause characterized by thrombocytopenia at birth that progressively improves and a lack of bilateral radius bones

9.37 Hemorrhagic Disease

Typically caused by a disturbance of the hemostatic system, leading to an increased bleeding tendency
Preliminary laboratory tests: PT/INR, aPTT, TT, platelet count (CBC) +/- platelet function analysis and bleeding time

Algorithmic diagnosis of hemorrhagic disease

1. aPTT and/or PT/INR?			
Abnormal		**Normal**	
2. Platelet count?		**2. Platelet count?**	
Normal	**Abnormal**	**Normal**	**Abnormal**
Factor deficiency	Combined factor deficiency and platelet or plasma abnormality	von Willebrand disease, hyperfibrinolysis, FXIII deficiency	Thrombocytopenia

Algorithmic diagnosis of plasma clotting disorders

1. PT/INR?			
<70%		**>70%**	
2. aPTT?		**2. aPTT?**	
Normal	**Abnormal**	**Normal**	**Abnormal**
Analyze: Factor VII	Analyze: • Factor X • Factor V • Factor II • Fibrinogen (I)	Analyze: • HMWK • Prekallikrein • Factors XII, XI, IX, VIII • vWF and activity	Clinically relevant factor deficiency excluded

Algorithmic diagnosis of thrombocytopenia

Confirmation in citrated blood	
Yes	**No**
Thrombocytopenia	**EDTA-induced Pseudothrombocytopenia**
Evaluate: • Exclusion of an underlying disease • Drug history • Differential blood count • Platelet Antibodies • Platelet function • Platelet secretion • Bone marrow histology	• Laboratory phenomenon • No further diagnostic work-up required

9.38   Disseminated Intravascular Coagulation (DIC)

AKA Consumptive coagulopathy:
An acquired coagulopathy based on systemic intravascular activation of the coagulation cascade with **thrombus formation in the microcirculation (small capillaries) and secondary hyperfibrinolysis** resulting in the **consumption of coagulation factors and platelets, hemorrhagic coagulopathy**, and the formation of microthrombi in organs with disturbance of vital functions (eg,- lungs' ARDS, kidney' renal failure)

More common underlying diseases that predispose to DIC:
Sepsis, Trauma (esp. extensive soft tissue injury, craniocerebral trauma, fat or bone marrow embolism), malignancies (esp. leukemia/lymphoma, highly proliferative solid tumors), aortic aneurysm, severe or large hematoma

Rarer underlying diseases that predispose to DIC:
Obstetric complications (placental abruption, amniotic fluid embolism), parasitemia (esp. malaria), hemolytic transfusion reactions, rhabdomyolysis

Typical course and laboratory parameters of DIC		
Parameter	Value	Change
Platelets	<100000	Decreased
aPTT	Extended >1.5x	Prolonged
PT	Suppressed (<40%)	Decreased
Fibrinogen	Absolute (<150 mg/dL)	Decreased
Antithrombin	<50%	Decreased
Factor V activity	<50%	Decreased
D-Dimer/FSPs	Up-trending	Increased
Soluble fibrin monomer (degradation)	Up-trending	Increased

Diagnostic laboratory panel	
Minimalist panel	Full panel
• PT, aPTT and CBC every 2 h • Fibrinogen • Antithrombin • Factor V activity	• PT, aPTT and CBC every 2 h • Fibrinogen • Antithrombin • Factor V activity • D-dimer • Soluble Fibrin

Phases in DIC	
Phase I	Compensated activation of the hematopoietic system triggering disproportionate formation of thrombin resulting in: • Incipient platelet decrease • Fibrinogen concentration increase or borderline normal • Increased activity of factors V and VIII • Consumption of AT and protein C • Increased concentration of activated coagulation products (soluble fibrin, prothrombin fragment, Thrombin-Antithrombin complex) • Shortened clotting times (PT, aPTT, and TT), due to fulminant activation of coagulation • Reduction of the fibrinolytic potential
Phase II	Congestive activation of the hemostatic system/measurable deficit of clotting potential The "consumption" is becoming apparent and concentrations of various coagulants is waning: • Platelet count continues to fall (thrombocytopenia) • Factor V is reduced • Factor VIII can be increased or normal • Fibrinogen normal or reduced • Reduced AT and protein C • Abnormal clotting times (PT decreased, aPTT/INR increased, TT prolonged) • Further increase in concentration of activated coagulation products and fibrinolysis • Soluble fibrin continues to increase

Phases in DIC (cont.)	
Phase III	Full DIC: Usually prevented with modern intervention if recognized in timely manner Severe generalized bleeding tendency associated with irreversible vascular occlusion causing organ damage → high mortality! • Often no measurable fibrinogen (defibrination syndrome) • Clotting times (PT, aPTT, TT) markedly extended (incoagulable due to in vivo defibrination) • Platelets, fibrinogen and factor V greatly reduced • Factor VIII is greatly reduced • For prolonged DIC, liver failure results in decreased production of other factors (particularly those not consumed by the initial DIC coagulopathy, eg, factor X) • Activation products of coagulation are greatly increased • Fibrin (ogen) degradation products greatly increased
Phase IV	Recovery of hemostasis (days to weeks) • First, normalization of acute phase reactant proteins; fibrinogen • Then, concentration of other factors increases • Decreased activated coagulation products and fibrinolysis • Normalization of the clotting times (PT, aPTT, TT) • Finally, normalization of platelet counts

Supportive therapy options (continuously consumed by DIC)	
• FFP (fresh frozen plasma) • Antithrombin • APC (Activated protein C) • Aprotinin	• Platelet transfusion • Fibrinogen • PPSB (Factor IX) • Heparin (reduce thromboembolic events)

Note: Treatment of DIC is generally supportive in nature, and largely relies on treatment of the primary disease or etiology (ie, - sepsis, malignancy).
There is no general treatment recommendation that fits all patient situations. However, treatment should be supportive in nature and based on close monitoring of the patient's clinical and laboratory status. Focus should be directed at treating the primary disease etiology for DIC as this will quell the systemic activation and consumption of coagulation factors

9.39　Thrombophilia

Increased tendency for venous and occasionally arterial thrombus formation

Suspect thrombophilia when/if:
- Patient is young (<45 years)
- Multiple recurrences
- Unusual site
- Multiple spontaneous abortions
- Conspicuous family history
- Paraneoplastic syndromes → exclude neoplasm with any unexplained venous thrombosis!

Types/etiologies of thrombophilia:
- Activated Protein C (APC) resistance (function test)/factor V Leiden mutation (genetic investigation)
- Prothrombin mutation (Factor II, **G20210A** polymorphism)
- AT deficiency
- Protein C deficiency
- Protein S deficiency
- Increase factor VIII
- Anti-phospholipid antibodies (lupus anticoagulants, anti-cardiolipin antibody)
- Homocysteinemia
- Dysfibrinogenemia

Diagnosis of thrombophilia	
First event	**Thrombosis**
• <45 year old 　- Recurrence 　- Atypical localization 　- Positive family history 　- Pregnancy 　- >2 abortions in history	ORDER "Advanced screening" panel: 　- APC resistance/factor V Leiden 　- Prothrombin mutation (**G20210A**) 　- AT 　- Protein C/protein S 　- Factor VIII 　- Anti-phospholipid antibodies
• 45-60 years old	ORDER "Basic screening": 　- APC resistance/factor V Leiden 　- Prothrombin mutation (**G20210A**)
• >60 years old	No need for thrombophilia screening with first event

9.40 Overview of Coagulation Testing

Panel	Δ	Causes of abnormal results
aPTT PT/INR platelet count	↑ NI NI	• Heparin anticoagulation (mild, can have mild TT prolongation) • Dilutional coagulopathy (massive transfusion /bolus) • von Willebrand disease • Antiphospholipid syndrome • Hemophilia A or B • Hemophilia inhibitor • Measurement errors due to high hematocrit (>60%)
aPTT PT/INR platelet count	↑ ↑ NI	• High dose heparin • Abnormal synthesis of prothrombin complexes (Factors X, IX, VII, II) in liver dysfunction, Warfarin therapy, or vitamin K deficiency • Fibrinogen deficiency/hyperfibrinolysis
aPTT PT/INR platelet count	↑ ↑ ↓	• Advanced DIC • Severe dilutional coagulopathy • Chronic liver dysfunction Suspicion of DIC or a dilutional coagulopathy should be considered if there is: • Fibrinogen deficiency (fibrinogen serves not only to plasma coagulation, but also conveys the platelet aggregation); • Prolonged thrombin time as a sign of secondary hyperfibrinolysis
aPTT PT/INR platelet count	↑ NI ↓	• Early DIC • von Willebrand disease type IIb • HIT Type II

Panel (cont.)	Δ	Causes of abnormal results
aPTT PT/INR platelet count	NI NI ↑	• Early DIC • Liver disease, minimal loss of synthetic function • HIT • ITP • TTP • HUS • HELLP syndrome • Displacement thrombocytopenia secondary to bone marrow infiltration or myelofibrosis • Bernard-Soulier syndrome • von Willebrand disease type IIb • Pseudothrombocytopenia by in vitro agglutination
aPTT PT/INR platelet count	NI NI NI	Differential diagnosis of bleeding with normal basic coagulation: • Platelet secretion or aggregation dysfunction • Factor XIII deficiency • von Willebrand disease (mild form without aPTT prolongation) • Overdose with low molecular weight heparin • Local primary cause ("surgical bleeding") In addition, isolated prolonged TT: • Heparin in therapeutic doses • Presence of fibrin products
aPTT PT/INR platelet count	NI ↑ NI	• Warfarin therapy • Vitamin K deficiency • Hepatic dysfunction • Pronounced fibrinogen deficiency or dysfibrinogenemia

aPTT
PT/INR
platelet count
	NI
	↑
	↓
		• Hepatic dysfunction (abnormal synthesis of prothrombin complexes)
		• DIC:
		  – Early stage of increased coagulability
		  – Stage of reactive fibrinolysis and increased coagulability (TT prolonged)
		  – Stage of increased coagulability with simultaneous heparin therapy (TT prolonged)

10 Transfusion Medicine

10.1 Blood Group Systems

ABO-system:

- Single most important blood group based on the presence or absence of **antigens A and B**, chr 9, Karl Landsteiner
- Present on RBCs, endothelial cells, (**all tissues of the body**) and found in soluble form in plasma and other body secretions in people known as secretors
  Three major antigens: A, B, H and two major antibodies: anti-A and anti-B
  Four phenotypes: A, B, AB, O
- H antigen is precursor, chr 19, present on 99.99% of RBCs, detected using *Ulex europeaus*
  Possible genetic combinations: HH, Hh (produce H Ag), or hh (**Bombay phenotype**, exceedingly rare, have Anit-H Ab, require H negative blood)
  Relative concentrations: O>A2>B>A2B>A1>A1B
- A and B genes do not directly produce antigens → produce an enzyme, glycosyltransferase → attaches a sugar molecule to H antigen responsible for specificity
  A: N-acetylgalactosamine
  B: D-Galactose
- O antigen → no transferase → only H antigen
- ABO Antibodies naturally occur in individuals who lack these antigens, **anti-A and anti-B**; IgM, present by 6 months, react at room temp.
  Subgroups A1, A2
  - Antisera specific for A1 (anti-A1 lectin) prepared dolichos biflorus
  - Anti-A → reacts with both A1 and A2
  - **A2 individuals can have Anti- A1**
  Even the **first incompatible transfusion is life-threatening,** leading to acute hemolysis
- Autosomal codominant inheritance of A and B, each are dominant over O
  Note: **"Acquired B"** antigen related to similar antigens on GI flora (E. coli), particularly seen after perforation or with large colon carcinomas leading to decreased integrity of bowel wall. Patient will look like they have B and Anti-B. Transient in nature, and elution (heat, acid) will cause Acquired B to not react

Blood group	Frequency	Subgroups
O (OO)	40%	–
A (AA, AO)	45%	A1: 80% (37% of total) A2: 20% (8% of total)
B (BB, BO)	10%	–
AB	5%	A1B: 80% (4% of total) A2B: 20% (1% of total)

	Group A	Group B	Group AB	Group O
RBC type	A	B	AB	O
Ab in plasma	Anti-B	Anti-A	None	Anti-A, Anti-B
Ag on RBC	A	B	A and B	H

Blood group	RBC antigen: reaction to test serum				Serum testing: agglutination of test RBCs			
	Anti-A	Anti-B	Anti-A1	Anti-H	A1	A2	B	O
O	–	–	–	+	+	+	+	–
A1	+	–	+	–	–	–	+	–
A2	+	–	-/+	+	–	–	+	–
B	–	+	–	–	+	+	–	–
A1B	+	+	+	–	–	–	–	–
A2B	+	+	-/+	+/-	–	–	–	–

Blood group	Compatible RBCs	Compatible FFPs
O	O	O, A, B, AB
A	A, O	A, AB
B	B, O	B, AB
AB	AB, A, B, O	AB

Rhesus system:
- Most complex, highly immunogenic, and significant clinical importance; chr 1
- IgG, reactive at 37°C (warm), enhanced with enzyme treatment
- Fischer and Race-5 antigens: D, C, E, c, e; 3 alleles: D, C/c, E/e
- In Caucasions: D-85%, C-70%, c-80%, E-30%, e-98%

- D is the most immunogenic followed by c, E, C, and e. In contrast to Cc and Ee, there is **no 'd' allele**, though we use that nomenclature for the absence of the D Ag for practical reasons. D is dominant, ie, Rh+ = genotype DD or Dd (Also Wiener- 5 antigens: Rho, Rh', Rh", hr', hr", and Rosenfeld - Rh1-Rh5)
- **Found exclusively on surface of RBCs, requires previous stimulus (transfusion)**
- If possible, always transfuse D compatible blood
- First Rh+ (DD, Dd) blood given to patient Rh- (dd) no reaction, however, second exposure will result in **marked acute hemolytic reaction** (can give Rh- person Rh+ blood one time if life or death situation, but that patient can never get Rh+ blood again causes severe hemolytic reaction). Also, don't give Rh- blood to Rh+ person if possible just to conserve Rh- stores
- **Can cross the placenta**, associated with **hemolytic disease of the newborn** (HDN), can lead to hydrops fetalis, **does not happen with first Rh+ pregnancy**, but will with subsequent ones without prophylaxis
- **Rh prophylaxis:** Pregnant Rh- woman given injection of IgG anti-D (standard dosage 200-300 mg) at ~28 wks of all gestations and after birth if Rh+ newborn
- Theory: Any D Ag that crosses the placenta into the mother's bloodstream will get bound by the Anti-D before the mother's immune system can react
- **Weak D (D^u):** weak or absent red cell agglutination by anti-D → detected only with use of anti-human globulin reagent (performed on all Rh- samples). Caused by 1 of 3 situations:
  - Less D antigen (quantitative)
  - Trans location to C Ag - Cepelli effect
  - Epitope missing - partial D (can produce Anti-D)

Partial D (variants): qualitative, modified D-antigen epitopes, freq ~0.04%. Patient may 'look' Rh+ but **can still have Anti D** if exposed to 'normal' D-Ag. Therefore, treat this patient as:
Donor: D-positive, Receiver: D-negative
Rh Null: Very rare disorder resulting from lack of all Rh antigens; leads to stomatocytosis, spherocytosis, ↑RBC K$^+$ permeability; must transfuse with Rh null blood

Weiner gene	Fischer antigen	Weiner gene	Fischer antigen	Frequencies
R^0	Dce	r	dce	Caucasians
R^1	DCe	r'	dCe	$R^1 > r > R^2 > R^0$
R^2	DcE	r"	dcE	African Americans
R^z	DCE	r^y	dCE	$R^0 > r > R^1 > R^2$

Approximate frequencies in United States					
Haplotype	Gene combo	Caucasian	African American	Native Americans	Asians
R^1	DCe	42%	17%	44%	70%
r	dce	37%	26%	11%	3%
R^2	DcE	14%	11%	34%	21%
R^0	Dce	4%	44%	2%	3%
r'	dCe	2%	2%	2%	2%
r"	dcE	1%	0	6%	0
R^z	DCE	0	0	6%	1%
r^y	dCE	0	0	0	0

	Caucasian	African American	Hispanic	Asian
O^+	37%	47%	42%	42%
O^-	8%	4%	4%	1%
A^+	33%	24%	29%	27%
A^-	7%	2%	2%	0.5%
B^+	9%	18%	9%	25%
B^-	2%	1%	1%	<1%
AB^+	3%	4%	2%	7%
AB^-	1%	<1%	<1%	<1%

Kell: Peptides found within the Kell protein (chr 7, CD238), a transmembrane zinc-dependent endopeptidase which cleaves endothelin-3; ~ 20 alleles (so-called para-Kell), the 2 main Ag: **K (Kell, K1)** and **k (Cellano, K2)**. All are codominant. Clinically K (Kell, K1) is the most important Kell antigen due to **Anti-K** immunogenicity, negated by enzymes (ZZAP, DTT). KK or Kk corresponds to Kell+ (~8% of Caucasian population), kk is Kell- (~92% of Caucasian population)

kk 92%, Kell negative:
Given the relative low prevalence of K, donor and recipient are usually compatible, aided by the fact that (like Rh) no response will occur with the first exposure (transfusion/pregnancy), however, subsequent exposures will lead to marked hemolysis. The relatively high antigenicity of K means that Kell+ preparations should NOT be given to Kell-recipients in order to avoid immunization
Note: KK individuals may have Anti-k (Cellano) antibodies, fortunately this represents <1% of the population

Kk >7%, Kell positive (heterozygous):
The heterozygous patient is considered Kell+ and may receive Kell-transfusions without risk. However, care must be taken to not give a Kell+ patient Kell-negative product (eg, FFP) that has Anti-K (Kell)
Note: The same risk of Anti-k Ab is present (see above) if given to KK individuals

KK <1%, Kell positive (homozygous):
Homozygous Kell+ patients should ideally only receive KK blood products to avoid Anti-k antibody formation; however, as these are normally not available, **heterozygous Kell+** products are preferred to reduce immunogenicity (decreased density of k-Cellano Ag)
Homozygous Kell-positive patients who have **already developed Anti-k (Cellano) Ab must receive homozygous Kell-positive blood products**. Given the extremely rare nature of KK, this is usually difficult and direct consultation with Transfusion Medicine is required. And as with Kk patients, care must be taken to not administer products that contain Anti-K (Kell)

Anti-K:
IgG, warm reacting, does not bind complement → extravascular hemolysis. The most frequent Ab after ABO and Rh, however, still rarely causes clinical issues and hemolysis is often mild. May cause HDN

Anti-k (Cellano):
Very rare due to the low prevalence of homozygous KK (<1%).
In the presence of Anti-k (Cellano), regional and possibly national cooperation must occur using specially frozen KK RBCs, or alternatively KK blood relatives, or autologous donation for planned procedures

McLeod syndrome:
Lack of kx (Mcleod gene) on X-chromosome; required for proper synthesis/presentation of Kell antigens; defect leads to poor clinical detection of Kell

Other systems:

Other warm-reacting antibodies that may be clinically significant (hemolysis, HDN)

Kidd:
- Jk^a and Jk^b: not very antigenic and are dosage dependent, 20-30% Caucasians Jk(a-), Jk(b-); 10-20% Blacks Jh(a-), 50-60% Jh(b-); enhanced by enzymes
- Note: Kidd is notorious for 'fading' with time, ie, a person who is exposed will make anti-Kidd, but over time it will become undetectable clinically, however, marked hemolytic reactions may occur with a new exposure (must make sure patients understand that they must ALWAYS tell clinicians they have anti-Kidd before they get transfusions)

Duffy: Fy^a and Fy^b, Fy^{a-b}- very rare in Caucasians, but present in 68% of African Americans (Duffy is receptor for plasmodium vivax infection, lack thereof provides resistance to malaria)

MNS: S, s and U, acquired IgG

Also: Lewis (Le^a and Le^b, IgM, 'shed' off RBC, usually clinically insignificant), Lutheran (Lu), P, BG and many others

10.2   Transfusion Medicine Testing

Type and screen: Patients blood is tested for ABO and Rh type and general screen is performed looking for RBC antibodies that formed during prior exposure (eg, pregnancy, transfusions), Coombs test, LISS

Type and cross (match): Patients blood is tested for ABO and Rh type, screened, and tested against samples from specific units of blood which then 'belong' to that patient. **Reserved for that specific patient and may be discarded if not used, so do not order lightly**

Cross-match (serological compatibility testing):

Serological testing between donor's RBCs and recipient's serum to ensure compatibility

Major cross-match:

- **Legally required before a blood transfusion** (except in emergency situations, see below)
- Ensures no transfusion reaction, especially important for irregular antibodies that are not routinely tested
- Incompatibility expressed by RBC agglutination in the test tube (Immediate Spin)
  - May be sole cross-match if screening negative; or may be done electronically)
- Particularly important if the recipient had a positive indirect Coombs test (ICT), meaning they have known antibodies

Minor cross-match:

Recipient red cells are tested against donor serum to detect donor antibodies directed against a patient's antigens. No longer routinely performed: the small amount of donor serum in a unit of RBCs will be diluted when transfused into the recipient

Emergency:

- Complete cross-match takes ~1 h, therefore, not always performed in emergency situations (ERs, Trauma, etc)
- Type-specific, uncross-matched blood can be requested. ABO/Rh compatible; less risk of serious transfusion reactions. Usually the lifesaving measure is more beneficial than the risk of an antibody mediated transfusion reaction
- Type O- blood often given when the recipient's blood group is unknown. However, blood grouping can be done quickly and easily (2-3 min) with appropriate reagents and trained staff

Immediate spin: (Performed bedside)

The recipient's serum is tested with the donor RBCs immediately before blood transfusion. Positive test will show agglutination

  - Ensures correct patient/unit correlation (prevents human/clerical errors)
  - Ensures the cross-match testing was correct, no suspected antibody-antigen reactions
  - **Mandatory minimum** crossmatch of all patients, should be performed even in emergency situations, if at all possible

- Always be performed by the medical staff actually doing the transfusion
- Always performed directly at the bedside (not in the ward, etc.)
- Immediately before transfusion
- Repeated for each new donor unit
- Document in patient's medical record

Antibody screening testing:

- Detects clinically relevant allo- and autoantibodies (present in ~2.5% of population) against RBCs at Room temp (cold, IgM), 37°C/LISS, and with Anti-Human Globulin (AHG)
- Patient's serum is incubated with several Type-O RBCs (2-3) that have been extensively antigen typed. FDA mandates antigens present must include: C, D, E, c, d, M, N, S, s, P1, Le^a, Le^b, K, k, Fy^a, Fy^b, Jk^a, Jk^b; not required, but generally performed: homozygosity for C, D, E, c, e, Fy^a, Jk^a
- Could not possibly cover all low-frequency antibodies, hence the need for cross-match
- **Low ionic strength solutions** (LISS, 0.2% NaCl) increases the attraction between positively charged IgG molecules and negatively charged RBCs, allowing shorter incubation time. In addition, **polyethylene glycol (PEG)** is a macromolecule additive that promotes antibody cross-linking further enhancing agglutination
- May include the addition of enzymes (papain, trypsin, bromelin) to affect immunogenicity, this can be helpful during identification, especially if several antigens are present

Enhanced by enzymes:

- RBCs have negative charge causing natural repulsion, enzyme modification reduces net charge facilitating agglutination by IgG
- ABO, Rh, P1, Kidd, I, Lewis

Inactivated by enzymes:

- Duffy, MNS
- In case of a positive reaction with one of the test cells, determination of the specific antibody ensues

- Validity of the screen is only 3 days (ie, **must be performed within 3 days of the scheduled transfusion**) if any of the following conditions exist:
  - Patient has been transfused in the last 3 months
  - Patient has been pregnant in the last 3 months
  - Patient's history is uncertain
  - Rare low frequency antibodies may not be detected; hence the screening test is not a **replacement for cross-match**

Screening Cells (Type O)	IS	37°C/LISS	AHG	CC
Cell 1	R	R	R	R
Cell 2	R	0	0	R
Cell 3	R	0	0	R
Auto	R	0	0	R

IS: Immediate Spin: Room temperature, detects 'cold' antibodies (IgM), usually not clinically important
37°C/LISS: Low ionic strength solution: Detects 'warm' antibodies (IgG)
AHG: Anti-human globulin: indirect antiglobulin test, ensures no IgG antibody binding
CC: Coombs control cells: Added to be sure the AHG works
Auto: Patient's own RBCs, if reactive may mean autoantibody/cold agglutinin present; **R:** Reactive: Agglutination occurred, antibody present

Antibody differentiation:
- If screening is positive, use of panels with 10 test cells to identify specific antibody(ies), basically, a more in-depth screening test, same procedure
- Incubation of patient's serum with the test RBCs, then compare the reaction pattern with the known antigenicity of the cells
- Reaction at 37°C/LISS or AHG must be considered clinically relevant
- A true allo-antibody if the patient lacks the corresponding antigen, hence the need to also run the patient's RBCs
- Detection of irregular immune antibody(ies) requires **education of the patient**, and documentation in the medical chart and on a blood group card which the patient can keep (in their wallet/purse)
- The patient may **only receive RBCs negative for that antibody(ies)** or risk a transfusion reaction

General rules:
- Rule out antigens: cross out antigens that did not react
  Note: Do not cross out heterozygous antigens that show dosage (E, e, MNS, Duffy (Fy), Kidd (Jk))
- Circle the antigens that are not crossed out
  The rule of three must be met to confirm antibody (p ≤5%)
  MUST be:
  - Positive with 3 cells with the antigen
  - Negative with 3 cells without the antigen
  - Not always positive with low frequency antigens (E, K)
- Consider antibody's usual reactivity (warm, cold)
- Look for a matching pattern
  Pay attention to reaction strength (1+, 2+, 3+), variation may allude to dosage or multiple antibodies

Reaction across the board may indicate anti-k or another high frequency antigen. Auto-control positive indicates autoantibody

Cell	D	C	E	c	e	f	M	N	S	s	P1	Le^a	Le^b	K	k	Fy^a	Fy^b	Jk^a	Jk^b	IS	37	AHG
1	0	+	0	+	+	+	+	+	+	+	+	+	0	0	+	+	+	+	0	R	-	-
2	+	+	0	0	+	0	+	0	+	0	+	0	+	0	+	0	+	0	+	-	-	-
3	+	+	0	0	0	0	+	0	+	0	+	0	+	+	+	+	0	+	0	R	-	-
4	+	0	+	+	0	+	+	+	0	+	+	0	0	0	+	0	+	+	+	R	-	-
5	0	0	+	+	+	0	+	0	+	0	+	0	+	0	+	0	+	+	+	-	-	-
6	0	0	0	+	+	+	+	0	0	+	0	+	0	+	0	+	0	+	0	-	-	-
7	0	0	0	+	+	+	+	+	0	+	+	0	+	0	+	0	0	0	+	R	-	-
8	0	0	0	+	+	+	+	0	+	0	+	0	+	0	+	0	0	+	0	-	-	-
9	0	0	0	+	+	+	0	+	0	+	0	0	+	0	+	+	+	+	+	R	-	-
10	0	0	0	+	+	+	0	0	+	0	0	+	0	+	0	+	0	+	0	-	-	-
Auto																				-	-	-

IS: Immediate Spin; **37: 37°C/LISS:** low ionic strength solution; **AHG:** Anti-human globulin, Indirect Coombs test
+: Antigen is present on that cell; **0:** Antigen is absent; **R:** The patient reacted, ie, the patient has an antibody to 1+ of those antigens
This case is Lea. All of the R's match up with this antigen, and it is cold reacting, so that also correlates

Direct antiglobulin test (DAT):
AKA Direct coombs test (DCT). In certain conditions in vivo IgG may bind to antigens on the RBC surface and their circulating RBCs will be coated with these allo-/auto-antibodies; most commonly **autoimmune hemolytic anemia**
Detection of antibody/complement proteins on the RBC membrane
Patient RBCs are washed (removing plasma) and then incubated with rabbit serum containing anti-human immunoglobulin (Coombs Reagent)
If antibodies are present, agglutination occurs → Positive

Indirect antiglobulin test (IAT):
AKA Indirect coombs test (ICT). Used in **prenatal testing and prior to blood transfusion**
Detection of unbound antibody present in patient's serum
Patient serum is incubated with washed RBCs of known antigenicity
The RBC's are washed again and unbound antibody is removed
Then, similar to DAT, anti-human antiglobulin (Coombs reagent) is added
If antibodies are now present on the RBCs, agglutination occurs → Positive

10.3 Transfusion Planning Timeline

Planned transfusion:
- Need 2 tubes of 10 mL of blood for: **blood grouping, antibody screen, cross-match**
- If irregular antibodies are detected (positive screen), then differentiation and finding compatible units may take several hours to days (if extremely rare)
- Request as early as possible!

Non-planned transfusions:
- In emergency situations in which there is no/minimal time for full work-up, do perform whatever you have the time for:
  - **Be sure to obtain 10-20 mL of blood prior to transfusion** for later blood typing and compatibility testing
- Only perform transfusions without proper testing when vitally indicated!

Time limit	Determination of	Supply with
>60 min	• ABO-blood grouping including serum ABO antibody • RhD typing • Cross-match and antibody screen	• Cross-matched ABO, Rh, and antibody identical RBCs • ABO identical FFP
45 min	• ABO-blood grouping including serum ABO antibody screen • RhD typing • Cross-match • Immediately start antibody screen	• Cross-matched ABO, Rh, and antibody identical RBCs • ABO identical FFP
30 min	• ABO-blood grouping including serum ABO antibody screen • RhD typing • Quick Cross-match (IS, LISS, IAT) • Immediately start antibody screen	• Quick cross-matched ABO and Rh identical RBCs • ABO identical FFP
10 min	• ABO-blood grouping including serum ABO antibody screen • RhD typing • Cross-match at bedside (IS) • Immediately start full crossmatch and antibody screen	• Un-cross-matched ABO and Rh identical blood (IS only) • ABO identical FFP
Immediately	For example, aortic aneurysm, trauma, massive acute GI bleed, etc.	

Basic approach to emergency transfusion	
Known blood group	• Uncross-matched ABO and Rh identical RBCs and ABO identical FFP • Immediately start cross-match and antibody screen
Unknown blood group	• Uncross-matched Type O Rh-negative RBCs and Type AB FFP (if available and absolutely necessary, or alternatively Type A*) • Immediately perform blood group testing and transfuse additional units with uncross-matched ABO and Rh identical RBCs and ABP identical FFP • Immediately start cross-match and antibody screen
General	**Immediate Spin: always perform bedside, regardless of the urgency!** • If ABO/Rh identical RBCs and/or ABO identical FFP unavailable, can use ABO/RH compatible products • Accurate labeling of samples and ensuring patient identity is essential! • Cross-match is only valid for 3 days, then must re-perform(also applies to already issued products that have not been transfused)

FFP: Fresh frozen plasma; IS: Immediate spin; LISS: Low ionic strength solution; IAT: Indirect antiglobulin test; *Will have Anti-B: ~12% of population have Type B blood (~20% of African Americans, ~25% of Asians); Type AB FFP is rare

11 Water and Electrolytes

11.1 Disorders of Water Balance

- As a result of changes in extracellular fluid volume: Hypovolemia, hypervolemia
- As a result of changes in osmolarity: Hypotonic, isotonic, hypertonic

11.2 Extracellular Space

- Interstitial space
- Intravascular space
- 'Third'-space (pleural, pericardial, and peritoneal fluids)

11.3 Intracellular Space

- Significantly different ion concentration compared to extracellular space
- Predominantly potassium, magnesium, phosphate, and intracellular proteins

11.4 Oncotic Pressure

AKA **Colloid osmotic pressure**
Reflects on the content and concentration of macromolecules, in particular, plasma proteins. In biological systems, the oncotic pressure is affected by the size of colloid particles such as proteins. Varies between plasma (25 mmHg) and interstitial space (2 mmHg)
Norm: In a supine individual, the plasma oncotic pressure should vary by ± 2 mmHg

11.5 Volume Status Evaluation

- Total protein concentration
- Hematocrit (red blood cell count)

11.6 Hypervolemia

Excessive total body volume, usually resulting in edema
- **Hypertonic:** Increased sodium compared to water (iatrogenic infusion of hypertonic saline or sodium bicarbonate solution; seawater ingestion)
- **Isotonic:** Equal proportion of sodium and water (excessive infusion of isotonic saline, decompensated congestive heart failure with edema, cirrhosis, nephrotic syndrome, impaired urinary sodium excretion)

- **Hypotonic:** "Water intoxication"; excess fluid with low percentage of sodium (infusion of sodium free solutions, such as pure water or decrease in water excretion [inadequate ADH secretion])

11.7   Euvolemic and Isotonic

Healthy individuals: Normal amount of fluid with a normal proportion of sodium

11.8   Hypovolemia/Dehydration

Decreased fluid volume leading to decreased skin turgor, oliguria, and orthostasis
- **Hypertonic:** Loss of water greater than loss of sodium, ie, volume depletion with an increased proportion of sodium (dehydration, fever, osmotic diuresis, diabetes insipidus)
- **Isotonic:** Water and sodium loss at equal proportions (extensive burns, hemorrhage, diarrhea, vomiting, adrenal insufficiency)
- **Hypotonic:** Loss of sodium is greater than loss of water, ie, volume depletion with a decreased proportion of sodium (diuretics, adrenal insufficiency)

11.9   Osmolarity

- Moles of solute/volume of total solution
- Usually expressed as mol/L or mmol/L

(Grams of solute x molar mass of solute)/liters of total solution

11.10   Osmolality

- Moles of solute/weight of solvent (in biological entities, solvent is water)
- Usually expressed as mol/kg or mmol/kg
- **Norm:** 285-295 mmol/kg

(Grams of solute x molar mass of solute)/kg of solvent

Note: Osmolarity is affected by changes in volume, temperature and pressure, whereas osmolality is not affected by temperature and pressure. Typically the osmolarity is slightly lower than osmolality because the total solvent weight excludes the weight of any dissolved solutes, whereas the total volume includes the solutes. However below ~500 mM, the difference is negligible and they are approximately equal

11.11 Increased Serum Osmolality

- Almost always secondary to hypernatremia
- Occasionally caused by an increase in glucose, urea or other small, osmotically active particle such as ethanol

11.12 Osmotic Gap

- The difference between actual versus expected osmolality with a given osmolar concentration of a solution; ie, the difference between the measured osmolality and the calculated osmolality
- Calculation of the osmotic gap is important for detection and monitoring of poisoning by various organic compounds (including ethanol, methanol, ethylene glycol, isopropanol, and dichloromethane). Because calculation of the osmotic gap does not include these compounds, poisoned individuals will have a greater difference in the expected versus the actual osmotic plasma concentrations
  $\uparrow$: Lactic acidosis; ketoacidosis; renal acidosis; alcohol poisoning; hemorrhagic shock

$$\text{Plasma osmolarity} = 2[Na^+] + [Glucose]/18 + [BUN]/2.8$$

Note: K^+ concentration is so proportionally low, not used in calculation

11.13 Anion Gap

Important for distinguishing the types of metabolic acidosis
Calculated from the concentration difference of sodium, chloride, and bicarbonate ions:

$$\text{Anion gap} = Na^+ \text{[mmol/L]} - (Cl^- \text{[mmol/L]} + HCO_3^- \text{[mmol/L]})$$

Norm: 8–16 mmol/L

$\uparrow$: Consumption of bicarbonate by increased serum anions (organic acids: lactate, ketone bodies)

Metabolic acidosis with normal anion gap: Loss of bicarbonate (due to a primary metabolic acidosis, primary respiratory acidosis with metabolic acidosis/alkalosis, bicarbonate excretors, or retention of chloride)

11.14 Sodium (Na$^+$)

- Body distribution: 98% extracellular, 2% intracellular. The extracellular concentration is at least 15-fold higher than intracellular concentration

Serum sodium concentration:
- Indirect measurement of free water content and the body's osmoregulation capacities
- Helps assess the total volume of extracellular spaces
- Does not provide information about total body sodium content

Ind:
- Disorders of fluid and electrolyte balance
- Imbalances with other serum electrolytes
- Acid-base disorders
- Renal failure
- Hypertension

Norm:
135-145 mmol/L	Adults (serum, plasma)
130-145 mmol/L	Children (serum, plasma)
40-300 mmol/day	Urine

↑:
- **Dehydration:** Hypernatremic hypovolemia
  - Decreased fluid intake and increased fluid loss: secondary to fever and diarrhea
  - Nephrogenic diabetes insipidus: ADH resistance, chronic pyelonephritis, renal cysts, nephrocalcinosis
  - Central diabetes insipidus: ADH deficiency, traumatic brain injury
- **Hyperhydration:** Hypernatremia with fluid overload due to excessive salt intake (iatrogenic, seawater intoxication), primary hyperaldosteronism (Conn's syndrome)

↓:
- **Pseudohypernatremia:** Euvolemia: suppression of plasma water excretion by high concentrations of plasma proteins and lipoproteins (hyperlipoproteinemia, hyperproteinemia) such as multiple myeloma and Waldenström gammaglobulinemia.
- **Hyperhydration:** Hyponatremia with hypervolemia: acute and chronic renal failure, congestive heart failure, acute myocardial infarction
- **Euvolemic hyponatremia:** SIADH, cerebral hemorrhage, meningitis, encephalitis, malignancy, tuberculosis, pneumonia
- **Dehydration:** hyponatremia with hypovolemia: vomiting, diarrhea, ileus, interstitial nephritis, mineralocorticoid deficiency (Addison's disease), diuretic therapy

Mat: Serum/plasma
Met: Flame-emission spectrophotometry, ion-selective electrode

↓ Na^+

Clinical symptoms:

The clinical symptoms of hyponatremia depend on the extent and rate of sodium wasting. Acute hyponatremia can result in a rapid increase in extracellular volume and may lead to cerebral edema. However, brain cells are able to release osmotically active substances such as potassium and calcium, limiting the degree of damage to the CNS with a sudden drop in sodium levels.
Patients may present with headache, lethargy, muscle cramps, seizures, neuropsychiatric symptoms such as disorientation and hallucinations, pyramidal symptoms, papilledema, and coma.

Treatment:

Treatment depends on the clinical symptoms of volume status
- Acute water intoxication without neurological or psychiatric symptoms, infuse 3%–5% (hypertonic) NaCl solution. Untreated patients may have up to 50% mortality rate
- Acute hyponatremia with normal extracellular volume: infuse 3%–5% (hypertonic) NaCl solution. The concurrent administration of loop diuretics is recommended because the shift in fluid from the intracellular to extracellular space can lead to a significant extracellular volume increase and provocation of underlying heart failure
- Hypervolemic hyponatremia: difficult to manage because most diuretics worsen the existing hyponatremia. Sodium infusion is contraindicated due to hypervolemia. However, increasing diuresis with a combination of furosemide (loop diuretic) and acetazolamide (promoter of bicarbonate excretion) is a possibility. Dialysis is the last resort solution

↑ Na^+

Clinical symptoms:

Patients may present with irritability, lethargy, seizures, neuropsychiatric symptoms, and coma. The severity of symptomatic hypernatremia correlates with the rate of sodium increase. Rapid increases in sodium concentration may lead to shrinkage of brain tissue, causing blood vessel laceration, meningeal bleeds (presenting with xanthochromasia upon analysis of CSF)

Treatment:

- Hypovolemic hypernatremia: Infuse with isotonic saline
- Hypervolemic hypernatremia: Avoid any saline intake. Treat with diuretics and D5W (5% glucose in water), taking caution not to decrease serum sodium concentration faster than 2 mmol/h

11.15 Potassium (K⁺)

- Potassium is present predominantly in ionized form
- The intracellular concentration is 40-fold higher than the extracellular concentration
- The concentration gradient is maintained by the Na/K-ATPase pump of the cell membrane
- Regulation of potassium homeostasis is established by the kidney, intestines, and protein/carbohydrate metabolism

Ind:
- Acute and chronic renal failure
- Acid-base disorders
- Ingestion of laxatives and diuretics
- Diabetes mellitus, insulin therapy
- Arrhythmia
- Hypertension

Norm: Serum: 3.6-5.2 mmol/L
Urine: 15-80 mmol/day

↑:
- Altered body distribution: Acidosis, diabetes mellitus, hemolysis, hyperkalemic periodic paralysis
- Increased total body potassium: Acute and chronic renal failure, hypoaldosteronism (isolated, Addison's disease), potassium-sparing diuretics (spironolactone)

↓:
- Altered body distribution: Alkalosis, insulin, catecholamines, hypokalemic periodic paralysis
- Decreased total body potassium:
  - Renal loss - hyperaldosteronism, diuretic use, renal tubular acidosis
  - Gastrointestinal loss - acute and chronic diarrhea, vomiting, gastric lavage, laxative abuse

Mat: Serum/plasma, urine

Met: Flame-emission spectrophotometry, ion-selective electrode

↓ K⁺

Clinical symptoms:

Patients present with tachycardia, extra-systoles, decreased reflexes, lethargy/paralysis, constipation (due to paralytic ileus), ECG abnormalities (ST segment depression, flat T waves, U waves). Patients on digitalis may experience these symptoms if they develop digitalis hypersensitivity

Treatment:

- Potassium-rich diet (bananas, fruit juices, dried fruit)
- Tablets (KCl), 1 tablet = 40 mmol. KCl tablet restores normal function with no significant risk of overdose, in the presence of normal renal function. Take with food along with adequate fluids
- In patients with gastrointestinal ulcers and/or malabsorption, KCl can be administered parenterally. Not to exceed 20 mmol/h. Administering at a rate greater than 40 mmol/h can lead to venous toxicity and potential cardiac arrhythmias

↑ K⁺

Clinical symptoms:

Patients present with cardiac manifestations including bradycardia, ECG disturbances showing conduction abnormalities (high T wave, AV blocks, bundle branch blocks, QRS abnormalities, QT interval shortening), asystole and ventricular fibrillation (in severe cases). Patients with Kussmaul respiration (metabolic acidosis) are already severe at presentation with a poor prognosis (absence of Kussmaul respirations is not a reliable clinical indicator of mild hyperkalemia)

Treatment:

- Insulin infusions with concurrent administration of glucose (eg, 500 mL 10% glucose solution with 10–20 IU of insulin for 1 h)
- Loop diuretics to promote forced diuresis
- Dialysis (in severe cases)

11.16 Chloride (Cl⁻)

- An anion present ~88% extracellular and ~12% intracellular
- Like bicarbonate (HCO_3^-), it serves to balance extracellular cations (Na^+ and K^+)
- Parietal cells of the gastric mucosa and sweat glands have a high chloride content
- Renal chloride excretion is largely influenced by dietary salt intake (NaCl)
- Shifts in Na^+ and Cl^- are often concomitant, whereas changes in Cl^- and HCO_3^- are not
- Most cases of hyperchloremia and hypochloremia are secondary changes associated with water and sodium balance

Ind:
- Acid-base imbalance
- Electrolyte imbalance
- Classification of metabolic acidosis
- Calculation of the anion gap

Norm: Serum: 95–110 mmol/L
Urine: 40–225 mmol/day

↑:
- Prolonged dehydration
- Diarrhea
- Bicarbonate losses leading to Cl^- increase (compensating for the loss of negative charge in serum)
- Renal tubular acidosis; chronic interstitial nephritis
- Use of carbonic anhydrase inhibitors
- Corticosteroids
- Chronic hyperventilation (respiratory alkalosis), eg, adjusting at high altitudes

↓:
- Heavy sweating
- Gastrointestinal losses (vomiting, diarrhea)
- Diuretics (ethacrynic acid, furosemide)
- Mineralocorticoid excess
- Excessive alkali substance intake
- Lactic acidosis and diabetic ketoacidosis
- Renal failure
- Respiratory insufficiency (chronic hypoventilation/hypercapnia)
- Selenium intoxication: can result in severe hypochloremia

Mat: Serum/plasma, urine

Met: Ion selective electrode volumetric titration, enzymatic metric complex

↓ Cl⁻ and ↑ Cl⁻

Changes in serum chloride concentrations usually parallel changes in sodium concentrations. Isolated deviations from the normal serum chloride concentration may be found in acid-base disturbances

Therapy in chloride deficient alkalosis:
Infuse isotonic 0.9% NaCl solution. Increase the RAAS activity to promote more sodium reabsorption; chloride will follow. Promote urinary excretion of bicarbonate to allow more chloride to balance out the negative charge in the serum

11.17 Calcium (Ca^{2+})

- 99% of total body calcium (approximately 1 kg) is stored in the skeleton; Extracellular Ca^{2+} varies dynamically with bone metabolism (osteoblastic and osteoclastic activities)
- Of serum Ca^{2+}, 50% is free, 35% is protein bound (mainly albumin); and 15% is ionically bound to anions such as bicarbonate and lactate
- The biologically active free fraction is most important in calcium homeostasis
- The degree of protein binding depends on the protein concentration and pH (protons displace binding site) → Acidosis leads to increased free Ca^{2+}; alkalosis leads to decreased free Ca^{2+}
- Regulated by PTH and vitamin D

Ind: Total calcium:
- Osteoporosis screening after 50 years of age
- Differential diagnoses of tetanic syndromes
- Differential diagnoses of spontaneous fractures, bone pain
- Nephrolithiasis
- Neuromuscular diseases

Ionized calcium: Acidosis, alkalosis, dysproteinemia, massive transfusion. Ionized calcium is a more sensitive measure than total calcium; sensitivity is 2-3 times higher for the aid of malignancy detection. However, ionized calcium is not available for testing at every laboratory

Norm: Total   Serum, Adults: 9.0-10.2 mg/dL
                       Serum, Children: 9.5-10.5 mg/dL
                       Urine: 20-300 mg/day
             Ionized   Serum, Adults: 4.7-5.3 mg/dL
                       Serum, Children: 4.9-5.5 mg/dL

↓:
- Hypoalbuminemia: cirrhosis, nephrotic syndrome
- Vitamin D deficiency: rickets, malabsorption (eg, gluten sensitive enteropathy), malnutrition
- Parathyroid hormone deficiency: hypoparathyroidism
- Kidney disease: renal failure (secondary hyperparathyroidism, renal tubular acidosis [bone loss])
- Other: Pseudohypoparathyroidism, osteoblastic metastases, acute pancreatitis, glucocorticoid excess, medications (loop diuretics, laxatives, anti-epileptics), plasmapheresis

Mat: Total calcium: serum/plasma; Ionized calcium: heparinized whole blood or plasma; urine

Met: Total calcium: photometry; Ionized calcium: ion-selective electrode

↓ Ca^{2+}

Clinical symptoms:

Patients may present with tetany, seizures (with retained consciousness), paresthesias, hand spasms, laryngospasm, hyperreflexia with Chvostek Sign (percussion of the facial nerve in cheek results in twitching of the mouth) and Trousseau signs (after applying a blood pressure cuff with the mean arterial pressure, producing spasms of the hand and forearm). QT-segment prolongation

Treatment:

- Acute (tetany): IV calcium; intubate patients with respiratory compromise
- Long-term therapy: Supplementation and vitamin D

↑ Ca^{2+}

Clinical symptoms:

Patients are often asymptomatic, but may present with nephrolithiasis, nephrocalcinosis, nausea, constipation, polydipsia, and polyuria. Hypercalcemic crisis can lead to fever, psychosis, confusion, somnolence/coma, arrhythmia, adynamia, and muscle weakness secondary to pseudoparalysis. QT-shortening

Treatment:

- Forced diuresis (5 L/day with normal saline solution, along with furosemide to prevent overload. Potassium supplementation is optional on a case-by-case basis)
- Cease calcium intake (watch for use of cardiac glycosides and thiazide diuretics)
- Bisphosphonates: treating tumor-induced hypercalcemia by inhibiting osteoclastic activity. Glucocorticoids, vitamin D antagonists
- Dialysis for emergent and persistently refractory cases

11.18 Phosphate (PO_4^{3-})

- Present in bones and teeth (85%), intracellular (14%), and extracellular space (1%)
- High-energy phosphates (eg, ATP) provide energy for metabolic reactions
- Also acts as a buffer in blood and urine
- Calcium and phosphate share common pathophysiological mechanisms. Levels are closely linked

Ind:
- Concomitant study to assess calcium metabolism
- Renal tubular defects with impaired phosphate resorption
- Vitamin D metabolism (Vitamin D resistance and rickets)
- Parenteral nutrition, chronic alcoholism
- Dialysis patients

Norm: Serum: 2.4–4.2 mg/dL
Urine: 0.4–1.4 g/day

↑: Chronic renal failure, hypoparathyroidism, pseudohypoparathyroidism, acromegaly

↓: Primary hyperparathyroidism, phosphate-binding antacid therapy, secondary hyperparathyroidism: hypocalcemia, vitamin D deficiency, malabsorption syndrome (vitamin D, calcium), rickets

Mat: Serum/plasma (fasting, process within 1 h of collection, to prevent spuriously elevated results from lysis of RBCs); urine

Met: Ascorbate is reduced to molybdenum blue by ammonium phosphate complex. The intensity of the resulting blue color is determined photometrically

↑ PO_4^{3-}

Clinical symptoms:

Patients may present with muscle weakness and pain. In severe cases may lead to respiratory failure. CNS symptoms such as disorientation, confusion, convulsions, and coma may be present in severe cases. Hematologic problems such as hemolytic anemia and dysfunctional neutrophils can also occur

Treatment:

- Mild hypophosphatemia with phosphate levels above 0.5 mmol/L do not require treatment
- Severe (even asymptomatic) hypophosphatemia should receive phosphate replacement
- Oral therapy is preferred over IV due to the risk of acute hypocalcemia.
- Tubular dysfunction involving phosphate transport: vitamin D supplementation is required

$\uparrow PO_4^{3-}$

Clinical symptoms:

Patients may present with calcium wasting (decrease in intestinal calcium absorption) or tumor calcinosis and pseudoxanthoma elasticum, cortical hyperostosis, and thyrotoxicosis (without calcium wasting). Ectopic calcification (can happen in any organ). And may result in acute or chronic renal failure

Treatment:

Acute hyperphosphatemia:
- Increase renal phosphate excretion by saline infusions
- Acetazolamide
- Administering bicarbonate inhibits renal phosphate resorption, but can induce symptoms of hypocalcemia

Chronic hyperphosphatemia:
- Decrease intestinal phosphate absorption
- Low phosphate diet and/or phosphate binders

11.19 Diagnose Water/Electrolyte Imbalance

In order to properly diagnose disorders of water and/or electrolyte balance, need to analyze all electrolytes in the serum and 24-h urine and correlate with the clinical picture

12 Urinary System

12.1 Urinalysis

A complete urinalysis has three components:
- Macroscopic assessment
- Dipstick analysis
- Microscopic examination

12.2 Macroscopic Assessment

Amount			
Normal	600–1800 mL/day	Oliguria	<400 mL/day
Anuria	<100 mL/day	Polyuria	>2500 mL/day

Color	
Clear	Polyuria, diabetes mellitus, diabetes insipidus
Dark yellow	Flavins (eg, high doses of vitamin B2), phenacetin
Yellow orange	Very concentrated urine, bilirubin, urobilin, fever
Blue-green	Biliverdin, pseudomonas infections (pyocyanin), methylene blue
Green	Bilirubin, pseudomonas infections (fluorescein)
Tan	Bilirubin/biliverdin, rhubarb (in acidic urine)
Red	Hemoglobin/RBCs, myoglobin, porphyrins, pyramidon, beetroot
Pink	Rhubarb (in alkaline urine)
Maroon	Methemoglobin
Brown-black	Methemoglobin, homogentisic (alkaptonuria, oxidation by atmospheric oxygen), melanin, porphyrins, L-dopa, methyldopa

Clarity
Normal urine is clear. Any clouding of fresh urine is abnormal.

Fresh urine
- **Cloudy:** Leukocytes, bacteria, yeast, sperm, cystine
- **Auburn:** (sediment) RBCs
- **Brown particles:** Bilirubin in infants
- **Milky:** Fat droplets (chyluria, lipiduria)

Clarity (cont.)

After prolonged standing, especially in cold:
- **Brightly colored**: Phosphates, carbonates in alkaline urine, urate, oxalates (rare)

After prolonged standing when warm
- **Cloudy**: Bacteria
- **After prolonged storage**: Phosphates, mucins, normal urothelial cells

Odor

The scent of urine becomes more noticeable when these substances have increased excretion:

- Ketones: Diabetes, starvation
- B vitamins: Oral intake
- Foods: Onions, garlic, asparagus, coffee
- Ammonium: Bacterial decomposition

The "three glass" test:
- Helps with the localization of bleeding site in clinical hematuria
- A voided urine is divided into three cups in sequential order (patient urinates and collects sample in three sequential containers)
  - First cup containing blood: bleeding in the urethral region
  - First and second cups containing blood: bleeding in the bladder area
  - All three cups containing blood: bleeding in the renal pelvis

12.3 Urine Dipstick Evaluation

- **Primarily utilized for detecting infection and bleeding, and monitoring diabetic patients**
- The initial tool for qualitative evaluation of urine glucose, protein, and bilirubin
- The reactive compartments are in stabilized form – When urine moistens the strip, the reagents dissolve, and the reactions proceed in proportion to the concentration of the substance being studied
- **Neither sensitive nor specific for distinguishing the different types of proteinuria** → A quantitative detection method must be performed

Ind: Screening: (eg, diabetes, inexpensive to perform)
- Kidney and urinary tract infection (detection of granulocytes)
- Hematuria, hemoglobinuria, myoglobinuria (reflex to microscopic examination)
- Monitoring blood sugar control in diabetics: glucose and possibly ketone bodies
- Detection of acidosis and alkalosis with a measurement of pH in the urine

Mat: Fresh urine

Met: Perform the analysis within 2 h of specimen collection:
- Close the container immediately after removing a dipstick
- Immerse the strip briefly (~1 sec) in the urine, otherwise reagents may be washed off
- The excess urine is removed, typically placed on paper towel
- After the appropriate reaction time, the results on the dipstick are compared (qualitatively) to the result references (usually present on the urine dipstick container)

Detectable items:
- pH, glucose, protein, specific gravity
- Hemoglobin, RBCs, WBCs
- Ketones, urobilinogen, nitrite
- Amylase
- Phenylpyruvic acid, cysteine, homocysteine, sulfite

12.4 Microscopic Examination

Ind:
- Routine examination of the urine
- Subsequent examination on positive test strip results
- Follow up of kidney disease

Mat: Random urine

Met: It is best to collect urine during the morning or at late night. Perform the microscopic examination within 4 h of specimen collection.

Norm:
Sediment:	<2 RBCs/HPF
	<5 WBCs/HPF
Minimal hyaline casts:	<15 squamous cells
	Semi-quantitative cell count
	<5 RBCs /µL
	<10 WBCs /µL

Casts:
- Clusters of cells as aggregates from the distal tubules and collecting ducts, especially after a wash/brushing
- Some are pathognomonic, as they can only arise from certain pathologically elevated cell counts or increased proteins within the tubules

Urine constituents	Disease states
Erythrocytes (RBCs)	Glomerulonephritis, tumors of the kidney and urinary tract, kidney and bladder stones
Leukocytes (WBCs)	Pyelonephritis, cystitis, prostatitis, urethritis, gynecological diseases
Waxy casts	Severe chronic renal failure, sometimes after acute renal failure
Bacteria	Urinary tract infections (UTIs)
Trichomoniasis	Usually in female patients
Fungi and yeast	More common in female patients

12.5 Urine pH

Ind: Nonspecific screening test for urinary tract infections
Acidosis and alkalosis
May be affected by long storage/transportation times

Norm: 4.6–8.0 (slightly acidic)

↑ Alkaline: Vegetarian diet

↓ Acidic: Meat-rich diet, degradation of endogenous protein, starvation, high fever

12.6 Glucose

Ind: Screening test for diabetes mellitus and renal glycosuria
Monitoring of therapy in diabetes mellitus

Norm: Random Urine: ≤150 mg/L
24 h Urine: ≤300 mg/day

Normal renal threshold: 1500–1800 mg/L

↑ Diabetes mellitus, diabetes with renal tubular damage, gestational diabetes (more pronounced during the last trimester)

12.7 Protein

Ind:
- Differentiation of various renal conditions
- Glomerular or tubular protein loss
- Infections of the urinary tract
- Orthostatic proteinuria
- Pregnancy monitoring

Pre-renal proteinuria

- Proteinuria secondary to a pre-renal etiology
- Increased formation and excretion of paraproteins; if Bence-Jones proteinuria is suspected, it is imperative to perform quantitative determination of urine protein (UPEP)

Urine proteins and possible causes	
Hemoglobin	Intravascular hemolysis
Myoglobin	Rhabdomyolysis
Ig light chain	Myeloma/plasmacytoma

Renal proteinuria

- Proteinuria secondary to intrinsic renal etiology
- **Glomerular proteinuria** → High molecular weight plasma proteins are excreted into the urine
  - Selective: Only albumin and transferrin (mainly albumin) pass through the basement membrane
  - Non-selective: In addition to albumin and transferrin, higher molecular weight proteins with a molecular weight up to 150,000 leak through the basement membrane, such as immunoglobulins
- **Tubular proteinuria** → Mainly low molecular weight proteins
- **Glomerular-tubular (mixed) proteinuria** → Patients with advanced renal damage

Differentiating causes of renal proteinuria

Compartment damaged	Main protein leaked
Glomerular, selective	Albumin
Glomerular, unselective	Albumin + Ig
Tubules	Alpha-1-microglobulin

Post-renal proteinuria:
- Proteinuria secondary to urinary tract etiology distal to the kidney
- Infection and bleeding (renal pelvis, urinary tract)

Differentiation by urine protein quotient:

Urine protein quotient	Renal	Post-renal
Alpha-2-macroglobulin/albumin (with albuminuria and hemoglobinuria, ≥100 mg/L)	Renal hematuria <0.02	Post-renal hematuria >0.02
IgG/albumin	• Renal proteinuria <0.2 • Selective glomerular proteinuria <0.03	• Post-renal proteinuria >0.2 • Non-selective glomerular proteinuria >0.03
Alpha-1-microglobulin/albumin	Pure glomerular proteinuria < 0.1	Glomerular and tubular mixed proteinuria >0.1

Norm: ≤150 mg/day

Morning urine: ≤30 mg/dL

Morning proteinuria has the greatest pathological significance, because ↑ protein excretion at other times may be caused by exercise or stress

Urine protein quotient	Renal
Physiological proteinuria	In newborns, after strenuous exercise, pregnancy
Orthostatic proteinuria	Albumin, transferrin, alpha-1 and gamma-globulins
Nephrotic syndrome	Mainly albumin is excreted (5-40 g/day)
Chronic pyelonephritis	Especially alpha-1, beta- and gamma-globulins
Inflammatory disorders	Alpha-1-globulin
Chyluria	High albumin and fibrinogen products
Glomerular damage	Albumin, transferrin, and possibly immunoglobulins
Tubular damage	Beta-2- and alpha-1-microglobulin, retinol-binding protein and N-acetyl-beta-D-glucosaminidase

Met: Measuring scattered light after precipitation, dye binding methods, copper-protein complex formation

Microalbuminuria:

In several studies a connection between microalbuminuria and cardiovascular risk factors (such as obesity, hyperlipidemia, smoking and alcohol consumption, hypertension and peripheral insulin resistance) has been observed. It is still unclear whether microalbuminuria should be used as an early indicator of glomerulonephritis and interstitial nephropathy, as a result of increased renal perfusion pressure, or as an expression of a pathological endothelial function. In any case, microalbuminuria is considered an additional cardiovascular risk factor

Classification of albuminuria:

	Normal	Microalbuminuria	Macroalbuminuria
Morning urine	<20 mg/L	20-200 mg/L	>200 mg/L
24-hour urine	<30 mg/day	30-300 mg/day	>300 mg/day

12.8 Bence-Jones Proteins

- Low molecular weight proteins pathologically excreted in the urine (Ig light chain = kappa and lambda)
- Occurs in ~80% of patients with myeloma, often with other paraproteins
- Can also been seen less frequently in Waldenström's macroglobulinemia or paraproteinemia
- Detected by using urine protein electrophoresis (UPEP) with immunofixation (sensitivity: 20-30 mg/L)

12.9 Erythrocytes (Red Blood Cells, RBCs)

Hematuria: Excretion of intact RBCs in the urine → gives it a reddish hue; Centrifugation of the specimen reveals a normal, clear colored supernatant
- Microscopic hematuria: Detectable only via microscopy or chemical testing
- Macroscopic (gross) hematuria: Blood volume of >1 ml/L (0.1% blood)

Ind: Screening test for hematuria

Norm: < 5/μL

Prerenal hematuria:
- Circulatory disorders (cardiovascular disease, renal vein thrombosis, arterial embolism)
- Coagulopathy (hemophilia, thrombocytopenia, platelet disorders)
- Medications (warfarin overdose, phenylbutazone)
- Essential hematuria

Renal hematuria:
- Primary renal disorders (nephritis, glomerulonephritis, pyelonephritis)
- Secondary renal damage (amyloidosis, tuberculosis, gout, Henoch-Schönlein purpura, lupus erythematosus)
- Tumors, cysts, hemangiomas, renal pelvic stones

Postrenal hematuria:
- Urinary calculi (most common)
- Tumors of the urinary tract
- Inflammation (cystitis, prostatitis, urethritis)

12.10 Myoglobin

Myoglobin = "muscle hemoglobin"; Myoglobulinuria: Myoglobin in the urine

Ind: Myopathies, rhabdomyolysis, performance evaluation in sports medicine

Norm: Not detectable in urine

↑ Muscle injury/necrosis, heavy physical exertion

Note: Myoglobinuria is almost always secondary to release from skeletal muscles, while myoglobinemia (myoglobin in the blood) may originate from the skeletal or cardiac muscle

12.11 Hemoglobin

Hemoglobinuria: Free hemoglobin in the urine hemoglobinuria; centrifugation of the specimen reveals a reddish-brown supernatant
- The sediment has no RBCs, but often hemoglobin casts
- The result of intravascular hemolysis and subsequent hemoglobinemia
- Not detectable microscopically

Ind: Screening test for hemoglobinuria

Norm: Not detectable in urine
Reabsorption capacity of the tubules is 1 g/L, normal value for serum free Hb is 50 mg/L

↑ **Prenatal intravascular hemolysis:**
- If exceeded the binding capacity of haptoglobin in the plasma
- If the renal tubular resorption of hemoglobin is exhausted

RBC hemolysis in urine:
- Especially with hypotonic urine
- Prolonged specimen standing, especially with alkaline urine

12.12 Leukocytes

White blood cells, WBCs

Ind: Screening test for kidney/urinary tract inflammation
Norm: <10/μL
↑
- Renal infections: pyelonephritis (acute and chronic), glomerulonephritis
- Urinary tract infections
- Medications (eg, aspirin, phenacetin)

12.13 Ketones

Ind:
- Suspected diabetes
- Acidosis
- Hypocaloric diet
- Eclampsia

Norm: Not detectable in urine
↑
- Diabetes (poorly controlled → hyperglycemia and ketoacidosis)
- Starvation (or generally decreased carbohydrate supply → increased fatty acid degradation → ketoacidosis)

Note:
- False negatives may be seen if specimen stands for too long → acetoacetic acid decomposes and is broken down by bacteria
- False positives may be seen during L-dopa

12.14 Bilirubin

- Degradation product of hemoglobin
- Conjugated primarily with glucuronic acid in microsomes of hepatocytes
- Conjugated form is water-soluble
- Unconjugated form is lipid-soluble, but not water-soluble
- Binds to elastic fibers of the skin and connective tissue, causing yellowing (>2 mg/dL serum levels)

Ind: Screening test for liver disease and biliary obstruction, however, of minor importance

Prod: From the degradation of hemoglobin, usually within the reticuloendothelial system: spleen and hepatic Kupffer cells

Norm: Virtually undetectable in the urine

↑ Intra- and extra-hepatic obstructive jaundice, icterus, acute or chronic hepatitis, cirrhosis
  - Bilirubin is detectable in the urine during the icteric phase of Dubin-Johnson syndrome

Met Urine dipstick detects the reaction of conjugated (water-soluble) bilirubin with a stabilized diazonium salt within a strongly acidic medium

Note • False negatives may be seen with high urinary ascorbic acid (Vitamin C) and nitrite concentrations or if sample has prolonged exposure to sunlight (photolysis of bilirubin)
  • False positives may be seen with drugs that alter the color of the reaction field

12.15 Urobilinogen

Breakdown product of bilirubin excreted in the urine

Ind: • Screening test of bilirubin levels (liver disease, bilirubin excretion disorders, extra- and intrahepatic cholestasis)
  • Differential diagnosis of kernicterus

Norm: ≤1 mg/dL

↑ Urobilinogen is increased when the enterohepatic circulation of bile pigments (functional capacity of the liver) is restricted or overloaded. A portal shunt can produce a similar picture
  • Increased hemoglobin degradation: Hemolytic anemia, pernicious anemia, intravascular hemolysis, polycythemia
  • Increased formation of urobilinogen in the intestine: Significant constipation, enterocolitis, ileus, increased fermentation
  • Increased urobilinogen production and resorption: Biliary tract infections

↓ Complete obstructive jaundice: lack of urobilinogen excretion

Bilirubin/uobilinogen in the urine with jaundice

Location	Bilirubin	Urobilinogen
Pre-hepatic	–	↑
Hepatic	+	↑
Post hepatic	+	↓

12.16 Nitrite

Ind:	Screening test for urinary tract infection (UTI)
Norm:	Not detectable in urine
↑	A test will be positive when all three conditions are met:

- Pathogens in the urinary tract reduce nitrate to nitrite
- Sufficient nitrate dietary intake
- Retention of urine in the bladder is sufficient (4-6 h)

Note A negative nitrite test is not sufficient to exclude a UTI
False negatives may be seen with urine ascorbic acid concentrations
>25 mg/dL or antibiotic treatment

12.17 Amylase

The determination of amylase in urine is not routinely performed, and should be accompanied by a serum amylase

Ind:
- Chronic hyperamylasemia
- Suspected macroamylasemia (plasma proteins-amylase complex formation leads to decreased renal amylase resorption; typically has a high plasma amylase with normal or reduced urine amylase)
- Detection or exclusion of renal insufficiency
- Suspected diabetic nephropathy

Prod Pancreas and salivary glands; the majority is secreted exogenously, only a small amount enters the bloodstream; excreted in the urine

Norm: <550 U/L

↑ Acute pancreatitis, chronic relapsing pancreatitis, parotid gland disorders/inflammation, acute alcoholism, ERCP, kidney failure

Note
- False negatives may be seen with high concentrations of bilirubin with bilirubinuria (alters the color of the reaction field)
- Highly buffered urine samples with skew pH values yielding unreliable results

12.18 Phenylketones

- Formed during the breakdown of phenylalanine
- Accumulation occurs in congenital metabolism disorder

Phe → / / →Tyr → dopamine, melanin, catecholamines, fumarate, acetoacetate

Ind:	Suspected phenylketonuria
↑	Phenylketonuria
Note	Since the introduction of screening test at birth, dipstick analysis for phenylketonuria is much less common

12.19 Cysteine and Homocysteine

Ind:	Suspected cystinuria or homocystinuria
	• Cystinuria: typically crystal formation in the urine
	• Homocystinuria: typically recurrent non-pigmented kidney stones (DDx: Marfan syndrome)
Norm:	Not detectable in urine
↑	Cystinuria or homocystinuria

12.20 Sulfite

Ind:	Screening test for sulfite oxidase disorders
Norm:	Rare, inborn error of sulfite metabolism
↑	Sample urine is dropped onto a test paper containing sulfite, a red color indicates the presence of sulfite (positive result)
Note.	False positives may be seen with cysteine and other compounds containing free SH groups or 2-mercaptoethanesulfonate
	False negative results may occur if specimen stands for too long

12.21 Urine Concentration

Norm:	500-1,000 mmol/kg
	Specific gravity: 1.003-1.035
Mat	Urine sample after a minimum of 12 h water deprivation

Met
- Using Urinstix: The test field "SG" not solely based on the specific gravity. A urine density is determined by urometer
- Using urometer: Takes specific measurements
- Concentration test: Significant part of the old water/thirst experiment in which the ADH secretion and effect is checked

Note   A known history of diabetes insipidus is a contraindication for a water deprivation test (may result in severe dehydration)

12.22 Clearance

Refers to the removal of a specific exogenous or endogenous substance from the blood as a measure of specific performance of excretion

Clearance = (Urine concentration × volume of urine)/plasma concentration × time

Renal clearance: A measure of renal function, measured by mL per minute (mL/min)

Substances that are excreted and not reabsorbed in the renal tubules can be measured and indicate the clearance of the substance. Substances that are secreted in the renal tubules (eg, mannitol, sodium thiosulfate, inulin, creatinine) can be used to measure tubular clearance. Substances that are secreted in the glomerulus (eg, p-aminohippuric acid) can be used to measure glomerular clearance.

At the onset of renal insufficiency, traditional measures of renal clearance by the administration of exogenous compounds are less effective. It is better to measure the increase in of compounds due to the lack of ability to effectively clear.

12.23 Glomerular Filtration Rate (GFR)

- Dependent on the effective filtration pressure and the filtration resistance of the glomerular basement membrane (factors: thickness, area, pore size)
- Determination is indirectly based on the clearance of substances that are exclusively and fully filtered, but not reabsorbed or secreted and are not metabolized in the kidney (eg, inulin, creatinine)
- The volume per unit time of glomerular filtrates

$$GFR = U \times V/P$$

U = urine concentration, V = urine volume; P = plasma concentration

GFR = urine concentration × urine volume/plasma concentration

Norm: 100-130 mL/min (affected by age, sex, and race)

12.24 Renal Blood Flow

Renal perfusion
- Refers to the amount of blood flowing through the kidneys per minute
- Calculated from the para-aminohippuric acid (PAH) clearance - (can be an issue in various nephrological conditions)

12.25 Creatinine

As creatinine phosphate: an energy reserve in muscle
- The daily produced amount is proportional to muscle mass
- The hourly amount excreted is fairly constant
- At high serum creatinine concentrations may also be secreted

Ind:	Screening test to evaluate renal function; follow-up of kidney disease; a parameter of renal function before, during, and after administering nephrotoxic drugs
Norm:	Serum: 0.6-1.2 mg/dL Urine: 15-25 mg/kg of patient/day
↑	Impaired renal function
Note:	Increased serum creatinine concentration (only when the GFR is reduced to ≤50%) → Mild impairment of renal function will not result in a change in the serum creatinine

12.26 Creatinine Clearance

Ind:	In normal and borderline elevated creatinine levels: • Therapy with nephrotoxic drugs; drugs with a narrow therapeutic index (dose adjustment is crucial) • Diabetes mellitus, hypertension, collagen vascular disease, hyperuricemia, increased muscle mass

Met
- Determine serum creatinine concentration
- Collect a 24-hour urine: Start in morning. First, empty the bladder and discard sample, noting the time. Then collect all urine until the same time the next morning. Collect the last sample at that time, emptying the bladder. Keep container refrigerated during and after collection, submit as soon as possible
- Determine urine creatinine concentration

Calculation of creatinine clearance:

$$CCr = (U_{Cr} \times U_{vol})/(SCr \times T_{Collection}) = mL/min$$

= Urine creatinine (mg/dL) × urine volume (mL)/serum creatinine (mg/dL) × collection time (min)

Since creatinine clearance is dependent on body mass, the clearance should be normalized to the specified standard of 1.73 m^2: body surface area of a 75 kg person

The body surface area (BSA) of the patient can be read on the basis of height and weight from corresponding tables or calculated:

Body surface area (m^2) = Weight $^{0.425}$ (kg) × Height $^{0.725}$ (cm) × 0.007184

Corrected formula for converting creatinine clearance to the standard body surface area:

C = Creatinine clearance x 1.73/BSA of patient

Norm: 80–160 mL/min/BSA (affected by age, sex, and race)

↑
- Increased muscle mass
- Acute ("crush-kidney") and chronic myopathies
- Paroxysmal myoglobinuria

↓
- Decreased muscle mass
- Renal failure

Note: With age, assuming that the kidneys function normally (not true most of the time), the creatinine clearance should decrease with decreasing muscle mass

Estimation of creatinine clearance in adults corrected for BSA (Cockcroft-Gault formula):

$$\text{Males: } C = \frac{(140 - Age) \times Body\ Weight\ (kg)}{72 \times Serum\ Creatinine\ (mg/dL)}$$

$$\text{Females: } C = 0.85 \times \frac{(140 - Age) \times Body\ Weight\ (kg)}{72 \times Serum\ Creatinine\ (mg/dL)}$$

12.27 Calculation of GFR

Glomerular filtration rate (MDRD formula)

- An alternate way of determining creatinine clearance is the so-called MDRD equation ("Modification of Diet in Renal Diseases")
- This formula takes into consideration the serum creatinine, urea nitrogen, albumin, age, gender and ethnicity
- Allows a quick and reliable indication of the renal excretory capacity without the time-consuming and potential inaccuracies of a 24 hour urine collection

$eGFR = 186 \times SCr-1.154 \times Age-0.203 \times (1.212$ if AA$) \times (0.742$ if female$)$

Or

$eGFR = 170 \times SCr-0.999 \times Age-0.176 \times (1.180$ if AA$) \times (0.762$ if female$) \times BUN-0.17 \times Albumin\ 0.318$

Note: The creatinine and blood urea nitrogen concentrations are both in mg/dL and the albumin concentration is in g/dL

As this formula does not adjust for BSA, it will underestimate eGFR for overweight patients and overestimate it for underweight patients

12.28 Cystatin C

- A low molecular weight protein consisting of 120 amino acids belonging to the family of cysteine proteinase inhibitors
- The formation rate is relatively constant, even in inflammatory states
- Filtered by the glomerulus, reabsorbed by the tubules, and is completely eliminated only by immediate removal
- Serum concentration is a marker for GFR; Decreased GFR → increase in serum cystatin C

Ind:	Assessment of GFR
Prod:	All cells
Norm:	0.6-1.5 mg/L
	Increases with age
	Independent of muscle mass and sex
↑	Decreased renal function
Mat:	Serum
Met:	Nephelometry/turbidimetry

Note: • Since the inter-individual variation of cystatin C concentration in the blood is lower than that of creatinine, it has a higher sensitivity and specificity, especially in patients with moderate GFR restriction and in marked creatinine increases

• A much better marker of GFR than creatinine and creatinine clearance in patients with decompensated cirrhosis

12.29 Phosphate Clearance

• Plasma volume of phosphate cleared per minute
• Not routinely performed
• Based on the serum and two urine samples, the volume of urine excreted during both collection periods is measured

Ind: Suspected tubular phosphate wasting syndromes or parathyroid disorders

Norm: 5.4–16.2 mL/min

↑   Primary hyperparathyroidism, hypocalcemia, rickets, Fanconi's syndrome, renal tubular acidosis, diabetes insipidus

Met   Determination of phosphate clearance (Cp) is performed in two one-hour collection periods according to the following test procedure:
Start time: The patient drinks 500 mL of tea
1st hour: The patient empties bladder into collection bottle, then drinks another 250 mL of tea
2nd hour: Patient voids into collection bottle
3rd hour: Draw blood for the determination of phosphate clearance
Calculated phosphate clearance:

$$Cp = \frac{\text{Urine Phosphate (mg/dL)} \times \text{Urine Volume (mL)}}{\text{Serum Phosphate (mg/dL)} \times \text{Collection Time (min)}}$$

↓   Acute and chronic renal failure, hypoparathyroidism, acromegaly

Note   Does not necessarily represent renal clearance (renal function often normal, eg, in primary hyperparathyroidism)

12.30 Urea (BUN)

Serum concentration increases only when the GFR is reduced to <50%.
When concentration is markedly increased it is often a marker of serious kidney
disease.

Ind: Calculation of the osmotic gap
   Estimation of the rate of metabolic states (anabolic, catabolic)

Norm: 6-25 mg/dL

↑
- Catabolic states
- High protein intake
- Dehydration
- Severe renal impairment

↓
- Severe liver disease
- Metabolic acidosis

12.31 Calculi (Stones)

- 10% of the population affected (in industrialized countries)
- Normally urine contains inhibitors of crystallization (glycoproteins, glycosaminoglycans, magnesium, citrate, pyrophosphate)
- Urinary calculi:
    - Calcium oxalate (envelopes)
    - Calcium phosphate (spheroids)
    - Magnesium ammonium phosphate/struvite/triple phosphate ("coffin lids")
    - Uric acid and urates (oval/elongated hexagons)
    - Cystine (hexagons)
    - Mixtures of these substances
- Causes: Lack of urinary crystallization inhibitors, decreased urine flow, increased renal excretion, extreme pH values

13   Gastrointestinal Tract

13.1   Gastric Secretions

13.1.1   Analysis

Func: Evaluation of the amount and acidity of the gastric fluids; rarely performed today, large normal variations

Ind: Suspected achlorhydria, pernicious anemia, gastric carcinoma or Zollinger-Ellison syndrome (ZES)

Norm: Parietal cells: hydrochloric acid, intrinsic-factor
Principal cells: pepsinogen
Mucous ells: pepsin resistant glycoproteins

Path: pH 1.5-3.5; 20-100 mL
Baseline:
1-5 mEq/h   Men
0.2-4 mEq/h   Women
Stimulation:
18-28 mEq/h   Men
11-21 mEq/h   Women

Met: Extraction of stomach secretions before and after maximum stimulation; 4 specimens taken q15 min for 90 min (1st two discarded)
- Basal secretion ⇒ basal acid secretion before stimulation (**4-6 h NPO**)
- Maximal secretion ⇒ acid secretion after stimulation
- Peak secretion (peak acid output) ⇒ adding the values of the two samples with the highest acid secretion and dividing by 2

13.1.2   Gastrin

Func: Peptide hormone that **stimulates gastric acid secretion (HCl) from parietal cells** (both directly and by binding CCK2 receptor on ECL cells of the stomach which release histamine then act in a paracrine to further stimulate parietal cell secreation) inducing insertion of $K^+/H^+/ATPase$ pump into the apical membrane
In addition, causes **pepsinogen secretion** from chief cells, **promotes stomach and LES contractions and relaxes the pyloric sphincter**, involved with relaxation of the ileocecal valve, induces pancreatic secretions and gallbladder emptying

Ind: **Severe peptic ulcer or reflux esophagitis, especially with associated diarrhea** (ZES), recurrent ulcers after partial gastrectomy, **suspicion of MEN I or IIa**

Prod: G-cells of the duodenum and gastric antrum, released into the bloodstream in response to vagal stimulation as well as through gastric distention, hypercalcemia, or partially digested amino acids
The secretion is inhibited when pH <2.5 in the antrum and by Somatostatin (also inhibits secretin, gastroinhibitory peptide, vasoactive intestinal peptide, glucagon, and calcitonin)

Norm: ≤200 pg/mL

↑ ↑↑↑: Gastrinoma (ZES), antrum remaining after gastric resection, autoimmune gastritis
↑↑: G-cell-hyperplasia, high-dose therapy with proton-pump inhibitors, after vagotomy, hyperthyroidism
↑: H2-Blocker-therapy, antacids, insulin, caffeine, catecholamines, mucolipidosis type IV
N–↑: Peptic ulcer

Mat: Fasting serum:
• Lundh test meal: high fiber
• Secretion test: secretin administered IV

13.1.3 Zollinger–Ellison syndrome (ZES) and gastrinoma

Gastrinoma: Gastrin producing pancreatic tumor often leading to ZES
Zollinger–Ellison syndrome: benign (adenoma) or malignant (carcinoma), non-insulin producing neoplasm of the pancreatic Delta cells with resultant increased gastrin (gastrinoma) leading to **peptic ulcers** due to massive hyperacidity of the gastric juice (stomach and duodenum, also esophagus and jejunum) that tend to perforate; also may lead to diarrhea with fatty stools and dehydration

13.1.4 Secretin provocation test

Func: Measurement of gastrin after secretin administration
Secretin is a peptide hormone that regulates secretions of the stomach and pancreas in order to regulate pH of the duodenum, also aids in water homeostasis throughout the body by acting on the hypothalamus, pituitary, and kidney; **inhibits gastrin release** from normal stomach **and gastric acid secretion** from parietal cells, however, **stimulates secretion from gastrinoma**; stimulates pancreatic centroacinar cell, intercalated duct, and duodenal Brunner's gland bicarbonate production; stimulates insulin, glucagon, somatostatin and pepsin release, enhances cholecystokinin, and promotes bile secretion

Ind: Suspected gastrinoma, post-operative monitoring of gastrinoma, increased basal gastrin

Prod: S-cells of the duodenum and jejunum (crypts of Lieberkühn)

Mat: Fasting serum

Met: Baseline gastrin level:
Clinical dose of 1–2 u/kg IV secretin
Gastrin level evaluation at 2, 5, 10, and 30 min
Increase $\geq$**100% from baseline $\rightarrow$ almost conclusive for gastrinoma** (false negative ~5%)
Low or no stimulation: Disorders with elevated basal gastrin (duodenal ulcer or gastric outlet obstruction)
Postoperative: no elevation

Note: Discontinue PPIs at least 1 wk prior to the investigation since these lead to increased gastrin

13.1.5 Pentagastrin stimulation test

Ind: Measurement of calcitonin after pentagastrin administration
Calcitonin: AKA thyrocalcitonin; polypeptide hormone produced primarily by parafollicular cells (C-cells) of the thyroid; it opposes PTH acting to reduce blood calcium, and is often elevated in medullary thyroid carcinoma (MTC) and C-cell hyperplasia; normal levels: <5 pg/mL (females), <10 pg/mL (males), may be higher in children <3 years
Pentagastrin is a synthetic polypeptide with the physiologically active C-terminal amino acid sequence of gastrin $\rightarrow$ stimulates secretion of gastric acid, pepsin, and intrinsic factor; it also stimulates calcitonin release in patients with medullary thyroid carcinoma (MTC) or C-cell hyperplasia of the thyroid, particularly useful when calcitonin is normal

Ind: Suspicion of medullary thyroid cancer (MTC), C-cell-hyperplasia, post-operative monitoring of MTC, family screening in MTC or MEN II

Met: Baseline calcitonin 10 min prior to and immediately before stimulation
Administration of 0.5 µg/kg IV Pentagastrin
Calcitonin level evaluation at 1, 3, and 5 min
MTC: Marked increase from baseline
Men: Baseline normal, increase >10-fold
Women: Baseline normal, increase >5-fold
Normal: Small increase from baseline
Men: Increase to <100 pg/mL
Women: Increase to <40 pg/mL
Note: May aid in tumor localization (primary or metastasis) with selective/multiple catheterization with multiple synchronous calcitonin determination

13.2 Exocrine Pancreas Function

13.2.1 Stool examination

Func: Collection of stool for the determination of:
Quantity: Mean value calculation from three consecutive 24 h-stools→ simple screening test for maldigestion and malabsorption
Fecal chymotrypsin (FCT): Low values indicate severe exocrine pancreatic insufficiency
Fat: Increased values indicate malabsorption (infection, reduced pancreatic lipase secretion)

Ind: Screening test for suspected exocrine pancreatic insufficiency and malabsorption

13.2.2 Chymotrypsin

Func: Digestive enzyme that cleaves proteins into peptides (esp. where the carboxyl side is large and hydrophobic - phenylalanine, tryptophan, tyrosine)

Ind: Screening test for suspected exocrine pancreatic insufficiency

Prod: Pancreatic acinar cells; activated by trypsin within the duodenum

↓ Severe exocrine pancreatic insufficiency, closure of the pancreatic duct, gluten-sensitive enteropathy, protein malnutrition

Mat: Preferred 1-2 g random stool sample, minimum 0.5 g; most useful if obtained on 3 different days

Met: Enzymatically

Prep: To determine the endogenous chymotrypsin production pancreatic enzyme preparations 5 days before being dropped off; abstinence from alcohol

Note: Falsely low results seen in diarrhea due to dilution. Little sensitivity for the diagnosis of chronic diarrhea or malabsorption syndromes. No validity in early forms of exocrine pancreatic insufficiency

13.2.3 Pancreatic elastase

Func: Pancreatic digestive enzyme released into the duodenum

Ind: Screening for suspected exocrine pancreatic insufficiency, monitoring of disease, (eg, chronic pancreatitis, cystic fibrosis, diabetis, cholelithiasis, papillary stenosis, pancreatic cancer); **"gold standard" of non-invasive pancreatic function tests** (sensitivity 93%, specificity 93%)

Norm: >200 mg/g stool

↓ 100-200 mg/g stool: mild to moderate pancreatic insufficiency
<100 mg/g stool: severe exocrine pancreatic insufficiency

Mat: Random 1 g stool sample, refrigerated if testing delayed

Met: Immunoassay
Note: Falsely low results possible with watery or small pulpy stools
- No influence of the measurement result by substitution therapy with pancreatic enzymes
- Pancreatic enzyme secretion test ⇒ previous gold standard; complicated method and expensive, no longer used routinely

13.2.4 Pancreoauryl test

Func: Pancreolauryl (Fluorescein-Dilaurate) is hydrolysed by pancreatic secretions (cholesterol ester hydrolase) resulting in free, water-soluble fluorescein, which is absorbed by the intestine and excreted in the urine

Ind: Screening test for suspected **exocrine pancreatic insufficiency**

Norm: Recovery of >30% of fluorescein

Mat: Urine, collected over 10 h after start of test (tablet ingestion)
Note: Must discontinue enzyme replacement therapy 3 days prior to test

Met: **Day 1:** Fluorescein-Dilaurate (Pancreolauryl) tablet along with a standardized breakfast
Day 2: Free fluorescein tablet along with a standardized breakfast (allows for correction for intestinal, hepatic, and renal function)
Photometric measurement of fluorescein concentration in urine
20%-30% Slightly decreased, retest recommended
<20% Evidence of exocrine pancreatic insufficiency
Note: Falsely low values (false positive) may be seen with incomplete urine collection and/or non-compliance with breakfast and/or Pancreolauryl capsules
Falsely high values (false negative) may be seen with pancreatic enzyme substitution

13.2.5 N–Benzoyl-L-Tyrosyl-p-Aminobenzoic-acid-test

NBT-PABA-Test

Func: Assessment of the PABA absorption

Ind: Screening test for suspected exocrine pancreatic insufficiency

Norm: Recovery of >50% of the injected PABA

Mat: Urine collected over 5 h after start of test
Note: Must be fasting for 12 h, with no food containing benzoic acid (preservative) for 48 h, and have empty bladder prior to testing

Met: Eat standardized breakfast (200 mL tea without sugar, 1 slice of bread with butter and jam), followed by 3 tbsp bentiromide (children <30 kg: 1 tbsp, between 30-45 kg: 2 tbsp), and then 500 mL tea
At 5 h eat another slice of bread with butter and jam
<40% Evidence of exocrine pancreatic insufficiency
Note: Falsely low values (false positive) may be seen in celiac disease and inflammatory bowel disease

13.2.6 Pancreatic enzyme secretion test

Func: Evaluation of the actual secretions of the pancreas

Ind: Screening test for suspected exocrine pancreatic insufficiency

Met: Using a duodenal tube, **secretions are tested before and after maximum stimulation of the pancreas.** Multiple determinations of the secretion volumes every 20 min along with determination of the enzyme and bicarbonate fractions

Slight insufficiency: volume and bicarbonate normal, enzymes partially decreased

Moderate insufficiency: volume and bicarbonate normal, all enzymes decreased

Severe insufficiency: All parameters decreased

Note: This test is very expensive and more invasive than newer assays

13.3 Small Intestine Function

Definitions:

Digestion: The mechanical and chemical breakdown of food into components small enough for absorption into the blood stream. Starts in the mouth with mastication (chewing - mechanical) and saliva (wetting - mechanical, salivary amylase - chemical, starts breakdown of starches). The food bolus then travels through the esophagus by peristalsis (mechanical) to the stomach where contractions (mechanical) and gastric juice (hydrochloric acid, pepsin, renin - chemical, starts breakdown of proteins) further breaking down the food particles. The resulting thick liquid food mixture (chyme) enters the duodenum where it mixes with the final set of digestive enzymes from the pancreas and bile from the gallbladder and is absorbed throughout the small intestine

Catabolism: The act of breaking down molecules in order to release energy. Lipids, nucleic acids, polysaccharides, and proteins are broken down into fatty acids, nucleotides, monosaccharides, and amino acids, respectively

Absorption: The passage of molecules (vitamin/nutrients/amino acids/ fatty acids) across the mucus membrane into the bloodstream. The majority (~95%) occurs in the small intestine (largely the jejunum, with the exception of iron - duodenum, B12 and bile - terminal ileum). The stomach will absorb water, some medicines, and alcohol and the large intestine absorbs residual water and minerals

Anabolism/assimilation: The opposite of catabolism. The synthesis of larger molecules from small units to aid in the building of organs/tissues

Steatorrhea: Greatly increased stool fat excretion (normal up to 7 g/day), seen in lipase deficiency, bile acid deficiency, abnormal intestinal colonization, acute diarrhea, malabsorption syndromes

13.3.1 Xylose tolerance test

Func: Verification of carbohydrate absorption capacity of the small intestine (intact renal function) based on 5 hour urinary values after oral load with 5 or 25 g D-xylose

Ind: Suspicion of **malabsorption**

Norm:
5 h urine	>20% of the administered dose of D-xylose
Serum q1 h	>21 mg/dL
Serum q2 h	>30 mg/dL

↓ Celiac disease, inflammatory bowel disease

Met: 25 g D-xylose in 500 mL (children 5g in 100 mL) of oral liquid, collect the urine over 5 h, blood sample after 60 and 120 min (in children only after 60 min)

Note: **Must be >12 h fasting**; start with empty bladder; falsely low values (false positive) in patients with renal impairment
Alternative: H_2-breath test (simple, faster, and cheaper) - increased exhalation of H_2 due to bacterial fermentation of undigested particles

13.3.2 Lactose-load test

Func: Evaluation lactose cleavage into glucose and galactose by intestinal lactase

Ind: Suspected **lactase deficiency** (bloating, diarrhea, and flatulence after consumption of dairy products)

Met: Met: 50 g of lactose in 400 mL of water in the morning on an empty stomach
Glucose determination after 30, 60, 90, and 120 min
Glucose elevated <20 mg/dL after 2 h: Positive result

Note: False negatives seen in diabetes, due to impaired glucose tolerance
False positives seen after gastric resection or with impaired intestinal motility
Alternative: H_2-breath test (Simple, faster, and cheaper) - After lactose ingestion, bacterial fermentation of undigested lactose in the colon leads to increased exhalation of H_2 (>20 ppm)

13.3.3 Schilling test

Vitamin B12 absorption test

Func:	Vitamin B 12 absorption test that can be performed in several stages to identify if a B12 deficiency is due to gastric damage (intrinsic factor deficiency) or intestinal damage (malabsorption)
Ind:	Suspected vitamin B12 deficiency due to pernicious anemia (loss of gastric parietal cells leading to decrease intrinsic factors)
Met:	Can be performed in three stages: with or without the addition of intrinsic factor, or after antibiotic therapy (metronidazole) for 5 days in cases of suspected bacterial overgrowth **Double labeling method:** Oral administration of isotope 57-marked vitamin-B12 bound to intrinsic factor with simultaneous free form isotope 58-marked vitamin B12 along with a flushing dose (1 mg) of unlabeled Vitamin B12 (IM injection); Then the isotope are measured in a 24h urine In healthy individuals **>9% of both fractions are eliminated** In the absence of endogenous intrinsic factor, **free vitamin B12** (58 fraction) is reduced (<5%), the **bound** (57 fraction) is **normally excreted** **In malabsorption,** however, **both groups are decreased**
Note:	**Falsely low** (false positive) levels seen with food intake before or during the first 3 h after testing, in renal insufficiency, or with bacterial overgrowth in the gut. Contraindicated in pregnancy

13.4 Fecal Occult Blood Test

Func:	Stool testing for the presence of not grossly visible blood
Ind:	Suspected intestinal blood loss, **screening test for colorectal cancers**
Met:	• Two different samples of stool for 3 consecutive days are spread on test paper (more samples better for sensitivity and specificity; may be done after DRE) • Hemoglobin peroxidase will be oxidized by H_2O_2/Guiac leading to a **blue discoloration** • The test is positive even if only one of the samples turns blue and must be investigated
Note:	Fiber-rich meals (whole wheat bread, vegetables, nuts) 3 days prior to testing; no red meat, limited vitamin C False positive: Hemoglobin or myoglobin rich diet False negative: High Vitamin C doses

13.5   Meconium Albumin Testing

Func: Detection of elevated concentrations of albumin in meconium (infant's first stools, 1–3 days postpartum, composed of materials ingested in utero: bile, intestinal epithelium, amniotic fluid, lanugo, mucus; high bile content leads to blacking-green color)

Ind: **Suspected neonatal cystic fibrosis (CF)**

↑   Significantly increased in cystic fibrosis

Note: Rarely used today due to low specificity and sensitivity; 15%–30% false negative results

Replaced with immunoreactive trypsin test (more reliable), or chloride sweat test (easily performed, though low sensitivity)

14 Cerebrospinal Fluid (CSF)

14.1 Macroscopic Examination

Normal cerebrospinal fluid is **clear and colorless**; cloudiness is most commonly due to an increased white blood cell (WBC) count

Spinning tissue clot: veil-like fibrin clot that may form in a standing CSF (24 h) in inflammatory conditions, especially in **tuberculous meningitis:** useful for diagnosis (spread on slides, air dry, Ziehl-Neelsen stain, etc.)

Blood in the CSF: Most often due to a 'traumatic tap,' ie, artificially induced bleeding from the puncture (later tubes more clear than first tube collected), but may be due to **subarachnoid hemorrhage:** all tubes collected are uniformly discolored, and there are hemosiderin-laden macrophages, erythrophagocytosis, and D-dimers

Xanthochromia: yellowing of the cerebrospinal fluid after centrifugation; see in **subarachnoid hemorrhage** (from hemoglobin metabolism, after ~12 h, lasts ~3 wk), **excessive protein** (>150 mg/dL), **severe jaundice**, carotenoids, melanin, rifampicin or delayed examination (>1 h)

14.2 Cells in the CSF

Norm: **Leukocytes**: ≤5/μL Adults
                        ≤30/μL Neonates
        Erythrocytes: Not detectable

Met: Mechanised cell counting is the norm, semi-quantitative test strip methods also available

Manual differentiation: perform within 60 min. Caution risk of infection! Fresh CSF is diluted with glacial acetic acid, in a filled Fuchs-Rosenthal counting chamber and viewed under a microscope. The counting chamber consists of 16 large squares, each of which is divided into 16 small squares, all identifiable leukocytes throughout the network are of the 256 small squares are counted. The chamber volume is 3 μL. For historical reasons, the cell number in the entire Fuchs-Rosenthal counting chamber often not divided by 3 and reported per μL, but reported without conversion as #/3 ("third cell")

In pathology the white blood cell count is given as a differentiation using colored smear or cytospin

Cell count	Bacterial meningitis: >1000/µL Viral meningitis: >100-1000/µL Tuberculosis: <400/µL
Cell type	Bacterial infections: Neutrophils/polymorphonuclear cells Viral infections: Lymphocytic/mononuclear cells Brain tumors/metastases: Pathological cells
Temp oral	Acute phase: granulocytes Subacute proliferative phase: lymphocytes, decrease in cell numbers Reparative: lymphocytic and monocytic cells

14.3 Normal CSF Differentials

Cell type	Neonates (%)	Adults (%)
Lymphocytes	10-40	30-90
Monocytes/macrophages	50-90	10-50
Neutrophils	0-10	0-6
Eosinophils	Rare	Rare
Ependymal	Rare	Rare

14.4 Meningitis CSF Differentials

Infection	WBC count	WBC type	Glucose	Protein
Bacterial	1,000-10,000	PMNs (lymphs - partially treated)	<40	>100
Viral	50-500	PMNs early, Lymphs later	NL (low- HSV)	20-100
Fungal/ mycobacterial	50-500	Lymphs	<50	20-100

14.5   CSF Protein

An increased protein concentration in CSF is a non-specific sign of a pathological process in the CNS

Norm: 15–45 mg/dL

↑:   Permeable blood–brain barrier: Most common; CSF serum albumin ratio should be <1:230
Meningitis, hemorrhage, CSF obstruction
Intrathecal immunoglobulin production: seldom >45 mg/dL; electrophoresis may help; also, if cell count is in the reference range, a CNS disorder is generally excluded
Multiple sclerosis: Increased intrathecal IgG (sensitivity ~90%) and oligoclonal bands on electrophoresis (2+ bands positive, sensitivity ~70%, specificity ~95%) or isoelectric focusing (4+ bands positive, sensitivity ~90%, specificity ~95%)
Cerebral adrenoleukodystrophy: Increased intrathecal IgA

Met: CSF protein is normally so minute it must be precipitated using trichloroacetic acid or sulfosalicyclic acid

Reference protein levels:

Bacterial meningitis:	>1000 mg/dL
Viral meningitis:	<100 mg/dL
Tuberculous meningitis:	<400 mg/dL
Compressions syndrome:	<4000 mg/dL
Polyradiculitis:	<2000 mg/dL

Reiber protein quotient graph:

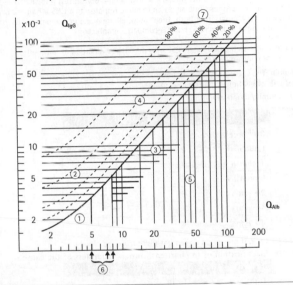

1	Normal range
2	Local IgG-synthesis without barrier disruption
3	Pure barrier disruption without local IgG-synthesis
4	Local IgG-synthesis with barrier disruption
5	Suspected errors in measurement or blood sample
6	Age-related limits of barrier disruption
7	Proportion of local IgG-synthesis of the total G in the CSF

Using the Reiber quotient graph (Reiber diagram) one can differentiate whether there is a pure barrier disorder (mainly non-inflammatory causes), a local immunoglobulin synthesis (mainly as an immune response to a CNS inflammatory process) or a combination of both. The ratio of albumin and immunoglobulins in the cerebrospinal fluid verses serum is compared graphically

May be done for any immunoglobulin (IgG, IgA, IgM, etc.)

Markedly increased blood in the CSF may make the evaluation of quotients difficult or impossible

Albumin The CSF-serum ratio of albumin thus represents a good parameter for
quotient estimation of barrier disruption

CSF albumin/serum albumin:

Norm:

Age	$Q_{Alb} \times 10^{-3}$
30th week	50
Childbirth	25
1 month	15
6 months	5
20 years	5
40 years	7
60 years	8

Prod: Liver. If present in CSF, it got there from the blood

Classification of the barrier disorders regardless of the cause

Severity	$Q_{Alb} \times 10^{-3}$
Light	To 10
Moderate	To 20
Heavy	Over 20

IgG   The CSF-serum ratio of IgG may be indicative of permeable blood brain
quotient barrier (albumin quotient will also be abnormal) or due to intrathecal synthesis

CSF IgG/serum IgG:

Prod: Activated B-cells/plasma cells: Normally only present in the blood
May have intrathecal synthesis (eg, MS, infection)

↑ Pathologically increased CNS Ig synthesis usually leads to oligoclonal immunoglobulins in the CSF, which are not present in the peripheral blood. They are found in 25%-40% of all CNS infections, but play a special role in the early diagnosis of **multiple sclerosis (MS)**. Electrophoresis (2+ bands positive, sensitivity ~70%, specificity ~96%) or isoelectric focusing (4+ bands positive, sensitivity ~90%, specificity ~95%) will show oligoclonal bands in the CSF. In MS, there is a polyspecific immune response, but there may also be a small diagnostically relevant amount of antibodies against measles, rubella and zoster, which is referred to as an "MAR" reaction

A distinction must be made from **monoclonal immunoglobulins (ie, multiple myeloma, Waldenstrom's macroglobulinemia)** and their possible detection within the CSF with a corresponding barrier disruption

14.6 CSF Glucose

Ind: Differentiate bacterial and viral meningitis, follow-up cerebral vascular accidents (CVA)

Norm: 45-75 mg/dL
~60% of the serum glucose

Eval: Acute **bacterial** meningitis: **glucose decreased**
Acute **viral** meningitis: glucose **normal**

Mat: Cerebrospinal fluid with simultaneous measurement of blood sugar

14.7 CSF in Nasal Secretions

Ind: • With rhinorrhea after head trauma it is necessary to distinguish between CSF and normal nasal secretions
• Glucose is very non-specific, but look for the amount normally in CSF (>nasal secretions)
• Protein electrophoresis to look for the twin transferrin/pre-albumin peak of CSF
• Asialated transferrin present is suggestive of CSF

	CSF	Nasal secretions
Glucose	>45 mg/dL	<10 mg/dL
Protein	40 mg/dL	300 mg/dL
Beta-trace-protein	>6 mg/L	<1 mg/L
Beta-2-transferrin	Detectable	Not detectable

14.8 Contraindications to Lumbar Puncture (LP)

Clinical situations where LP should only be performed if absolutely necessary and with appropriate precautions
- Increased intracranial pressure (ICP):
  - Rationale: May result in uncal herniation
  - Exception: Therapeutic use to reduce ICP
  - Prior to LP:
    - CT brain, especially when patient >65, reduced consciousness, recent history of seizure, neurological signs
    - Ophthalmoscopy for papilledema
- Coagulopathy:
  - Thrombocytopenia (<50 × 10^9/L)
- Infections:
  - Skin infection at puncture site
  - Sepsis
- Hypertension with bradycardia and deteriorating consciousness
- Spine deformities (eg, scoliosis)

15 Pleural, Peritoneal and Synovial Fluid

15.1 Pleural Effusion

Specimen: Pleural effusion, serum

Light criteria is used to classify pleural effusion as transudative or exudative based on comparison to serum

Other pleural fluid findings that support exudate. Specific gravity >1.1016, cholesterol >45 mg/dL, fluid bilirubin:serum bilirubin >0.6

Transudate (Cardiac)	Substance being measured	Exudate (Parapneumonic or malignancy)
<3 g/dL	Total protein effusion	>3 g/dL
<0.5	Total protein effusion/serum	>0.5
<200 U/L	LDH effusion	>200 U/L
<0.6	LDH effusion/serum	>0.6
<60 mg/dL	Cholesterol	>60 mg/dL

Specimen: Pleural effusion, serum

Parapneumonic	Substance being measured	Malignancy
Positive	Bacteria	Negative
Negative	Tumor cells	Positive
<3 µg/L	CEA	>4.5 µg/L
<20.9 µg/L	CYFRA 21-1	>20.9 µg/L
<4.6 mg/L	Beta-2-microglobulin	>7.2 mg/L

Etiology: Differential diagnosis of an effusion via the presence/absence of the following: bacteria, cholesterol, triglycerides, lipase, pancreatic amylase, salivary amylase, CEA, NSE, CYFRA 21-1, beta-2-microglobulin, ANF, tumor cells

- **Transudate:**
  - Usually cardiac-related heart failure (right > left), pericardial effusion), but also hypoproteinemia (cirrhosis, nephrotic syndrome), pulmonary embolism (1/3) and hypothyroidism

- **Exudate:**
  - **Neutrophils:** infectious (eg, pneumonia, tuberculosis [TB], **empyema** [>100,000 PMNs/mL, pH<7.2]), pleuritis, sympathetic pleurisy (eg, pancreatitis), pulmonary infarction
  - **Eosinophils: Prior tap,** parasites, **Churg-Strauss** syndrome, lymphoma
  - **Lymphocytes:** TB (particularly when few mesothelial cells)
  - **Mesothelials:** Noticeably scant in TB and RA
  - **Rarely:** Trauma, malignant tumors (especially lung, breast, mesothelioma), pulmonary embolism (2/3), collagen vascular disease (esp **rheumatoid arthritis** [RA, pH <7.2, LDH >700, glucose <30, rheumatoid factor-IgM with anti-IgG activity]), asbestos, post-MI (**Dressler's syndrome**), uremia, ovarian fibromas (**Meigs' syndrome**)
- **Chylous:**
  - Chylomicrons in the effusion, evident as creamy top layer if allowed to stand
  - True chylothorax is cause by thoracic duct lymphatic drainage; majority due to malignancy (lymphoma, lung carcinoma), trauma, and surgery. Rarely associated with infection, sarcoidosis, and lymphangioleiomyomatosis (LAM)
  - Pseudochylous result from accumulation of lipids from cell degradation; TB, RA, myxedema
- **Amylase:**
  - Esophageal perforation, malignancy, pancreatitis (classically left-sided)

Note: Low glucose and low pH usually indicates empyema, malignancy, or RA. Low pH alone is usually esophageal perforation

15.2 Ascites

Specimen: ascites, serum

Criteria similar to pleural effusions (light). The serum-ascites albumin gradient is helpful for distinguishing portal hypertension (seen in cirrhosis, gradient >1.1 g/dL) from other causes (gradient <1.1 g/dL)

Portal HTN	Substance being measured	Malignancy infection
>11 g/L	**Albumin difference** (Serum minus ascites)	<11 g/L
<160 U/L	**LDH** (Ascitis)	>160 U/L
<0.6	**LDH-quotient** (Ascitis/serum)	>0.6
<250/µL	**Neutrophils** (Ascitis)	>250/µL

Specimen: Ascites

Infection	Substance being measured	Malignancy
<45 mg/dL	**Cholesterol**	>45 mg/dL
<100 mg/L	**Fibronectin**	>100 mg/L
>250 µL	**Neutrophils**	<250 µL
Positive	**Bacteria**	Negative
Negative	**Tumor cells**	Positive

Diagnostic peritoneal lavage: Helpful after trauma to decide if exploratory laparotomy is necessary. Positive if: >15 mL frank blood, RBC >100,000/mL, WBC >500/mL, similar fluid in chest tube or Foley catheter, bacteria present on gram stain

15.3 Synovial Fluid

Not part of routine clinical work-up. Generally performed to look for **infection**, but may also be done in effusions due to arthritis

Mucin clot test: Not routinely performed anymore. Used to evaluate if there is inflammation by adding acetic acid which under normal conditions leads to congealing ('clot') of hyaluronic acid. When inflammation is present the hyaluronic acid is degraded and there is poor clot formation

Septic arthritis: LDH often >250 mg/dL

Lupus and RA: Complement is low

Crystals:
- **Monosodium urate:** Seen in **gout**; needle shaped, 2-20 μm in length; strongly negatively birefringent (yellow when light polarized; parallel and blue when perpendicular)
- **Calcium pyrophosphate: Pseudogout**, AKA calcium pyrophosphate deposition disease (CPPD); rods or rhomboids, 2-20 μm; weakly positively birefringent
- **Hydroxyapatite:** Small, non-birefringent crystals that are detectable with Alizarin red S stain
- **Corticosteroid:** Blunt jagged crystals with variable birefringence seen after steroid injections

Clinical	WBC count	PMN%	Serum-synovial glucose gradient	Gross
Normal	0-150	<25	0-10	Clear-straw color
Non-inflammatory	0-3000	<25	0-10	Clear-straw color
Inflammatory	3000-75000	30-75	0-40	Opaque and turbid
Septic, urate and rheumatoid arthritis	<100000	>90	30-100	Purulent yellow

16 Musculoskeletal System

16.1 Bone Matrix

Osteoid: (organic matrix formed by osteoblasts)
- Contains mainly collagen type I (characterized by a high proline and hydroxyproline)
- Scaffolding upon which the mineralization is deposited
- Inside of the canaliculi: Osteoid synthesis by osteocytes

Apatite crystals: (mineral portion, also formed with help of osteoblasts)
- Arranged parallel to the collagen fibers consisting of calcium phosphate ($Ca_3(PO4)_2$), calcium hydroxide ($Ca(OH)_2$), calcium fluoride (CaF_2), calcium carbonate ($CaCO_3$), and calcium chloride ($CaCl_2$)

16.2 Bone Formation Markers

Func: Alkaline phosphatase, osteocalcin, and procollagen as markers of bone formation

Ind: Osteoporosis, tumor-associated bone destruction, Paget's disease, hyperparathyroidism, growth disorders, rickets

Mat:
- Serum (total AP, bone AP, osteocalcin, PICP [P1CP], PINP [P1NP])
- Determination of the total AP from plasma also possible

Met:
- RIA: Bone-AP, osteocalcin, PICP
- Photometry: Total AP

16.2.1 Alkaline phosphatase (AP)

Func: A hydrolase enzyme that removes phosphate groups (dephosphorylation). Most effective in an alkaline environment (basic)

Ind: Diseases associated with **increased osteoblastic activity**, hepatobiliary disease

Prod: Osteoblasts, hepatocytes, especially adjacent to the biliary canaliculi, placenta

Norm:	40–120 U/L	Men
	35–120 U/L	Women
	130–560 U/L	Children (4–15 years)
	50–400 U/L	Children (16–18 years)

Note: Females are generally lower than males. Elderly females tend to have slightly higher levels. Pediatric reference values should be used to interpret values in children and adolescents

↑   **Bone metastases** (commonly prostate, breast, lung cancer), **primary bone tumors** (sarcomas, multiple myeloma, some benign lesions), **fractures**, post bone surgery, bone necrosis, osteomyelitis, osteomalacia, vitamin D overdose, rickets, Paget's disease (greatly increased), (pseudo)hyperparathyroidism, acromegaly, hyperthyroidism, pregnancy (3rd trimester, placental origin)

Also: **Liver disease or injury** (toxicity, drugs, tumors), **obstructive jaundice**, cholangitis

↓   Penicillamine and theophylline

Int: Among bone diseases, Paget's disease has the highest level (10–25x) of AP due to the hyperactivity of osteoblasts trying to rebuild bone that is being resorbed by the uncontrolled osteoclast activity. Extremely high levels are also seen in bone forming tumors. Mild to moderate increases are seen in osteomalacia and rickets. Levels in hyperparathyroidism (primary and secondary) vary based on amount of skeletal involvement. Levels are usually **normal in osteoporosis**

AP elevation often >3x in extrahepatic biliary obstruction (eg, stones, cancer) than in intrahepatic obstruction. Levels may reach 12 times the upper limit of normal and return to normal after removal of the obstruction. In cholestatic liver disease AP is similar to, but slightly less than GGT. If both GGT and ALP are elevated, the liver is the likely source.

16.2.2 Bone specific alkaline phosphatase

Func: A glycoprotein enzyme found on osteoblasts. Levels reflect osteoblast activity (bone formation).

Norm:

≤20 µg/L	Men
≤14 µg/L	Women (premenopausal)
≤22 µg/L	Women (postmenopausal)
25-220 µg/L	Infants (<? years)
30-175 µg/L	Children (2-13 years)
10-80 µg/L	Children (14-17 years)

Note: Falsely high levels may be seen with significant elevations of liver-derived AP due to cross-reactivity

↑ Paget's disease, bone tumors/metastasis, osteomalacia, hyperparathyroidism (esp. with skeletal involvement), growth spurts, fractures

↓ Hypoparathyroidism, chronic or high-dose steroid use

16.2.3 Osteocalcin

AKA bone gamma-carboxyglutamic acid-containing protein (BGP)

Func: Important non-collagen protein in bone matrix whose production is dependent on vitamin K and 1,25-dihydroxy vitamin D3. Released into the circulation during bone resorption, therefore is a **marker of bone turnover**

Due to a protease cleavage site between amino acids 43 and 44, intact osteocalcin is unstable. The cleavage results in an N-MID fragment that is much more stable. Both intact osteocalcin (aa 1-49) and the large N-MID fragment (aa 1-43) are found in the blood and recent studies have shown them to have a hormone affect causing increased insulin release from pancreatic beta cells and adiponectin release from adipocytes - increasing sensitivity to insulin. There is also evidence that osteocalcin enhances the production of testosterone, playing a role in male fertility

Ind: **Monitoring anti-resorption treatment** in osteoporosis or Paget's disease; **suspected disease with increased bone turnover** (metastasis, Paget's disease, primary hyperparathyroidism, renal osteodystrophy)

Prod: Osteoblasts

Norm: 10-45 ng/mL

↑	Metabolic bone diseases with increased bone formation and resorption: high-turnover osteoporosis, osteomalacia, rickets, hyperparathyroidism, renal osteodystrophy, hyperthyroidism, fractures, acromegaly, and bone metastasis, Paget's disease
↓	Low-turnover osteoporosis, hypoparathyroidism, hypothyroidism, growth hormone deficiency, rheumatoid arthritis
Mat:	Serum/plasma, fasting, preferably in the morning (highest levels)
Met:	Immunoassay
Int:	Anti-resorptive therapy (bisphosphonates, hormone replacement): a decrease ≥20% from baseline after 3-6 months Hyperparathyroidism/hyperthyroidism: with 'cure,' should have a return of normal within 3-6 months **Note**: Measurements of bone turnover markers are not useful for the diagnosis of osteoporosis; diagnosis is made on the basis of decreased bone density with or without fracture Osteocalcin levels may not be accurate in patients on vitamin D3 therapy or with D3 deficiency/abnormality, those on high-dose biotin (>5 mg, wait 8 h between dosage and blood draw), or those treated with mouse antibodies, or with high titers of streptavidin or ruthenium antibodies **Falsely high** levels may be seen in renal insufficiency due to decreased excretion **Falsely low** levels may be seen with delayed processing or insufficient cooling

16.2.4 Procollagens I (PICP, PINP)

Func:	~90% bone matrix proteins are type I collagen. Osteoblasts synthesize a precursor procollagen that is cleaved by specific proteases and releases PICP and PINP into the system. Cleavage of PICP is required for fibril formation. PINP may be retained (type I pN-collagen) **PICP:** Carboxy-terminal propeptide of type I procollagen (P1CP) **PINP:** Amino-terminal propeptide of type I procollagen (P1NP)
Ind:	Indirect marker of osteoblast activity: Limited specificity as a marker of bone formation: type I collagen is also synthesized in skin and connective tissue
Prod:	Both are equimolar to type I collagen. Varies slightly based on age and sex 20-105 ng/mL

↑ Osteoblast hyperactivity; any disorder with increased bone formation

Note: Falsely high levels possible in wound healing processes due to increased fibroblast activity

Higher stability against heat and degradation than other markers

16.3 Bone Resorption Markers

Func: Pyridinium crosslinks, hydroxyproline, acid phosphatase as markers of bone resorption

Bones are continuously remodeled through a process of bone formation and resorption. This helps keep normal structure and aids in mineral homeostasis (eg, Ca^{2+}). ~90% of the protein matrix of bone is type I collagen, crosslinked at the N- and C-terminal ends. Osteoclasts cause bone resorption by secreting a mixture of acid and neutral proteases thereby degrading the collagen fibrils into their molecular fragments

Ind: Tumor-induced bone destruction, monitoring of Paget's disease and osteoporosis

Mat: Serum (acid phosphatase)

24 h-urine (Pyridinium crosslinks, hydroxyproline - a collagen-free diet must be strictly adhered to)

Met: • Photometry: Hydroxyproline, total-acid phosphatase
• HPLC after acid hydrolysis (pyridinoline and deoxypyridinoline)
• Immunoassay: free deoxypyridinoline in the urine and blood

16.3.1 Pyridinium crosslinks (PyD, DPyD)

Func: ~90% of the protein matrix of bone is type I collagen, crosslinked at the N- and C-terminal ends. Pyridinoline are "crosslinks" of bone and cartilage collagen. Deoxypyridinoline is a specific "cross-link" from bone collagen

Ind: Monitoring anti-resorptive therapy (bisphosphonates, HRT); Diagnosis of conditions with increased bone turnover

↑ Osteoporosis, hyperparathyroidism, Paget's disease, bone metastases, multiple myeloma, Cushing's disease, acromegaly

Mat: Serum/plasma: ß-CrossLaps (fasting blood sample clock between 8-9 am)
Urine: Pyridinium Crosslinks (10 mL of the second morning urine, protected from light). No specific dietary requirements. Very pronounced diurnal rhythm - Spot urine samples should be obtained between midnight and 2:00 am

Met: HPLC, Immunoassay

Note: Increased pyridinoline with normal deoxypyridinoline may indicate increased degradation of non-bone collagen (cartilage, arthritis)

16.3.2 Hydroxyproline (OH-proline)

Func: Major component on collagen, important for stability (stereoelectronic effects) and allows the sharp twists of the protein helix. Produced from the hydroxylation of the amino acid proline by prolyl hydroxylase

Ind: Disorders of skin and musculoskeletal system (fairly specific for collagen in general, but not bone specifically)

Prod: Released in the degradation of type I collagen by osteoclasts

↑ High collagen or bone turnover - Paget's disease, multiple myeloma, primary hyperparathyroidism, osteoclast activity due to bone metastases (much higher than increase due to osteoclast activity by osteoblasts)

↓ Hypothyroidism, growth restriction, rickets, chronic connective tissue destruction

Note: Falsely high values: dermatological disorders, renal insufficiency, arthritis, hydroxyproline-rich food (gelatin, meat)
Only one-tenth of hydroxyproline will be protein bound and excreted in the urine. Free hydroxyproline is subject to tubular reabsorption

16.3.3 Tartrate resistant acid phosphatase (TRAP)

Func: Part of a group of isoenzymes (acid phosphatases) fairly specific for bone

Prod: Predominantly osteoclasts - particular the ruffled border, but also macrophages and neurons

↑ Diseases of increased osteoclastic activity, metabolic bone disease, osteoporosis, osteoclastoma, Gaucher's disease, hairy cell leukemia, HIV encephalopathy

Mat: Serum (be sure to avoid hemolysis or coagulation - but don't use heparin or oxalate tubes)

Note: **Falsely high levels:** Hemolysis (RBC-AP) or coagulation (platelet-AP)
Falsely low levels: Heparin and oxalate as anticoagulants (inhibition of AP)

16.3.4 Type-I collagen telopeptide (CTx)

Func: Collagen fibrils are linked via adjacent helical regions by the carboxy- and amino-terminal ends of the alpha 1 and alpha 2 AP. During osteoclast bone resorption the collagen fibrils are degraded into their molecular fragments including C-terminal telopeptide releasing the alpha form. In older bone, the alpha form of aspartic acid present in CTx converts to the beta form (beta-CTx), which then can serve as a specific marker of mature type I collagen degradation

ICTP: Carboxy-terminal networked type-I collagen

INTP: Amino-terminal networked type-I collagen

↑ Disease of increased bone resorption (eg, Paget's disease, bone metastasis, metabolic bone disorders, hyperparathyroidism)

Mat: 10 mL of a 24 h urine
Note: Random urine show marked fluctuation

16.4 Laboratory Findings

Bone disorders	Serum			Renal excretion		
	Ca^{2+}	P	AP	Ca^{2+}	P	OH-proline
Primary hyperparathyroidism	↑↑	Nl-↓	↑	Nl-↑		↑↑
Osteoclastic neoplasms (eg, myeloma/plasmacytoma)	↑	Nl-↑	Nl-↑	↑	Nl-↑	↑↑
Paget's disease	Nl-↑		↑↑			↑↑
Osteoporosis	Nl-↓		Nl-↑	↑		Nl-↓
Osteomalacia (malabsorption, vitamin-D-deficiency)	Nl-↓	Nl-↓	↑	Nl-↑	↓	Nl-↓
Osteomalacia (renal loss or insufficiency)	Nl-↓	↑	Nl-↑	↓	↓	Nl-↑
Osteoblastisc neoplasms	↓	Nl-↓	↑↑	Nl-↓	Nl-↓	↑

17　Hormones

17.1　Thyroid and Parathyroid

17.1.1　Thyroid stimulating hormone (TSH, Thyrotropin)

Func: A 2 subunit glycoprotein (related to FSH, hCG, LH via alpha subunit) that stimulates release of T_3 and T_4 from the thyroid and can lead to thyroid hypertrophy with chronic elevations. Useful in evaluating thyroid function and differentiating primary (thyroid) hypothyroidism (TSH ↑) from secondary (pituitary) and tertiary (hypothalamus) hypothyroidism (TSH ↓)

Ind: Suspected hypo- or hyperthyroidism; suspected TSH-producing pituitary adenomas; thyroid replacement monitoring

Prod: Synthesized in the anterior pituitary gland and released in response to TRH (synthesized in the hypothalamus and secreted into the bloodstream) and via negative feedback of fT_3 and fT_4

Norm: 0.3-5.0 mIU/L

↑
- Primary hypothyroidism: T_3 and T_4 ↓
- Secondary hyperthyroidism (rare): T_4 ↑

↓
- Primary hyperthyroidism: T_3 and T_4 ↑ (may be high nl)
- Secondary hypothyroidism: T_3 and T_4 ↓
- Tertiary hypothyroidism: T_3 ↓
- Medical suppression: T_3 and T_4 nl

Mat: Serum

Met: Immunoassay

Note: TSH will remain increased for several weeks with T_4 substitution, even if T_3 has reached euthyroid status. TSH will remain low for several weeks after treatment of hyperthyroidism, even if T_3 has reached euthyroid status. In primary hyperthyroidism a high-sensitivity TSH assay is used to detect the extremely low levels (sensitivity down to 0.002 mIU/L). Chronically ill patients may have falsely low or falsely normal levels. Some patients have circulating antibodies which can interfere with the assay

17.1.2 Thyroxine (T4)

Func: A prohormone for T3, primarily protein bound in the blood (~99.9%), therefore the proportion of free T4 (fT4), the biologically active form, is relatively low. Contains 4 iodine atoms

Ind: Suspected hypo- or hyperthyroidism (in conjunction with TSH), therapeutic monitoring

Prod: In the thyroid, secreted in response to TSH

Norm: • 5.0-12 mcg/dL Total
• 0.8-1.8 ng/dL Free

↑ Hyperthyroidism, high-dose thyroid replacement medication

↓ Hypothyroidism, anti-thyroid therapy (if T3 normal: euthyroid)

Mat: Serum

Met: Immunoassay

Note: fT4 better suited for monitoring and diagnosing thyroid disorders than total T4 if TBG is altered. T4 increases in hyperthyroidism before T3. False values may be seen with autoantibodies, heparin, or free fatty acids. Phenytoin competes for TBG bindings sites leading to an increased fT4

17.1.3 Triiodothyronine (T3)

Func: Main acting thyroid hormone (lower levels, but more active than T4), regulates many metabolic and neural actions; >99% is protein bound, <1% is free (fT3) and biologically active. Contains 3 iodine atoms

Ind: Total T3 used in suspected thyroid disorder (along with TSH and T4); fT3 is often a second or third order test to confirm thyroid dysfunction or if binding proteins are altered (pregnancy, hormone replacement, steroids, dysalbuminemia)

Norm: • 80-190 ng/dL Total
• 2-3.5 pg/mL Free

↑ Hyperthyroidism, thyroid replacement medication, T3 toxicosis

↓ Hypothyroidism, antithyroid therapy, chronically sick or hospitalized patients (sick euthyroid)

Mat: Serum

Met: Immunoassay

Note: Levels will be affected in binding globulin alterations. Levels are low in sick patients, so not a good marker for hypothyroidism on its own

17.1.4 Free thyroid hormone (fT3, fT4)

Func: Only free (unbound) thyroid hormones are biologically active

Ind: Suspicion of hypo- or hyperthyroidism

Norm: 2-3.5 pg/mL fT3
0.8-1.8 ng/dL fT4

↑ Hyperthyroidism

↓ Hypothyroidism

Mat: Serum

Met: Immunoassay

Note: The advantage of free hormone determination is the independence of binding globulin influences

17.1.5 Thyroid binding globulin (TBG)

Func: Transport protein for T3 and T4, along with thyroid binding prealbumin (TBPA) and thyroid binding albumin (TBA); >99% of total T3 and T4 protein bound
Thyroid gland will try to adjust hormone production accordingly for TBG levels

Ind: Suspected congenital TBG disorder; when total thyroid hormone levels do not correlate with clinical findings

Prod: In the liver

Norm: 13-30 mg/L

↑ Pregnancy, OCPs, hormone replacement, acute intermittent porphyria, genetic variance

↓ Liver disease, steroids/glucocorticoids, nephrotic syndrome, genetic variance

Mat: Serum

Met: Immunoassay

Note: Patient may be euthyroid with TBG deficiency and low total T4, or high TBG and total T4
The total T4/TBG quotient can help determine if elevations are compensated

17.1.6 Thyroid releasing hormone (TRH)

Func: Regulator for the biosynthesis and secretion of TSH

Ind: Suspected pituitary or hypothalamic insufficiency, suspected TSH secreting tumors, suspected hormone resistance, borderline thyroid dysfunction

Specific testing performed to test TSH secretion after TRH administration; TSH response is extreme in primary hypothyroidism, absent in secondary hypothyroidism, and delayed in tertiary hypothyroidism. Patients with primary hyperthyroidism do not respond to a TRH stimulation test

Prod: Hypothalamus

↑ **Increase <2 mIU/L:** missing or decreased TSH increase
- fT4 and T3 normal: Incipient thyroid autonomy/deferred hyperthyroidism, early form of Graves' disease, treatment with thyroid hormone preparations
- fT4 and T3 increases: Clinically evident hyperthyroidism or adequate treatment with thyroid hormone preparations
- fT4 and T3 decreased: Can indicate secondary hypothyroidism

Increase 2–25 mIU/L: TSH-increase
If fT4 and T3 are in the reference range, a pituitary-thyroid loop malfunction is excluded

Increase >25 mIU/L: an excessive TSH-increase
- fT4 and T3 normal: Latent hypothyroidism, iodine deficiency
- fT4 and T3 decreased: Hypothyroidism

Met: TRH administration → Detecting TSH-increase (∧-TSH)
1. Initial blood TSH concentration
2. TRH administration (dosage depends on the selected route):
   - IV: 200–400 mcg, re-check TSH after 30 min
   - Nasal: 2 mg, re-check TSH after 2 h
   - Oral: 40 mg, re-check TSH after 3–4 h

Note: Contraindicated: Known TRH hypersensitivity reaction
Specific TRH test rarely performed today due to improvements in determining TSH

17.1.7 Calcitonin

Func:
- Polypeptide hormone that helps **regulate blood calcium levels** by **reducing bone resorption** by osteoclasts; small role compared to PTH and vitamin D (not useful for diagnosis calcium metabolism disorders); **Reduces phosphate levels** in the blood by **inhibition of reabsorption** in the proximal kidney tubules
- ~30% of those with familial MTC syndromes (MEN II or fMTC) will have normal basal calcitonin levels, calcium infusion test will stimulate abnormality; though largely replaced by RET mutation identification
- After MTC tumor resection levels fall to undetectable within several weeks. Persistent elevation indicates incomplete excision (incomplete excision, lymph node or distant metastasis); and a new rise typically indicates recurrence (may be at surgical location or distant metastasis)

Ind: Suspected C-cell hyperplasia/medullary thyroid carcinoma (MTC), MEN II (Sipple's syndrome) or familial MTC syndrome (~95% have RET proto-oncogene mutations), pheochromocytoma, rarely islet cell tumors

Prod: Parafollicular C-cells of the thyroid gland, secretion stimulated by hypercalcemia, pentagastrin, GI tract hormones

Norm: Basal Levels:
<18 ng/L	Men
<10 ng/L	Women

Peak Calcium Infusion Test Levels:
≤130 ng/L	Men
≤90 ng/L	Women

↑ Benign: Renal failure, lymphocytic (Hashimoto) thyroiditis, hypercalcemia, hypergastrinemia, pregnancy

Malignant: **Medullary thyroid carcinoma**, neuroendocrine tumors (small cell carcinoma, carcinoid), pheochromocytoma, lung, breast or pancreatic carcinoma, Zollinger-Ellison syndrome, pernicious anemia

Mat: Serum/plasma

Met: Immunoassay

Note: Falsely high levels: renal impairment, calcitonin therapy, antibody interference

17.1.8 Parathyroid hormone (PTH)

Func:
- Polypeptide hormone with multiple forms, only 2 of which are metabolically active (those with N-terminus, whole molecule and PTH-N). ~90% of circulating total PTH is inactive PTH-C (half-life ~30 h). Active forms have half-lives of ~5 min
- Increases blood calcium levels via bone demineralization, increases calcium absorption in GI tract, increases calcium reabsorption in the kidney, and increases renal synthesis of 1,25-dihydroxy vitamin D which also increases GI tract calcium absorption
- Reduces blood phosphate levels by inhibiting reabsorption in the proximal kidney tubules
- Is also regulated by serum calcium level via a negative feedback loop
- **Hyperparathyroidism:** Hypercalcemia, hypophosphatemia, hypercalciuria, hyperphosphaturia, dehydration, renal stones, HTN, osteoporosis/bone lesions, possibly neuromuscular issues and altered mental status. Most often primary (adenoma). Also secondary and tertiary forms; and rare calcium receptor mutations leading to lack of feedback inhibition
- **Hypothyroidism:** Hypocalcemia - petechial, perioral tingling, weakness, tetany (Trousseau sign - carpal spasm with inflated blood pressure cuff; Chvostek's sign - facial spasm with zygomatic tapping), hyperactive reflexes, cardiac arrhythmias/intermittent prolonged QT/ Torsades de pointes. Most commonly due to surgical removal (thyroidectomy), but may be autoimmune, or rare aplasia or activating calcium receptor mutation

Ind: Disorders of calcium and phosphate metabolism (hyper-/hypocalcemia) suspected hyper-/hypoparathyroidism, renal insufficiency, nephrolithiasis, malabsorption, malnutrition

Prod: In the parathyroids (4 glands on the posterior thyroid); secretion stimulated by hypocalcemia; secretion inhibited by hypercalcemia and vitamin D; rapidly broken down in the blood and excreted in urine

Norm: 10-65 ng/L

↑	**Hyperparathyroidism:** Primary hyperparathyroidism (usually an adenoma, rarely hyperplasia, and very rarely parathyroid carcinoma) Secondary hyperparathyroidism (often due to renal failure, calcium and/or vitamin D-deficiency) Note: Renal failure: Elevations of 2-3x is 'normal' due to accumulation of PTH-C fragments
↓	Primary hypoparathyroidism (usually post-thyroidectomy, rarely autoimmune, aplasia [DiGeorge syndrome], calcium receptor mutation) Secondary hypoparathyroidism (usually due to malignant hypercalcemia, rarely excessive vitamin D, milk-alkali syndrome, hyperthyroidism)
Mat:	Serum/plasma; rapidly processed Note: Patients on high-dose biotin should wait at least 8 h after last dose
Met:	Immunoassay, electrochemical-illuminescence
Note:	An appropriately low PTH with hypercalcemia and hypophosphatemia suggest paraneoplastic parathyroid-related protein secretion (common N-terminus with active PTH) PTH secretion is inhibited by low Mg^{2+} levels, can mimic hypoparathyroidism Elevated PTH with low Ca^{2+} suggests PTH resistance/infectivity (if normal renal function) Test interference may occur with antibodies (circulating mouse antibodies, anti-ruthenium, or anti-steptavidin)

17.2   Adrenal Cortex

17.2.1   Cortisol

Func:	Steroid hormone, main glucocorticoid, acts like a gene transcription factor playing a role in metabolism vascular tone maintenance, suppresses immune system, stimulates gluconeogenesis, and elicits the stress response. Protein bound to transcortin (corticosteroid binding globulin, CBG), only free form is metabolically active

Cushing's syndrome: Cortisol increased; weight gain, 'moon' facies, buffalo hump, abdominal striae, hirsutism in women, hair loss in men, irritability, depression, memory and attention deficits, osteoporosis, diabetes, HTN, amenorrhea/decreased fertility, hypercholesterolemia; "Disease" refers to pituitary cause (ACTH producing adenoma), ~70% of non-medication induced cases; Can be distinguished from adrenal causes by measuring ACTH - lower in syndrome, higher in disease; may also be a paraneoplastic syndrome

Addison disease: Cortisol reduced (along with other steroid hormones); abdominal pain, weakness, fever, weight loss, nausea, vomiting, diarrhea, craving salty foods, hyperpigmentation (due to increased ACTH, not seen in secondary or tertiary); "Crisis:" marked hypotension, coma; chronic primary adrenal insufficiency (dysgenesis, autoimmune, infection, surgery); may be secondary - ACTH deficiency (pituitary) or tertiary - CRH deficiency (hypothalamic)

Ind:	Suspected hyper- or hypocortisolism
Prod:	Adrenal cortex (zona fasciculata), synthesized from cholesterol; secretion stimulated by corticotropin (ACTH - from pituitary [ACTH stimulated by CRH from hypothalamus]); negative feedback through hypothalamus/anterior pituitary loop; excreted by the kidney

Norm:

Serum	Total	
	5-20 µg/dL	Morning
	4-11 µg/dL	Late afternoon
	Free	
	0.1-1.8 µg/dL	Morning
	0.05-0.5 µg/dL	Late afternoon
Urine	Free	
	5-50 µg	24 h
	1-120 µg/g	Random

↑ Hypercortisolism (Cushing); pseudo-Cushing: alcohol abuse, pregnancy, drugs (cortisone, anticonvulsants); increased CBG (OCPs, hormone replacement), stress

↓ Adrenocortical insufficiency - may be primary, secondary (pituitary), or tertiary (hypothalamus), decreased cortical binding globulin (liver disease, hyperthyroidism, androgen therapy)

Mat: Serum/plasma; 24 h urine - preferred screening test for Cushing; limited use in adrenal insufficiency

Met: Immunoassay; liquid chromatography/mass spectrometry

17.2.2   Adrenocorticotropic hormone (ACTH, Corticotropin)

Func:
- A polypeptide hormone that stimulates the release of corticosteroids (cortisol) from the adrenal glands
- An elevated ACTH in hypocortisolism indicates primary adrenal insufficiency; however, a low ACTH would indicate a central cause (pituitary or hypothalamus)
- A low ACTH in hypercortisolism indicates adrenal primary, ectopic cortisol production, or medications; whereas a high ACTH indicates an ACTH or rare CRH secreting lesion
- Very rarely an ectopic ACTH is produced which is metabolically active but not detectable on the assay
- Has same precursor molecule as melanocyte stimulating hormone (MSH) leading to increased pigmentation with chronic elevation

Ind: Suspected adrenal insufficiency/hypocortisolism; hypercortisolism (DDx: ACTH-dependent vs. ACTH-independent)

Prod: Anterior pituitary; secretion stimulated by CRH from the hypothalamus; negative feedback by cortisol

Norm: 8–60 ng/L Morning

↑   ACTH secreting pituitary tumor (Cushing's disease), ectopic ACTH production (paraneoplastic syndrome), Addison's disease (primary adrenal insufficiency, loss of feedback inhibition), stress, CRH secreting tumor (paraneoplastic or hypothalamic - rare), pseudo-Cushing's: alcohol abuse, pregnancy

↓   Primary Cushing's syndrome (adrenal overproduction of cortisol), cortisol producing tumor, hypopituitarism, hypothalamic insufficiency (decreased CRH), OCPs

Mat: Serum/plasma, early morning (6–8 am)

Met: Radioimmunoassay

17.2.3   Dexamethasone suppression test

Func: An exogenous steroid that suppresses ACTH via negative feedback of the pituitary thereby suppressing cortisol secretion

Ind: Used to diagnosis specific type of hypercortisolism (Cushing's syndrome - primary adrenal vs. disease - pituitary)

Met: Both low-dose and high-dose variants; dexamethasone administered at night then cortisol is measured next morning

> **Low-dose:** 1-2 mg given, single dose
> Normal: Cortisol suppression
> Cushing's syndrome: Cortisol unchanged
> Cushing's disease: Cortisol unchanged

False negatives (lack of suppression) may be seen in morbid obesity, chronic renal failure, pregnancy, estrogen therapy, OCPs, severe depression or anxiety

> **High-dose:** 8 mg given over a day (2 mg q 6 h), or single 8 mg dose given at night (higher doses up to 32 mg are sometimes given)
> Normal: Cortisol suppression
> Cushing's syndrome: Cortisol unchanged
> Cushing's disease: Cortisol suppressed (negative feedback achieved), >90% of pituitary-based causes will decrease 50%
> Ectopic production: No cortisol or ACTH suppression

Dexamethasone suppression test		
ACTH	Cortisol	Most likely
↓	Not suppressed by low-or high-dose	Primary adrenal Cushing's syndrome
Nl-↑	Not suppressed by low-or high-dose	Ectopic ACTH
↑	Suppressed by high-dose, but not low	Cushing's disease (Pituitary, rarely hypothalamic)

17.2.4 Corticotropin releasing hormone test

Func:
- CRH is a polypeptide hormone that stimulates the secretion of ACTH (which, in turn, stimulates cortisol secretion)
- **Primary adrenal insufficiency:** High baseline ACTH which elevates after CRH administration; cortisol is low before and after
- **Secondary adrenal insufficiency:** Low baseline ACTH which does not elevate after CRH administration; cortisol levels are not affected
- **Tertiary adrenal insufficiency:** Low baseline ACTH which shows prolonged elevation in response to CRH administration, cortisol levels elevate
- Cushing's syndrome/ectopic ACTH: No response to CRH
- Cushing's disease: Elevation of ACTH and cortisol

Ind: Hyper- or hypocortisolism: differentiation between primary (adrenal), secondary (pituitary), and tertiary (hypothalamic); hypothalamic insufficiency

Prod: In the hypothalamus

Met: Serum/plasma levels of ACTH and cortisol are measured after CRH administration

Note: Expensive

17.2.5 ACTH test

Func: Clinical examination of adrenal cortical function by administering ACTH and determining corticosteroids in plasma and/or urine (especially serum cortisol, or 17-hydroxycorticosteroid in urine)
ACTH IV bolus leads to immediate increase in adrenal steroid biosynthesis by binding to its specific receptors in the adrenal cortex

Ind: **Suspected adrenocortical insufficiency or decreased responsiveness to ACTH**
Short ACTH Test:
1. Baseline blood levels obtained prior to testing
2. Administer 25 IU ACTH IV
3. Blood levels re-evaluated 1 h after injection
Long ACTH Test:
1. Baseline blood levels obtained prior to testing
2. Administer 50 IU ACTH IV over 8 h
3. Blood levels re-evaluated at 4, 6, and 8 h after the start of infusion
The long test shows limited benefit compared with the short test and is rarely performed
- Cortisol ↑↑: Patients with Cushing's syndrome
- Normal: Increase of cortisol levels to >200 µg/L excludes adrenal insufficiency
- No increase: Adrenal insufficiency, long-term hypopituitarism or steroid therapy, adrenal carcinoma

Note: **Care must be taken to avoid acute Addisonian crisis**

17.2.6 Adrenal androgens (DHEA, ANDRO)

Func:
- **Dehydroepiandrosterone (DHEA):** Steroid hormone produced from cholesterol. Weak androgen with a high rate of degradation. Primary precursor of natural estrogens. Total blood levels approximately 300-fold lower than that of the DHEAS
- **Dehydroepiandrosterone-sulfate (DHEA-S):** Sulfate ester of DHEA converted by sulfotransferase primarily in the adrenal glands, liver, and small intestines. ~300 x more abundant in blood than non-sulfated form. **Non-virilizing, no diurnal variation,** mainly dependent on the mechanism of sulfate synthesis
- **Androstenedione (ANDRO):** AKA 4-adrenostenedione, 17-ketoestosterone. Precursor to testosterone as well as estrone and estradiol. Sometimes used as athletic or body building supplement - banned by sport/Olympic organizations

Ind:
- **Suspected adrenal neoplasm**
- Hirsutism/virilism
- Androgen insensitivity syndromes
- Differentiating adrenal/ovarian testosterone increases

Prod: Zona reticularis of adrenal cortex (innermost layer)

↑
- DHEA/DHEA-S: Adrenal neoplasms (adenoma, carcinoma), hirsutism, virilization, obesity
- ANDRO: hirsutism, polycystic ovaries, androgen-producing tumors, pregnancy, adrenal hyperplasia, Cushing's syndrome, obesity

↓ Depends on the hormone: eg; hypopituitarism, exogenous glucocorticoid administration, adrenal insufficiency, ovarian failure

17.2.7 17-Hydroxyprogesterone

Func: Precursor of 21-hydroxylated steroids and interacts with progesterone receptors

Ind:
- Suspected steroid biosynthesis disorders, particular 21-hydroxylase
- Precocious puberty, virilization, hirsutism, growth disturbances
- Suspected androgen-producing tumors

Prod: Adrenal and ovary (corpus luteum); derived from progesterone via 17-hydroxylase or 17-hydroxypregnenolone

Norm: 20-100 ng/dL   Women - Follicular phase (pre-ovulation)
100-300 ng/dL   Women - Luteal phase (post-ovulation)
5-50 mg/dL   Women - Post-menopausal
10-200 ng/dL   Men
5-100 ng/dL   Prepubertal children
<700 ng/dL   Infants <28 days - normalize around 6 mos

↑   21-hydroxylase synthesis disorders, adrenocortical hyperplasia with hypercortisolism, pregnancy (third trimester)

17.2.8 11-Deoxycortisol (Cortodoxone)

Func: A steroid hormone involved in the synthesis of cortisol via 11-β-hydroxylase or oxygenation; can also be converted to androstenedione; also functions as a weak glucocorticoid

Ind:
• Suspected secondary or tertiary adrenal insufficiency
• Differentiating adreno-genital syndromes

Prod: Can be synthesized from 17-hydroxyprogesterone

↑   11-β-hydroxylase deficiency (leads to HTN), Cushing's
↓   Adrenal insufficiency

17.3 RAAS and ADH

Renin-angiotensin-aldosterone system and antidiuretic hormone

17.3.1 Renin (Angiotensinogenase)

Func:
• An important member enzyme of the renin-angiotensin-aldosterone system and thus the **regulator** of **blood pressure and water-electrolyte balance (blood volume)** leads to formation of angiotensin I
• Renin formation is increased in reduced kidney perfusion, sodium deficiency, sympathetic innervation and by various hormones

Ind:
• Differentiating hyperaldosteronism
• Suspected renal hypertension
• Differentiating hypokalemia

Prod: Juxtaglomerular apparatus of the kidneys

Norm:	Renin	Renin activity*
Lying:	3–19 ng/L	0.5–4 ng/mL/h
Upright:	5–40 ng/L	2–5-fold increase

* Highly affected by age and sodium status - higher levels in deficiency

↑
- Secondary hyperaldosteronism
- Renal artery stenosis (renal hypertension)
- Addison's disease (adrenal insufficiency)
- Bartter syndrome
- Renin-producing tumors (very rare)

↓
- Primary hyperaldosteronism (Conn's syndrome)
- Corticosteroid therapy
- Heavy black licorice consumption (Glycyrrhiza glabra root)

Mat: Serum/Plasma

Met:
- Direct measurement: Renin concentration
- Plasma renin activity: Detection of angiotensin I production

17.3.2 Aldosterone

Func: A mineralocorticoid synthesized primarily through the renin-angiotensin system; important in maintenance of blood volume via Na^+ absorption, K^+ secretion, water re-absorption in the renal tubules

Ind:
- Differentiating arterial hypertension, renovascular hypertension
- Primary or secondary hyperaldosteronism
- Sodium/potassium disorders
- Suspected Bartter syndrome

Prod: Zona glomerulosa of the adrenal cortex (outermost layer); released in response to volume depletion (hemorrhage, dehydration), hypotension, renal hypoperfusion, and hyponatremia; also ACTH, serotonin, thyroxine, ammonia, estrogens

Norm:	Serum
Lying down	29–145 ng/L
Upright	65–285 ng/L
	Urine
Normal diet	6–25 µg/24 h
Low-salt diet	17–44 µg/24 h
High-salt diet	0–6 µg/24 h

↑ Primary (Conn) and secondary hyperaldosteronism

↓
- **Primary hypoaldosteronism:**
  - Generalized adrenal insufficiency (Addison, Waterhouse-Friderichsen syndrome)
  - Isolated hypoaldosteronism and/or enzyme disorders (deficiencies in corticosteroid synthesis)
- **Secondary hypoaldosteronism:**
  - Suppression of the renin-angiotensin system (Liddle's syndrome, Pseudo-Conn's syndrome)
  - Suppression by iatrogenic glucocorticoids

Mat: Serum, heparin, plasma, 24-h-sammelurin

Met: RIA

Note: Measure between 8-9 am; discontinue ACE-inhibitors and diuretics (spironolactone) 2 wks prior to performing this test
- **Falsely low levels:** Inhibition of the RAAS by beta-blockers, central alpha-receptor agonists, antacids, corticosteroids
- **Falsely high levels:** Medications: stimulation of the RAAS by sympathomimetics, diuretics, and laxatives. EDTA-Plasma: 10%-20% may have non-specifically increased values

17.3.3 Angiotensin converting enzyme (ACE)

Func:
- **Peptidyl dipeptidase:** Key enzyme within the renin-angiotensin system: Conversion of **angiotensin I to angiotensin II, a more potent vasoconstrictor**
- **Inactivation of bradykinin vasodilatators:** While plasma ACE levels are not involved in these reactions, its pathophysiological importance is unclear. Increased ACE activities in the plasma are described in a number of diseases, in particular, **sarcoidosis**

Prod: Localized production by the luminal surface of the vascular endothelial cells, but also by cells of the mononuclear-phagocyte system

Ind:
- Suspected sarcoidosis
- Assessing the granulomas in sarcoidosis
- Monitoring of disease and therapy response prognostic testing in sarcoidosis

↑ 25% of all increased ACE levels can be attributed to: Gaucher disease, silicosis, asbestosis, hyperthyroidism, diabetes mellitus with retinopathy, cirrhosis of the liver, lymphangiomyomatosis, berrylliosis, chronic fatigue syndrome

↓   Possible dysfunction of the various microvasculatures, such as in the case of toxic lung damage or hypothyroidism. However, the significance of low serum ACE levels is not completely known

Mat: Serum, plasma

Disease	Aldosterone	Cortisol	Renin
Primary aldosteronism (Conn)	↑	NL	↓
Secondary aldosteronism	↑	NL	↑
Adrenal insufficiency (Addison)	↓	↓	↑
Hypercortisolism (Cushing)	↓	↑	↓

17.3.4 Renin-aldosterone-orthostatic-test

Func: Review of the sensitivity of the zona glomerulosa to angiotensin II

Ind: Diagnosis of **primary hyperaldosteronism** (Conn's syndrome)

Norm: **Increase of renin, aldosterone and 18-OH-B by 150%-300%** over basal levels

- **Adrenal adenoma:**
  - Increased aldosterone and 18-OH-B baseline levels
  - Renin values are low to low-normal
  - Under orthostatic increases in aldosterone, 18-OH-B and renin levels are resistant to decrease or increases in levels
- **Adrenal hyperplasia:**
  - Aldosterone levels are high-normal to increased
  - 18-OH-B levels are normal, renin levels are low to low-normal
  - Under orthostasis, there is a marked increase in aldosterone and 18-OH-B, with a slight increase in production of renin

Met: 1. Collect first sample at bedtime, 8 h before morning test
       2. Collect morning sample between 7-9 am to determine serum **renin, aldosterone**, and 18-OH-B levels
       3. Have patient **walk around for 2 h** without interruption, then collect another sample
       4. Re-determine the (stimulated) **renin, aldosterone**, and (sitting) **18-OH-B-levels**

Note: Antihypertensive medications such as beta-blockers, ACE-inhibitors, diuretics. Spironolactone can interfere with the test and should be discontinued 2 weeks prior

17.3.5 Captopril test

Func: Captopril is analogue of angiotensin I (the C-terminal end) with
competitive inhibition of the "converting enzymes" (ACE-inhibitor)
Measure the subsequently affected plasma aldosterone levels secondary
to a reduction of angiotensin II-concentration after administration of an
ACE-inhibitor

Ind:
- Differential diagnosis of primary versus secondary hyperaldosteronism
- Suspected renovascular hypertension (eg, renal artery stenosis),
  perfusion at a stenotic site within a vessel is correlated by higher
  renin levels

Res:
- **Primary hyperaldosteronism:** (Conn's syndrome)
  - Increased basal aldosterone levels
  - No suppression of aldosterone production 2 h after taking captopril
  - Renin secretion remains suppressed
- **Secondary hyperaldosteronism:**
  - Increased basal aldosterone levels
  - Significant waste of the aldosterone, concentration measured 2 h
    after taking captopril
- **Renovascular hypertension:** (renal artery stenosis)
  - Baseline renin and aldosterone concentration usually increases
  - Increase in the renin concentration on more than 200% of expected
- **Essential hypertension:**
  - No significant increase in renin concentrations (<150 %)

Met:
- Collect first sample at bedtime, 8 hours before morning test
- Collect next sample in the morning between 7-9 am to determine
  baseline renin and aldosterone concentrations
- Administer 25 mg captopril PO, before bed, the following night
- After 2 hours, measure the stimulated renin and aldosterone
  concentrations

Note: Do not take ACE inhibitors 2 weeks prior to the test

17.3.6 Antidiuretic hormone

ADH, Arginine vasopressin

Func: Peptide hormone: Nonapeptide with a S-S-bridge between the first and sixth cysteine residues
- **Antidiuretic effect:** increase in the permeability of the convoluted tubules and distal membranes for water, resulting in an antidiuretic effect via **increased absorption of water** from the distal tubules and collecting ducts
- **Vasopressor effect:** Arterial vasoconstriction → increase in blood pressure

Ind:
- Suspected **diabetes insipidus** (hypotonic polyuria)
- Suspected **Schwartz-Bartter syndrome** = SIADH (syndrome of inappropriate ADH secretion)

Prod: Synthesized in the **hypothalamus**, on the supraoptico-hypophysial tract within the neurohypophysis where it is then transported further downstream

Norm. <1.0 pg/mL

↑
- **Renal diabetes insipidus** (ADH receptor defect)
- Schwartz-Bartter syndrome **(SIADH)**
- Cirrhosis
- Drug stimulation of ADH release (nicotine, morphine, clofibrate, tricyclic antidepressants, vincristine, vinblastine, cyclophosphamide)

↓
- **Central diabetes insipidus**
- Pharmacological inhibition of ADH release (alcohol, phenytoin, chlorpromazine)
- Pregnancy (increased degradation within the placenta)
- Alcoholism
- Nephrotic syndrome

Mat: Serum/plasma

Met: Immunoassay

Note:
- Obtain venous access 30 min prior to sample collection
- When suspecting diabetes insipidus, do the water deprivation test to confirm diagnosis

17.3.7 Water deprivation test

Func: Examination of the concentrative renal function by stimulating ADH in the setting of dehydration

Ind:
- Confirmatory test for suspected diabetes insipidus (polyuria >5 L/24 h)
- DD diabetes insipidus vs polydipsia (eg, psychogenic)

In diabetes insipidus: Uosm <300 mosmol/L, while the plasma osmolarity increases >295 mosmol/L – In this case, do the desmopressin or ADH test

Norm: ADH secretion leading to increase in urine osmolarity
Positive test
- Weight loss >3%-5%
- Increases in serum sodium
- Spontaneous increase of voided urine osmolality is an indicator of adequate concentrating ability by the kidney

Distinguishing central and nephrogenic diabetes insipidus from psychogenic polydipsia: When performing a water deprivation tests, urine osmolality remains low. In central diabetes insipidus, ADH levels are low, but urine osmolality increases with administration of desmopressin

Met:
- Absolutely no drinking of liquids during the test
- Determine the basal levels: urine (osmolality, specific weight), serum (osmolality, sodium; chloride, glucose, hematocrit, ADH)
- Monitoring of vital signs during the test period
- Determining the values in the test: body weight, urine values (voided volume, osmolality, specific weight), serum values (osmolality, sodium). Optional serum values: urea, chloride, glucose, hematocrit, ADH)
- Collect for extended time intervals, usually at least 6 h, max 24 h

17.3.8 Desmopressin test (DDAVP test)

Func: 1-Desamino-8-D-Arginine-Vasopressin = desmopressin (the synthetic analogue of vasopressin)
Measure the increase in urine osmolarity after exogenous administration of ADH-like compound

Ind: Polyuria >5 L/h
Differentiating central, nephrogenic, and psychogenic diabetes insipidus

Met: 1. Fully empty the bladder
2. Give of 2 µg desmopressin IV (preferred) or 20 µg desmopressin nasal
3. Collect urine in 15 min
- Diabetes insipidus can be excluded in the water deprivation test. DDAVP not necessary
- Central diabetes insipidus: immediate decline of diuresis with increase in the urine osmolarity from <300 to >750 mosmol/kg
- Renal diabetes insipidus: unaffected by DDAVP. No change in urine osmolarity

17.3.9 Salt loading test

(Hickey-Hare test, or Carter-Robbins test)

Func: ADH stimulation with infusions with hypertonic sodium chloride with subsequent increase in serum osmolarity

Ind: Another test to distinguish central and nephrogenic diabetes insipidus

Norm: Decrease in urine output with subsequent concentration of the urine
- **Central diabetes insipidus** - ADH is missing
- **Renal diabetes insipidus, primary polydipsia** rapid increase in ADH until the physiological maximum value is reached

CI: Hypertension, congestive heart failure

Note: The salt loading test can also aid the diagnosis of **primary hyperaldosteronism:**
- Normal: Suppression of aldosterone in the serum/plasma to <85 ng/L
- No adequate suppression of aldosterone: primary hyperaldosteronism

17.4 Growth Hormone

17.4.1 Growth hormone (GH, Somatotropic hormone)

Func: **Essential for the normal vertical growth**
Decreased production leads to dwarfism. Increased production leads to acromegaly and/or gigantism
Used today by the food industry to stimulate protein synthesis, lipolysis, and gluconeogenesis

Ind:
- Detection of defects of growth hormone secretion
- DD of pituitary adenomas: Hypopituitarism, short stature, tall stature, gigantism, acromegaly, hypoglycemia
- Suspected ectopic GH, or GHRH-production (very rare)

Prod:	Synthesized by the alpha cells of the anterior pituitary, release regulated by somatotropin-releasing-factor (SRF = GRH, GRF) and somatostatin
Norm:	<4 µg/L Adults Higher values in infants and children Note: Reference range dependent on assay used
↑	Acromegaly, secretion pituitary adenomas
↓	Hypopituitarism
Mat:	Serum/Plasma
Met:	RIA and other assays
Note:	Falsely high results may be seen with stress and hypoglycemia Falsely low results may be seen in poorly controlled diabetes mellitus • Obtain venous access 30 min before blood collection • After approximately 20 min, measure growth hormone for 10 µg/L increases • Approximately 1 h after sleep, growth hormone should be over 15 µg/L

17.4.2 Growth hormone releasing hormone test (GHRH Test)

Func:	Measure GH response to the hypothalamic releasing hormone
Ind:	**Suspicion of GH-deficiency or anterior pituitary insufficiency** (usually in combination with deficiency in other hormones)
Met:	1. IV Access 30 min prior to start of test 2. Determination of the basal GH concentration at 0 and 30 min 3. GHRH injection (dosage: 1 µg/kg IV) 4. Measure GH levels after 15, 30, 45, 60, and 90 min after the injection
Res:	Norm: GH increase to >10 µg/L GH deficiency: less than normal increase in growth hormone (diagnosis is not exclusively made by this criteria)
Note:	Flushing may be seen with 20% of the patients

17.4.3 Oral glucose challenge

Func:	After glucose intake GH falls in normal subjects, often to <1 µg/L, within the first 60 min, and returns to normal when the blood sugar levels fall This complete suppression is absent in growth hormone excess
Ind:	**Suspected growth hormone excess** - autonomous secretion (acromegaly, gigantism)

Met: 1. Collect blood sample (determine baseline GH and glucose)
2. Administration of **75 g of glucose** in 400 mL of water PO
3. Collect samples after 30, 60, 90 and 120 min for determination of GH and glucose
Exclusion of autonomous GH secretion: Response is normal with GH <1 µg/L

17.4.4 Insulin hypoglycemia test (IHT)

Func: Hypoglycemia usually leads to an increase in growth hormone and ACTH secretion

Ind: • Suspected isolated **growth hormone deficiency**
• Suspected **ACTH deficiency**

Met: 1. 12 h fasting
2. Determination of GH and glucose 15 min and immediately before testing
3. Administer 0.1 IU short acting insulin per kg of body weight IV
4. Collect blood sample after 15, 30, 45, 60, 90 and 120 min to determine GH and glucose
The test is valid when blood glucose drops to 50% of the initial or below 40 mg/dL

Res: Growth hormone increase:
<5 mg/L: Growth hormone deficiency
5–10 mg/L: Partial growth hormone deficiency, severe or chronic underlying disease
>10 mg/L: No growth hormone deficiency

Note: Care must be taken to avoid hypoglycemic shock and appropriate measures (medical staff present, IV access) must be taken prior to testing

17.4.5 Arginine loading test

Func: GH stimulation test

Ind: Suspicion of growth hormone deficiency

Norm: GH increase to >10 µg/L or at least the 3- to 4-fold after 30–60 min

Met: 1. Establish IV access 30 min before the test
2. Measure GH levels 30 min and immediately before the start of test
3. Infusion of 0.5 g/kg L-arginine/HCl over 30 min
4. Measure GH concentration 30, 45, 60, 90, 120 min

17.5 Prolactin

17.5.1 Prolactin

Ind: Differential diagnosis of abnormal uterine bleeding, galactorrhea, hirsutism, hypogonadism in men

Prod: Primarily in the anterior pituitary gland; production increased from 8 weeks gestation with **direct effect on** the female **breast tissue and milk production**
Normally antagonized by prolactin inhibiting factor (PIF) from the hypothalamus - likely the same with dopamine

Norm: 3.0 -14.7 µg/L   Men
3.8 - 23.2 µg/L   Women, Luteal phase

↑   Prolactinoma, cerebral convulsions, PIF deficiency, functional hyperprolactinemia, severe renal impairment, drug effect, stress

↓   Hypopituitarism, overdose of dopamine agonists/prolactin-lowering agents

Mat: Serum/plasma

17.5.2 Metoclopramide test

Func: Diagnosis of the hyperprolactinemia due to the ability of **metoclopramide to release prolactin**
Perform this test under stress-free conditions and in the luteal phase (in women

Ind: **Latent hyperprolactinemia**

Norm: Increases are <200 µg/L with a normal baseline
- **Latent hyperprolactinemia:** increase >200 µg/L with a normal baseline
- **Overt hyperprolactinemia:** increase >200 mg/L in already elevated baseline

Met: 1. Blood sample for the determination of baseline prolactin levels
2. 10 mg metoclopramide on a venous access
3. Recheck prolactin levels after 25 min

Note: **Contraindications:** Severe renal impairment, methemoglobinemia
Side effects: Dizziness, transient hypotension, ataxia

17.5.3 TSH releasing hormone test (TRH test)

Func: Prolactin stimulation test via TRH

Ind: Borderline elevated prolactin levels suggest overt prolactin hypersecretion beyond latent hyperprolactinemia

Norm: Women before menopause: Prolactin increases at slightly higher levels
Men and postmenopausal women: lower increase in prolactin levels
- **Prolactin levels increase to the 2- to 5-fold: true increase; prolactinoma unlikely**
- **Missing prolactin increase response:** Suspicion of **prolactinoma, hyperthyroidism**, as well as suppression of thyroid hormones, glucocorticoids, and dopamine agonists

Met: 1. Establish IV access 15 min prior to start of test
2. Obtain samples for serum prolactin levels 10 min before and at the time of administration of TRH
3. Administer 200 µg TRH IV
4. Obtain sample for serum prolactin level 30 min after TRH administration

Note: The TRH-test to prolactin stimulation is less preferred over the metoclopramide test
Contraindications: Known hypersensitivity reaction to TRH
Side effects: Nausea, dizziness, abdominal pressure, sensation of warmth in the lower abdomen

17.6 Sex Hormones

17.6.1 17-Beta-estradiol (E2)

Func: The most potent endocrine estrogen of ovarian origin, mainly present in the maturing ovarian follicles under FSH stimulation
Main effects: endometrial proliferation, vaginal and breast tissue changes, prevention of osteoporosis, reduction of cardiovascular risk, and regulatory effect on pituitary gland and hypothalamus

Ind:
- Follow up with treatment for hormonally-induced sterility
- Assessment of ovarian disorders
- Tumor diagnostics (rare)

Norm:	30-300 ng/L	Women, Follicular phase
	100-600 ng/L	Women, Ovulation phase
	100 - 300 ng/L	Women, Luteal phase
	<10 ng/L	Women, Post-menopausal
	<55 ng/L	Men

↑ Peri-ovulatory phase, drug-induced polyovulations, excessive administration, estrogen producing tumors (granulosa cell tumors, thecoma)

↓ • **Primary ovarian failure:** Loss of endocrine ovarian function by functional or morphological changes of the ovary (eg, postmenopausal)
  • **Secondary ovarian failure:** Loss of time coordinated stimulation of the ovaries (eg, hypopituitarism, oral contraceptives)

17.6.2 Progesterone

Func: Steroid hormone important in the biosynthesis of corticosteroids and sex hormones; causes the **decidualization of the endometrium** in the luteal phase and maintains pregnancy

Ind: Ovulation detection, suspected tumors (hydatidiform moles, choriocarcinomas, thecomas)

Prod: Produced primary by the corpus luteum of the ovaries and in the placenta

Norm:	<1.5 µg/L	Women, Follicular phase; Men
	2.0-25 µg/L	Women, Luteal phase
	<1 µg/L	Women, Post-menopausal

↑ Ovarian tumors (thecoma, choriocarcinoma), hydatidiform mole, androgen insensitivity syndrome, hyperstimulation

↓ Ovulation disorders, hypogonadism

17.6.3 Luteinizing hormone (LH)

Func: Pituitary gonadotropin in **women, induces ovulation**
Serum LH levels are increased (LH peak) at 14 day of the menstrual cycle, preceding luteinization
In men: stimulation of the testicular supporting cells and regulation of testicular steroid biosynthesis

Ind: Women: Developmental disorders, DD of ovarian failure (hyper- or hypogonadotropism), determination of the LH mid-cycle
Men: Developmental disorders, DD of hypogonadism (hyper- or hypogonadotropism), infertility, disorders of spermatogenesis

Prod: Synthesized and released by the anterior pituitary, release stimulated by LH-releasing hormones from the hypothalamus

Norm:

3-15 IU/L	Women, Follicular phase
20-200 IU/L	Women, Ovulation phase
5-10 IU/L	Women, Luteal phase
>20 IU/L	Women, Post-menopausal
<15 IU/L	Men

↑   Women: Primary ovarian failure, pre-ovulatory gonadotropic disease, polycystic ovarian disease
       Men: Testosterone ↑: Androgen insensitivity
                 Testosterone ↓: Primary testicular insufficiency, hypergonadotropic hypogonadism

↓   Women: Secondary ovarian failure, ovulation inhibitors
       Men: Testosterone ↑: Exogenous testosterone intake
                 Testosterone ↓: Secondary testicular insufficiency, hypogonadotropic hypogonadism

17.6.4 Follicle stimulating hormone (FSH)

Func: A glycoprotein **required for follicular development and spermatogenesis**, as well as development of the seminiferous tubules; serum levels in men and women are roughly equal (Increases after menopause in women)

Ind: Women: Developmental disorders, ovarian failure, determination of menopause status
Men: Developmental disorders, differential of hypogonadism (hyper- or hypogonadotropism), infertility, disorders of spermatogenesis

Prod: In the anterior pituitary gland, stimulated by FSH-releasing hormone from the hypothalamus; excreted by the kidney

Norm:

2-10 IU/L	Women, Follicular phase
8-20 IU/L	Women, Ovulation phase
2-8 IU/L	Women, Luteal phase
>20 IU/L	Women, Post-menopausal
<15 IU/L	Men

↑   Women: Primary ovarian insufficiency
          Men: Primary hypergonadotropic hypogonadism, tubular damage,
          disorders of spermatogenesis

↓   Women: Secondary ovarian insufficiency, ovulation inhibitors
          Men: Secondary hypogonadotropic hypogonadism

17.6.5 Gonadotropin releasing hormone test (GnRH Test)

Func: GnRH is a peptide hormone formed in the infundibulum of the
hypothalamus; stimulates gonadotropin (LH and FSH) release from the
anterior pituitary (via the portal circuit); required for normal female and
male fertility; a primary decrease leads to a primary amenorrhea;
gonadotropin stimulation test

Ind:
- Differential of **hypogonadism** in men and women: hypothalamic vs.
  pituitary
- Differential of **pituitary adenomas** (endocrine active/inactive)
- Differential of low-normal and abnormally low gonadotropins
- Differential of late or precocious puberty

Norm:

LH Increase	FSH Increase	
>20 IU/L	5–10 IU/L	Women, Follicular phase
>40 IU/L	5–15 IU/L	Women, Ovulation phase
>30 IU/L	5–10 IU/L/L	Women, Luteal phase
2–4x	1.5–3x	Men

Baseline values within reference ranges, true increases in the baseline
levels after stimulation

- Pituitary insufficiency: missing and/or significantly reduced FSH and
  LH release
- Polycystic ovarian disease: Increased LH with normal FSH (increased
  LH:FSH ratio); Increased LH production after stimulation
- Defects of spermatogenesis: increase in FSH release
- Androgen deficiency in men: increase in LH release
- Hyperandrogenic ovarian failure: baseline and subsequent increase in
  LH
- Low FSH- and LH-production for the following disorders and after
  taking certain medications: Late puberty, anorexia nervosa,
  malnutrition, severe liver and renal impairment, drugs (such as
  anabolic steroids, H2-blocker, dopamine, and various psychotropics)

17.6.6 Human chorionic gonadotropin (HCG)

Func:
- **Stimulation of the corpus luteum to increase progesterone synthesis**
- The role of the HCG during gestation is primarily to preserve the function of the corpus luteum, preventing menstrual breakdown

Ind:
- **Detection of pregnancy, diagnosis of spontaneous abortion**
- **Germ cell tumors** (markers of testicular and ovarian tumors)
- **Trophoblastic tumors** (HCG levels increased 40%-80%)

Norm: <5 IU/L   Men and premenopausal women
<10 IU/L Postmenopausal women

↑ Pregnancy levels:
- 3 weeks: ≤50 IU/l
- 4 weeks: ≤400 IU/L
- 7 weeks: 5000-90000 IU/L
- 13 weeks: 40000-140000 IU/L
- Second trimester: 8000-100000 IU/L
- Third trimester: 5000-65000 IU/L
- Testicular tumors (seminomas, teratomas)
- Gestational trophoblastic disease (hydatidiform mole, choriocarcinoma)
- Extra-gonadal tumors (very rare, pancreas, breast)

↓
- Ectopic pregnancy (<80% with respect to the normal values of pregnancy)
- Imminent spontaneous abortion

Mat: **Serum**: increased as early as 1 week post-conception
Urine: increased as early as 2 weeks post-conception

Met: EIA

17.6.7 Alpha-fetoprotein (AFP)

Func: Fetal albumin, gradually replaced by adult human albumin after birth; glycoprotein of the alpha-1-group

Ind: Suspicion of neural tube defects, germ cell tumors, liver cirrhosis

Norm: ≤10 ng/mL

↑
- **Pregnancy**: Continuously, from conception to 24 weeks gestation, with continual rise until birth, then levels decrease
- **Prenatal diagnosis of neural tube defects** (high maternal serum and amniotic AFP)
- Ectopic pregnancy
- **Cirrhosis** and other liver disorders
- **Yolk sac tumors** (sensitivity of only 50%-80%)
- **Hepatocellular carcinoma**
- Renal insufficiency - postmenopausal women undergoing dialysis

Mat: Serum, pleural fluid, ascitic fluid, cerebrospinal fluid

Met: Immunoassay

17.6.8 Testosterone

Func: **Primary male sexual hormone, androgenic steroid hormone**
Primary physiological function: development of the primary and secondary sexual characteristics; anabolic effects on energy levels and libido

Ind: Primary testicular failure, congenital hypogonadism, secondary testicular insufficiency, impotence

Prod: In Leydig cells of the testes, ovary, and adrenal cortex

Norm:
2.5-9.5 µg/L   Men
0.5 -1.2 µg/L   Boys, prepubertal
<0.8 µg/L   Women

↑
Women: Adrenal or ovarian hyperandrogenism (eg, congenital adrenal hyperplasia, androgen insensitivity syndrome, Cushing's syndrome, polycystic ovary syndrome, ovarian tumors), androgen-producing adrenocortical carcinoma, precocious puberty
Men: Exogenous testosterone intake, androgen-producing testicular tumors, androgen resistance, androgen receptor defects, androgen-producing adrenocortical carcinoma

↓
Women: Primary and secondary gonadal insufficiency (prepubertal, postmenopausal), antiandrogenic medication, contraceptives, estrogen medication, Addison's disease, bilateral adrenalectomy, liver cirrhosis, drug abuse, anabolic steroids, severe malnutrition, anorexia

↓	**Men**: Primary hypergonadotropic hypogonadism (eg, anorchia, castration, Klinefelter's syndrome), secondary hypogonadotropic hypogonadism (hypopituitarism); prepubertal, anabolic steroids, synthetic androgens supplementation, liver cirrhosis, drug abuse, severe malnutrition, anorexia
Mat:	Serum/plasma; best measured in the morning
Met:	Immunoassay

17.6.9 Sex hormone binding globulin (SHBG)

Func:	**Transporter of testosterone in serum** (as well as other sex hormones including estrogens) - only 2% free testosterone in serum
Ind:	To study the shift in equilibrium between the free testosterone and bound testosterone, suspected androgen deficiency, and various gonadal disorders
Prod:	In the liver
Norm:	10-50 nmol/L Men
	20-140 nmol/L Women (non-pregnant)
↑	Testicular and ovarian tumors, pregnancy, estrogens, OCPs, cirrhosis, hyperthyroidism, virilism
↓	Hypothyroidism, Cushing's syndrome, hyperandrogenism, hyperprolactinemia, severe obesity, glucocorticoid administration
Mat:	Serum
Note:	Levels change with increasing age

17.6.10 HCG test

Func:	HCG stimulates (LH-like) Leydig cell testosterone production
Ind:	• Suspected **Leydig cell insufficiency,** assessment of the testicular secretory reserve
	• Differential of **undescended testis vs. anorchia**
	• Search for extraneous testicular tissue
Norm:	2-fold increase in testosterone levels:
	• Sub-normal increase: Limited function of Leydig cells
	• Very low baseline, lack of stimulation: Anorchia, impaired testosterone synthesis biofeedback
Met:	1. Measure baseline testosterone concentration
	2. Give 5,000 IU HCG IM
	3. Measure testosterone concentration at 48 h, and/or 72 h

17.7 Catecholamines, Serotonin, and Metabolites

17.7.1 Plasma catecholamines

Ind: Suspected **pheochromocytoma**

Norm: Under resting conditions
10-80 ng/L   Adrenaline
100-600 ng/L Noradrenaline
10-150 ng/L Dopamine
The normal ranges in children are approximately 50% lower

↑
- Increased sympathetic activity/high sympathetic tone, stress, hypoglycemia
- **Noradrenaline** >2000 pg/L at rest is highly suggestive of **pheochromocytoma**
- Predominantly elevated **dopamine** is highly suggestive of **neuroblastoma or malignant pheochromocytoma**

Mat: Serum/plasma

Met: HPLC, electrochemical detection
Obtain venous access 30 min before blood collection while patient is supine, then allow patient to sit up. Increases in the plasma catecholamine levels by 50%-100% may be seen

Note: The baseline measurement of plasma catecholamine concentration is less sensitive and specific than the 24 h urine concentration

17.7.2 Urine catecholamines

Ind: Suspected **catecholamine-producing tumor**

Norm: ≤ 27 μg/d   Adrenaline
≤ 97 μg/d   Noradrenaline
≤ 500 μg/d   Dopamine
Children are the low normal range

↑
- Catecholamine-producing tumors (eg, pheochromocytoma, neuroblastoma), highly likely if >3-fold increase
- Essential hypertension (up to 2- to 3-fold increase)
- Stress, physical stress, hypoglycemia

Mat: 24 h urine

Met: High-performance liquid chromatography (HPLC), electrochemical detection

17.7.3 Urine catecholamine metabolites

Func:
- **Vanillylmandelic acid (VMA):** Metabolite of adrenaline and noradrenaline
- **Homovanillinic acid (HVA):** Metabolite of dopamine

Ind:
- VMA: Adrenaline- and noradrenaline-secreting tumors (**pheochromocytoma**)
- HVA: Dopamine-secreting tumors (**neuroblastoma**)

Mat: 24 h urine

Note: Lower specificity and sensitivity than selective catecholamine testing

17.7.4 Clonidine test

Func: Clonidine inhibits the central sympathetic nervous system, **suppressing catecholamine release**

Ind: **Suspected pheochromocytoma (more specific than catecholamines in the urine)**

Norm: <50% fall in catecholamine levels after 3 h: pheochromocytoma unlikely
Pheochromocytoma: >90% fall in catecholamines (less reliable in non-catecholamine secreting tumors, such as primarily dopamine-secreting)

Met:
- Obtain venous access 30 min prior to start of test
- Measure baseline catecholamines within 10 min
- Administer 300 μg clonidine by mouth
- Measure catecholamines after 3 h, (optional: 1 and 2 h)

Note: **Contraindicated in hypotension**

17.7.5 5-Hydroxyindoleacetic acid (5-HIAA)

Ind:
- Suspected **neuroendocrine tumor (carcinoid)**
- Suspected 'carcinoid' syndrome - flushing, diarrhea, edema, asthma
- Therapeutic monitoring

Prod: Byproduct of serotonin metabolism

Norm: <8 mg/24 h
Carcinoid syndrome: >15 mg/24 h

↑ Neuroendocrine tumors, carcinoid syndrome

Mat: Urine

Note:
- Falsely high values may be seen in tryptophan/serotonin-containing foods (bananas, nuts, tomatoes, plums, pineapple, cocoa, nicotine, caffeine), medications (reserpine, amphetamines, acetaminophen/paracetamol)
- Falsely low values may be seen in renal impairment, alcohol, exposure of specimen to light, medications (ACEIs, MAOIs, L-dopa, methyldopa, imipramine, isoniazid)

17.7.6 Serotonin (5-hydroxytryptamine, 5-HT)

Func:	**Monoamine neurotransmitter:**

- ~90% of serotonin is located in the enterochromaffin cells of the GI tract - helps regulate intestinal movements
- Also present in platelets - helps with vasoconstriction and clotting

Ind:	Suspected **'carcinoid syndrome'**	
Prod:	Modified from the amino acid tryptophan	
Norm:	<2 µmol/L	Serum
	<1 µmol	24 h Urine
↑	Carcinoid syndrome	
Mat:	Serum, urine	

Note:
- **Falsely high values** may be seen with MAOIs, reserpine, nicotine
- **Falsely low values** may be seen with alcohol, L-dopa, methyldopa

17.7.7 5-Hydroxytryptophane (5-HTP)

Func:	The serotonin precursor molecule
Ind:	Suspected **'carcinoid syndrome'**
Prod:	From tryptophan
Norm:	<0.7 µmol/24 h
Mat:	Urine
Note:	**Neuroendocrine tumors**, in particular well-to-moderately-differentiated foregut types (carcinoid, atypical carcinoid), may lack dopa-decarboxylase resulting in an inability to convert 5-HTP into serotonin - leads to an increased 5-HTP and serotonin in blood and urine, due to platelet and kidney conversion, respectively. 5-HIAA is usually normal or borderline. Occasionally there are isolated 5-HTP increases

18 Blood Gas Analysis

18.1 Pulse Oximetry

Func: Transcutaneous hemoglobin saturation measurement (SaO_2); in healthy patient may be used to **estimate arterial pO_2**

Ind: Suspected unstable patient oxygenation. Typically done in ER's for initial evaluation, and on medical wards, ICU's, or during procedures to monitor patient's oxygen saturation
Evaluate need for/effectiveness of supplemental oxygen

Norm: 95%-99%
88%-94% COPD, hypoxic drive issues

Mat: A sensor placed on a part of the patient's body with thin epidermis (eg, fingertip, earlobe, or foot in infants)

Met: **Transmissive pulse oximetry:** Light of two wavelengths (red: 600-750 nm, infrared: 850-1000 nm) is passed through the patient and the changing absorbance at each wavelength is measured by a photodetector. Oxygenated hemoglobin (O_2Hb) absorbs more infrared and allows red to pass, whereas the opposite occurs for deoxygenated Hb. This measurement excludes venous blood, skin, bone, muscle, fat, and (in most cases) nail polish
Reflectance pulse oximetry: Does not require a thin epidermis so may be done on the feet, forehead and chest. However, there are limitations such as vasodilation and pooling of venous blood in the head due to compromised venous cardiac return (eg, congenital heart disease, Trendelenburg position), may cause a combination of arterial and venous pulsations in the forehead region and lead to falsely low SaO_2

Note: Used to monitor oxygenation, but cannot determine oxygen metabolism, CO_2, pH, or bicarbonate (HCO_3^-). Oxygen metabolism can be measured via expired CO_2 monitoring. Also, though it is possible to detect hypoventilation using pulse oximetry, this mechanism is impaired by supplemental oxygen
Falsely low levels: Incorrect sensor placement, hypoperfusion (vasoconstriction from cold temperature or vasopressors), or markedly callused skin
Falsely high levels: Hb has an ~200x higher affinity for carbon monoxide (CO) than O_2, but will 'read' as a high SaO_2 despite the patient actually being hypoxemic

Note:
- **Methemoglobin (metHb):** Hb with ferric (Fe_3^+) rather than ferrous (Fe_2^+) iron. The ferric form has a decreased oxygen binding ability, but this leads to an increased affinity for bound oxygen by the ferrous iron on the remaining heme molecules (tetrameric hemoglobin unit) leading to an overall reduced oxygen delivery to tissues. Treated with supplemental oxygen and methylene blue (1-2 mg/kg administered IV over 5 min followed by saline flush) restoring iron to its reduced state
- **Methemoglobinemia:** Congenital or acquired; levels >1%. Symptoms: 3%-15%: Slight skin and blood discoloration (pale, gray, blue); 15%-20%: Cyanosis, though patients often asymptomatic; 25%-50%: Headaches, dyspnea, lightheadedness, weakness, palpitations; 50%-70%: Abnormal cardiac rhythms, altered mental status, seizures, coma; >70% - Usually fatal
- **Circulatory insufficiency:** During decreased blood flow or anemia (decreased hemoglobin) tissues may suffer hypoxia despite normal oxygen saturation
- **Cyanide poisoning:** Reduces oxygen release from Hb. Reading is accurate, but tissue will become hypoxic

18.2 Arterial Blood Gas Analysis

Func:
Generally performed on arterial blood for the purpose of analyzing the partial pressure of oxygen (pO_2) and carbon dioxide (pCO_2), bicarbonate (HCO_3^-), acidity (pH), and often oxyhemoglobin saturation (SaO_2Hb - normal, ferrous, Fe^{2+}), carboxyhemoglobin ($SaCOHb$), and methemoglobin ($SaMetHb$ - cannot bind O_2, Ferric, Fe^{3+})
Acid-base balance: Normal pH is 7.35-7.45, a lower pH implies increased acid (acidosis, eg, CO_2), an increased pH implies increased base (alkalosis, eg, HCO_3^-). The respiratory system is one of the main ways that pH levels are maintained along with renal excretion and liver metabolism

Ind:
Often performed on critically ill patients, ICUs, to determine gas exchange across alveolar membranes and/or metabolic dysfunction. In cases of suspected acid-base disorder(s), used to determine the severity (compensated/decompensated) and the cause (metabolic/respiratory/combined)
- **Pulmonary disorders:**
    - Obstructive and restrictive ventilation impairment
    - Diseases of the lung, bronchi, alveoli

- **Metabolic disorders:**
  - Comatose states, fever, sepsis, intoxication, diabetes
  - Circulatory insufficiency
  - Renal failure, renal tubular disorders
  - Adrenal dysfunction
  - Electrolyte imbalance, particularly hypo-and hyperkalemia
  - GI disease with vomiting, diarrhea, gastric drainage
- **Basic tests:**
  - Blood Gas Analysis: pO_2, pCO_2, pH, HCO_3^-, base excess
  - Electrolytes: Na^+, K^+, Cl^-
- **Further work-up:**
  - Respiratory: Lactate, arteriovenous variation
  - Metabolic: Lactate, creatinine, urea

Mat:
- The most accurate results: **arterial blood** from the **brachial**, **radial** (most common) or **femoral** artery
- When arterial blood cannot be obtained, may use **capillary blood** (fingertip, earlobe, or heel stick) carried out under induced increased blood flow via warming or medical vasodilation, though values are not as accurate
- May be **performed on venous blood for comparison purposes**.
- May only use **heparin as anticoagulant**, because all other anticoagulants lead to changes in acid-base parameters
- **Syringe or capillary must be filled, free of air bubbles**

Met: pH, pO_2, and pCO_2 are measured using specific electrodes; HCO_3^- and oxygen saturation are calculated

Note: Contact with air may cause falsely high pO_2 and falsely low pCO_2

Normal adult values				
	Unit	Arterial	Venous	Interpretation
pH		7.35–7.45	7.35–7.43	pH <7.35: Acidemia pH >7.45: Alkalemia
H^+	nmol/L	35–45	43–50	H^+ >45: Acidemia H^+ <35: Alkalemia
pO_2	mmHg	75–100	36–44	Low PaO_2: Hypoxemia; PaO_2<60: Should give supplemental O_2; Note: A low PaO_2 is not required for the patient to be hypoxic
	kPa	10–13	4.8–6	
pCO_2	mmHg	35–45	37–50	Indicator of production/ elimination; during normal metabolism, determined solely by ventilation High pCO_2: hypercapnia/ respiratory acidosis: hypoventilation or hypermetabolic disorder Low pCO_2: Hypocapnia/ respiratory alkalosis: hyperventilation
	kPa	4.7–6.0	4.9–6.7	
HCO_3^-	mmol/L	21–26	21–28	Low HCO_3^-: Metabolic acidosis High HCO_3^-: Metabolic alkalosis
Base excess	mmol/L	-2 to +2.5	-2 to +2.5	A calculated value that isolates the non-respiratory portion of pH change; Used to assess metabolic acid-base disorders
tCO_2	mmol/L	22–30	22–30	Total CO_2 = (HCO_3^-) + (pCO_2 x 0.226 mmol/kPa)
SaO_2	%	95–99	70–80	Percent of Hb with bound O_2
CaO_2	mL/L	180–230	130–180	O_2 concentration: Amount dissolved in plasma and bound to Hb CaO_2 = (pO_2 x 0.003) + (SaO_2 x 1.34 x Hb)

18.3 Acid–Base Disorders

Acidemia: Blood pH <7.35
Acidosis: General term referring to a condition that leads to a decreased pH (though pH may be normal if mild disorder or if compensated)
Alkalemia: Blood pH >7.45
Alkalosis: General term referring to a condition that leads to an increased pH (though pH may be normal if mild disorder or if compensated)
Respiratory acidosis: pCO_2 >45 mmHg; CO_2 acts as a weak acid (carbonic acid) and can affect pH in large concentrations
Hypoventilation/poor pulmonary circulation causes retention of CO_2 by the lungs (ie, ↑ CO_2) leading to ↓ pH; Initially, this change will be buffered by plasma proteins, but the body will then try to maintain pH balance by increasing respiratory rate (tachypnea) if possible or by metabolic means
Respiratory alkalosis: pCO_2 <35 mmHg; Hyperventilation causes ↓ CO_2 leading to ↑ pH
Note: Care must be taken during mechanical ventilation to not over (hyper) or under (hypo) ventilate the patient
Metabolic acidosis: Caused by an increase in acid or a loss of base; all metabolic acidotic disorders have ↓ HCO_3^- and ↓ base excess leading to ↓ pH
Mechanisms include:
• Excessive formation of keto or lactic acids
• Reduced renal excretion of H^+
• Increased GI base loss (diarrhea)
The body will try to compensate by adjusting the respiratory rate accordingly, but oftentimes it is not sufficient for the level of disruption
Metabolic alkalosis: Caused by an increase in base or a loss of acid; all metabolic alkalotic disorders have ↑HCO_3^- and ↑ base excess leading to ↑pH
Mechanisms include:
• Addition of base through bicarbonate salts or metabolizable acids
• Renal tubular function disruption by diuretics, potassium deficiency, mineralocorticoids
• GI acid loss (vomiting)

Compensation: The respiratory pathway will try to compensate for pH change within a matter of hours (2-4); however, if this mechanism is not enough, then metabolic mechanisms ensue

A simple disorder is when there is only one primary acid-base disturbance with or without associated compensation

- Compensation of primary respiratory disorders involves alterations of renal excretion of HCO_3^-
- Compensation of primary metabolic disorders involves alterations of pulmonary excretion of CO_2 via respiratory rate

A complex disorder involves several acid-base disturbances, typically without compensation

Bicarbonate: HCO_3^-; a base that helps buffer excess H+ in acidemia; As a part of metabolic compensation it takes hours to several days to take effect. Thus when an ABG reveals an elevated HCO3- the problem has most likely been present at least several days

In respiratory acidosis HCO_3^- levels rise, in order to neutralize the excess acid; the opposite happens in respiratory alkalosis

Note: In a patient with a normal pH, $\uparrow CO_2$, and $\uparrow HCO_3^-$ there is full compensation. The **CO_2 must be lowered slowly** to avoid a metabolic alkalosis and a decrease in respiratory drive ($\rightarrow$ decreased pO_2)

- As a general rule of thumb **"metabolically together"**: Meaning in **metabolic disturbances** the **changes of pH, HCO_3^-, and pCO_2** are in the **same direction**
- Compensation is not possible in combined respiratory/metabolic acidosis or combined respiratory/metabolic alkalosis

Acid homeostasis: Based on the Henderson-Hasselbach equation. The body will try to maintain a normal pH by varying this equation. pK is a constant (6.1), base is typically HCO_3^-, acid is PaCO_2, the ratio of these must be maintained at ~ 20:1

Note: Should technically include K^+, but concentrations are so low in comparison to Na^+ the difference is infinitesimal

$$pH = pK + log\ (base/acid)$$
$$pH = 6.1 + log\ (HCO_3^-/dissolved\ CO_2)$$

Anion gap:

Func: The calculated difference between cations and anions in the serum. This gap helps to identify the cause of the metabolic acidosis

$$Anion\ gap = Na^+ - (Cl^- + HCO_3^-)$$

Norm: <12 mEq/L

Hyperchloremic metabolic acidosis: Patients with a normal anion gap often have a decreased HCO_3^- as the primary etiology, as Cl^- is the other major anion this leads to Cl^- elevation

Normal anion gap: FUSEDCARS: **F**istula (pancreatic), **U**retero-enterostomy, **S**aline administration, **E**ndocrine (hyperparathyroidism), **D**iarrhea (vomiting causes hypochloremic alkalosis), **C**arbonic anhydrase inhibitors (acetazolamide), **A**mmonium chloride, **R**enal tubular acidosis, **S**pironolactone; also TPN, Addison's disease, alcoholic ketoacidosis (if combined with metabolic alkalosis)

Increased anion gap: MUDPILES: **M**ethanol, **U**remia (renal failure), **K**etoacidosis (**D**iabetic, EtOH – unless combined with metabolic alkalosis), **P**araldehyde/**P**ropylene glycol, **L**actic Acidosis, **E**thylene glycol, **S**alicylate (aspirin), also iron, isoniazid, cyanide, and rhabdomyolysis

Falsely low anion gap: Hemorrhage, nephrotic syndrome, intestinal obstruction, cirrhosis, multiple myeloma with paraproteinemia

Hypoalbuminemia– albumin is negatively charged and leads to retention of the other anions when it is decreased, therefore for every 1 g/dL drop in albumin there is a 2.5 mEq change in anion gap (correct for albumin if levels are abnormal **[+ 2.5 (4 – albumin)]**

Osmolal gap: The difference between measured serum osmolality and calculated serum osmolarity

Osmolal gap = Osm (measured) − $(2Na^+ + Glu/18 + BUN/2.8)$

Algorithm for simple disorders

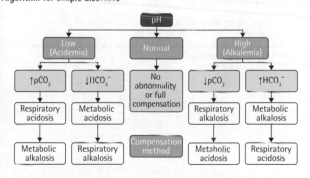

Acid base normogram

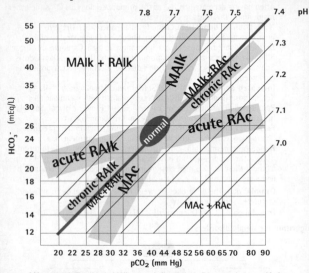

MAc = metabolic acidosis, MAlk = metabolic alkalosis, RAc = respiratory acidosis, RAlk = respiratory alkalosis

Alkalosis					pH normal			Acidosis				
pCO_2 or HCO_3^- normal?					pCO_2 or HCO_3^- normal?			pCO_2 or HCO_3^- normal?				
Yes		No			Yes	No		Yes		No		
CO_2 ~ BiC ↑	BiC ~ CO_2 ↓	BiC ↑ CO_2 ↑	BiC ↑ CO_2 ↓	CO_2 ↓ BiC ↓	NI	BiC ↓ CO_2 ↓	CO_2 ↑ BiC ↑	CO_2 ~ BiC ↓	BiC ~ CO_2 ↑	BiC ↓ CO_2 ↓	BiC ↓ CO_2 ↑	CO_2 ↑ BiC ↑
Met. alk.	Resp. alk.	Met. alk.	Met. + resp. alk.	Resp. alk.	Nls	Met. acid. or resp. alk.	Resp. acid. or met. alk.	Met. acid.	R-Ac.	Met. acid.	Met. + resp. acid.	Resp. acid.
-	-	Part comp	CDO	Part comp	-	Full compensation		-	-	Part comp.	CDO	Part comp.

	HCO_3^- ↓	HCO_3^- normal	HCO_3^- ↑
pCO_2 ↑	Combined metabolic and respiratory acidosis	Respiratory acidosis	Metabolic alkalosis and respiratory acidosis
pCO_2 normal	Metabolic acidosis	Normal	Metabolic alkalosis
pCO_2 ↓	Metabolic acidosis and respiratory alkalosis	Respiratory alkalosis	Combined metabolic and respiratory alkalosis

	pH	pCO_2	HCO_3^-	BE
Met. acidosis	↓ - Normal	Normal - ↓	↓	Negative
Met. alkalosis	↑ - Normal	Normal - ↑	↑	Positive
Respiratory acidosis	↓ - Normal	↑	Normal - ↑	Positive
Respiratory alkalosis	↑ - Normal	↓	Normal - ↓	Negative

Metabolic acidosis	
Increased anion gap (>12)	**Normal anion gap (<12)**
Methanol	Carbonic anhydrase inhibitors
Uremia	Saline IV rehydration
Ketoacidosis	GI (pancreatic fistulas, diarrhea)
Propylene glycol/paraldehyde	Ammonium chloride (NH_4Cl)
Lactic acidosis	Total parenteral nutrition
Ethylene glycol	Renal tubular acidosis (RTA)
Salicylates	Uterostomy
Cyanide	Spironolactone
Isoniazid	Addison's disease
Rhabdomyolysis	Hyperparathyroidism
Increased osmolar gap	
Increased anion gap (>12)	**Normal anion gap (<12)**
Methanol	Isopropyl alcohol
Ethylene/propylene glycol	Mannitol/sorbitol/glycerol
Paraldehyde	Acetone
+/- Ethanol	+/- Ethanol

19 Antibodies

Suspected disorder	Antibody(ies)	Explanation
Autoimmune hemolytic anemia (AIHA)	Anti-erythrocyte	Warm and cold erythrocyte Ab
Chronic active hepatitis	SMA ("classical CAH") ANA LKM SLA AMA	Smooth muscle antibodies" Antinuclear Ab Liver-kidney microsomal Ab Soluble liver antigen Ab Anti-mitochondrial Ab
Chronic polyarthritis	RF	Rheumatoid factor (IgM against IgG)
Ulcerative colitis	pANCA	Perinuclear anti-neutrophil Cytoplasmic Ab (Myeloperoxidase)
Diabetes mellitus Type I	ICA IAA GADA IA-2A	Islet cell Ab (80%) Insulin Ab (30%-100%) Glutamate decarboxylase Ab (70%-80%) Tyrosine phosphatase IA-2A Ab (50%-70%)
Dressler's syndrome	Anti-myocardial	Autoimmune pericarditis, typically post MI
Dermatitis herpetiformis	Anti-reticulin Anti-gliadin Anti-endomysium	Dermatitis, often associated with (subclinical) gluten sensitive enteropathy (90%)
Gluten sensitive enteropathy	Anti-gliadin Anti-endomysium	IgA-gliadin Ab IgA-endomysium Ab
Anti-glomerular basement membrane disease (Goodpasture syndrome)	GBM	Anti-glomerular basement membrane
Lymphocytic thyroiditis (Hashimoto)	Anti-TPO Anti-TG Anti-TSHr	Microsomal Ab (95%) Thyroglobulin Ab (70%) TSH receptor Ab (≤10%)

Suspected disorder	Antibody(ies)	Explanation
Graves' disease	Anti-TSHr	TSH receptor Ab (active: 80%-100%, remission: 10%-30%)
	Anti TPO	Microsomal Ab (60%-70%)
	Anti-TG	Thyroglobulin Ab (10%-20%)
Immune thrombocytopenic purpura (ITP)	Anti-platelet	Platelet membrane glycoproteins IIb/IIIa or Ib/IX Ab
Addison's disease	Anti-21-hydrolylase	Adrenocortical Ab (Autoimmune cases)
Lambert-Eaton syndrome	Anti-Ca^{2+} channel	Presynaptic disorder of ACh release
Myasthenia gravis	AchR	Acetylcholine receptor Ab
	SKM	Skeletal muscle Ab
Polyarteritis nodosa	pANCA	Perinuclear anti-neutrophil Cytoplasmic Ab (Myeloperoxidase)
Primary biliary cirrhosis	AMA	Antimitochondrial Ab
Pemphigus vulgaris	EICA	Epidermal intercellular Substance Ab (Desmoglein)
Pemphigoid	EBMA	Epidermal basement membrane Ab
Pernicious anemia	PCA	Parietal cell Ab
	IFA	Intrinsic factor Ab
Polymyositis/ Dermatomyositis	ANA	Antinuclear Ab (50%)
	Jo1	Histidyl tRNA synthetase Ab (54%)
	PM1	ANA subtype: non-histone protein
	SKM	Skeletal muscle Ab
	Mi2	PM 10%, 20% DM

Suspected disorder	Antibody(ies)	Explanation
Primary Sjögren syndrome	ANA	Antinuclear Ab
	SS-A (= Ro)	Soluble substance A = Robert Antigen
	SS-B (= La)	Soluble substance B = Lane Antigen
Progressive systemic scleroderma (PSS – Diffuse, limited – CREST syndrome)	ANA	Antinuclear Ab
	ACA	Anticentromere Ab (70%; no SCL-70)
	SCL-70	Anti-topoisomerase Ab (40%)
Rheumatic fever –Skin, tonsillitis, renal and/or cardiac involvement	ASL/ASO	Antistreptolysin-O Ab
	Anti-Hyaluronidase	
	ADB	Anti-DNAse B Ab
	ASA	Anti-sarcolemmal Ab (Tropomyosin, Myosin)
SHARP syndrome	ANA	Antinuclear Ab
	U1RNP	Ribonucleoprotein-Ab
Systemic lupus erythematosus (SLE)	ANA	Antinuclear Ab (95%)
	Anti-dsDNA	Double stranded DNA Ab (60%-90%)
	Anti-Sm	Ribonucleoprotein-Ab (Smith antigen)
	Anti-Histone	Histone Ab
	APA (ACLA, LA)	Anti-phospholipid Ab (Anticardiolipin, Lupus Anticoagulant)
Pseudo lupus	AMA	Anti-mitochondrial Ab
Drug-induced lupus	Anti-Histone	Histone Ab
Gastritis type A	PCA	Parietal cell Ab
Granulomatosis with polyangiitis (Wegner's granulomatosis)	Anti-Histone	Histone Ab

Suspected disorder	Antibody(ies)	Explanation
Vitiligo	Anti-melanocyte	Antinuclear Ab (95%) Double stranded DNA Ab (60%-90%) Ribonucleoprotein-Ab (Smith antigen) Histone Ab Anti-phospholipid Ab (Anticardiolipin, Lupus anticoagulant)

19.1 Antibodies in Detail

Antinuclear antibodies (ANA)

The group includes all of the auto-Ab against nuclear antigens in the cell nucleus

Ind	Autoimmune disease, rheumatic disease; serositis (eg, pericarditis, pleuritis), recurrent thrombophlebitis, recurrent spontaneous abortion, unexplained fever			
↑	Positive ANA results indicate an autoimmune disease - the higher the titers→ more likely			
	Systemic lupus	95%	Autoimmune hepatitis	60%-100%
	Drug-induced lupus	95%	Primary biliary cirrhosis (PBC)	40%
	Cutaneous lupus	20%-60%	Viral hepatitis	30%
	SHARP syndrome	95%	Alcoholic cirrhosis	30%
	Limited systemic scleroderma (CREST syndrome)	95%	Alveolitis/ pulmonary fibrosis	20%-60%
	Sjögren syndrome	50%-95%	Thyroiditis	20%-40%
	Polyarteritis nodosa	20%	Leukemia	30%-70%

↑ (cont.)	Autoimmune hemolytic anemia	50%	Malaria	30%
	Felty's syndrome	60%-95%	Pregnancy	<10%
	Rheumatoid arthritis	20%-50%	Pregnancy with complications	0%-50%
	Norm <60 years	≤8%	Norm >60 years	≤30%
Ø	A negative titer makes many autoimmune disorders unlikely (eg, systemic lupus erythematosus, other connective tissue diseases).			
False	False negative: Immunosuppressive therapy			

Double stranded DNA antibody (dsDNA Ab)

Ind	• Systemic lupus erythematosus (practically diagnostic of SLE) • Suspected SLE and negative screening on ANA (rare)
↑	• Systemic lupus erythematosus in the active stage - 70%-95%, esp with nephritis • Rarely other immunopathies: RA - usually treatment related, Viral - HIV, parvo-B19, BK; transient, myeloma, autoimmune hepatitis
Ø	• Healthy normal subjects: no detectable anti-dsDNA • No evidence of anti-dsDNA in drug induced LE

Single stranded DNA antibody (ssDNA Ab)

Ind:	Drug-induced lupus Juvenile rheumatoid arthritis Suspected collagen vascular disease
↑	• In general, relatively low diagnostic significance • An interesting feature of ANA-negative tissue diseases: ssDNA Ab 10%-20% • Active lupus (>80%) • Drug-induced lupus • Juvenile rheumatoid arthritis (35%-50%) • Autoimmune hepatitis, almost all collagen vascular diseases
False	False positive: inflammatory processes, tumors

Extractable nuclear antigens (ENA)

Ind	• Drug-induced lupus
	• Juvenile rheumatoid arthritis
	• Suspected collagen vascular disease
↑	• In general, relatively low diagnostic significance
	• An interesting feature of ANA-negative tissue diseases: ssDNA Ab 10%–20%
	• Active lupus (>80%)
	• Drug-induced lupus
	• Juvenile rheumatoid arthritis (35%–50%)
	• Autoimmune hepatitis, almost all collagen vascular diseases
False	False positive: inflammatory processes, tumors

ENA subgroups:

Anti-Sm Ab	
Smith antibodies are directed against small nuclear ribonucleoproteins whose function is to "splice" the primary RNA transcripts into mature messenger RNA	
Ind	• Suspected systemic lupus erythematosus
	• Differentiation of ANA with coarsely granular or speckled fluorescence pattern
↑	SLE
Note	Sm-Ab are largely specific to SLE, however, the diagnostic sensitivity is 10%–30% lower

U1-snRNP Ab	
Antibody against small nuclear ribonucleoprotein particle	
Ind	• Suspected connective tissue disease (esp. MCTD, SHARP syndrome)
	• Also, SLE, systemic sclerosis, rheumatoid arthritis, polymyositis
↑	• Mixed connective tissue disease (U1-snRNP Ab obligatory)
	• SLE (25%–40%, often with Anti-Sm Ab)
Note	In contrast to Anti-Sm Ab, U1-RNP antibodies recognize only the class U1-snRNP

Anti-SSA Ab

Anti-Ro antibody (Robert antigen, named after prototype patient Robert)

Ind	• Suspected primary or secondary Sjögren's syndrome • Suspected SLE (even in the absence of detection of ANA) • Suspected subcutaneous/cutaneous lupus • Suspected congenital heart block/neonatal lupus
↑	Sjögren's syndrome (65%), systemic LE (35%), Scleroderma (25%), SHARP syndrome (60%)
Note	Anti-SSA Ab can cross placenta→ associated with severe congenital cardiac disorder

Anti-SSB Ab

Anti-La Ab (Lane antigen, named after prototype patient Lane)

Ind	• Suspected primary Sjögren's syndrome • Suspected SLE • Suspected congenital heart block/neonatal lupus
↑	Sjögren's syndrome (65%), systemic LE (15%)

Anti-SCL 70 Ab

Antibody against DNA topoisomerase I

Ind	• Suspected systemic sclerosis • Subtyping and prognostic assessment in systemic sclerosis or scleroderma associated early symptoms • Differentiation of ANA with associated fine granular, chromosomal fluorescence patterns
↑	Progressive systemic sclerosis (70%), limited systemic sclerosis (CREST syndrome - 20%)
Note	• Occur most often in variants of scleroderma • Antibodies against SCL70 and centromere should both be determined

ACA

Anti-centromere antibody

Ind	• Antibodies against the centromere region of chromosomes • Are mainly directed against 3 proteins: CENP-A, CENP-B, CENP-C • Most affected patients respond with at least 2 of these antigens, and almost always CENP-B

ACA (cont.)	
↑ (cont.)	• Suspected systemic sclerosis or CREST syndrome • Subtyping and prognostic assessment in systemic sclerosis or early scleroderma associated symptoms such as such as the Raynaud phenomenon
Note	In limited systemic sclerosis (CREST syndrome) Ab detection in 40%-80% (especially interesting because anti-SCL-70 Ab are often negative)

Anti- histone Ab	
Ind	• Suspected drug-induced lupus • Suspected systemic lupus • Differentiate chromosome-associated antinuclear antibodies
↑	Drug-induced LE (95%), systemic LE (30%), rheumatoid arthritis (15%)

Anti-PM/SCL Ab	
Antibody against polymyositis/scleroderma antigen	
Nuclear complex of 11-16 polypeptides of unknown function	
Ind	• Suspected systemic sclerosis • Suspected poly- or dermatomyositis • Suspected scleroderma and Myositis-overlap syndrome • Differentiation of ANA with homogeneous, nucleolar fluorescence pattern
↑	Especially in polymyositis-scleroderma overlap syndrome

ACPA	
Anti-cytoplasmic antibodies	
Ind	• Polymyositis, dermatomyositis, DD: Rheumatoid arthritis with associated polymyositis or dermatomyositis • Anti-synthetase syndrome (sub-form of polymyositis)
↑	**Jo-1 Ab:** Auto-antibodies to histidyl-tRNA synthetase (polymyositis - 54%, dermatomyositis - 40%, myositis - 6%, and other collagen diseases; over 50% of the Jo-1 positive patients have or develop an interstitial pulmonary fibrosis) **Non-Jo-1 Ab:** Auto-antibody to aminoacyl-tRNA synthetase (dermatomyositis > polymyositis; myositis, pneumonitis, interstitial lung disease, Raynaud's syndrome, arthritis)

APA		
Anti-phospholipid antibodies		
Heterogeneous group of autoreactive immunoglobulins: including lupus anticoagulant, anti-cardiolipin, anti-beta-2-glycoprotein I (β2-GPI)		
Ind	• Suspected primary antiphospholipid syndrome • Suspected SLE • Recurrent spontaneous abortions • Unexplained thrombembolic events • Unexplained thrombocytopenia • Unexplained prolonged activated PTT • Suspected secondary anti-phospholipid syndrome (in SLE and collagen vascular disorders)	
↑	**Anti-phospholipid syndrome (APLS)** • Disease with recurrent arterial and venous thrombosis, spontaneous abortion, and thrombocytopenia with simultaneous detection of persistently elevated anti-phospholipid antibody titers • Increases are also found in **collagen disorders, malignancies, hematopoietic system diseases, multiple sclerosis, myasthenia gravis, and temporarily after viral and bacterial infections**	
Note	Laboratory diagnosis when there is a suspicion of anti-phospholipid syndrome: • Lupus Anticoagulant; Different phospholipid-dependent screening tests with associated confirmatory tests should be performed; Russell's viper venom time (RVVT), clotting time, or a lupus-sensitive PTT • Anti-cardiolipin (IgG, IgM): Important autoantibodies in antiphospholipid syndrome • Anti-Beta-2-glycoprotein I (IgG, IgM): A cofactor of anti-cardiolipin Ab; In a small proportion of patients only anti-beta-2-GPI Ab detected Anti-phospholipid antibodies are also encountered in 5% of healthy normal population, however, usually remain asymptomatic. In case of positive results, laboratory analysis needs to be repeated every 4-6 weeks in order to clarify whether persistently increased autoantibody titers are present	

ANCA	
Antineutrophil cytoplasmic antibodies	
Ind	Suspicion of primary vasculitis
↑	• **Cytoplasmic ANCA (cANCA):** Proteinase 3 Granulomatosis with polyangiitis (Wegner's granulomatosis), Churg-Strauss syndrome, possibly cutaneous necrotizing glomerulonephritis • **Perinuclear ANCA (pANCA):** Myeloperoxidase (rarely lactoferrin, elastase, and cathepsin) Microscopic polyangiitis, anti-glomerular basement membrane disease (Goodpasture's syndrome), Churg-Strauss syndrome, hydralazine-induced glomerulonephritis, hydralazine-induced lupus, rheumatoid arthritis, ulcerative colitis, autoimmune hepatitis, primary sclerosing cholangitis, Felty's syndrome • **Atypical ANCA:** Bacterial permeability increasing factor (BPI), myeloperoxidase, and other unknown antigens Cystic fibrosis, inflammatory bowel disease, primary sclerosing cholangitis, primary biliary cirrhosis, autoimmune hepatitis, rheumatoid arthritis, systemic lupus

Sens:	Sensitivity of ANCAs	cANCA (%)	pANCA (%)
	Granulomatosis with polyangiitis (Wegner's granulomatosis)	85	10
	Microscopic polyarteritis	45	45
	Churg-Strauss syndrome	20	60
	Polyarteritis nodosa	5	15

AMA	
Anti-mitochondrial antibodies	
	There are 9 subtypes (M1–M9) against various mitochondrial antigens. Of particular significance are antibodies against the M2 antigen, which are detectable in almost all cases of primary biliary cirrhosis

M1: Cardiolipin	M5: Outer membrane
M2: Branched-chain alpha-keto acid dehydrogenase	M6: Outer membrane
	M7: Sarcosine dehydrogenase
M3: Outer membrane	M8: Outer membrane
M4: Sulfite oxidase	M9: Glycogen phosphorylase

AMA (cont.)	
Ind	• Suspected primary biliary cirrhosis • Suspected autoimmune hepatitis
↑	Markedly - Primary biliary cirrhosis: Anti-M2 (high specificity), anti-M4, anti-M9 • Autoimmune hepatitis: Anti-M2 • Syphilis: Anti-M1 • Systemic lupus erythematosus: Anti-M5 • Drug induced lupus: Anti-M3 • Overlap syndrome of primary biliary cirrhosis and chronic active hepatitis: Anti-M4 • Cardiomyopathy: Anti-M7 Nonspecific positivity may be seen in individuals in contact with patients with primary biliary cirrhosis

Anti-SLA Ab	
Soluble liver antigen autoantibodies	
Ind	Suspected autoimmune hepatitis
↑	Autoimmune hepatitis type 3

Anti-TPO Ab	
Antibodies against microsomal thyroid antigen – thyroid peroxidase	
Ind	• Suspected lymphocytic thyroiditis (Hashimoto's) • Suspicion of Graves' disease • Suspected postpartum thyroiditis • Suspected cytokine-induced thyroiditis • Primary myxedema
↑	• Lymphocytic thyroiditis (Hashimoto's): 60%-90% • Atrophic autoimmune thyroiditis: 40%-70% • Graves' disease: 60%-70% • Primary myxedema: 40%-70% • Postpartum thyroiditis: 50%-70% • Subacute thyroiditis de Quervain: ≤5% • Autonomous thyroid: 5% • Normal/euthyroid goiter: 5%

Anti-TG Ab

Thyroglobulin autoantibodies

Thyroglobulin: a glycoprotein involved in thyroid hormone synthesis
Antibodies against thyroglobulin occur in destructive processes of the thyroid with "leakage" of thyroglobulin

Ind	• Suspected autoimmune diseases of the thyroid gland, esp lymphocytic thyroiditis (Hashimoto's) • Monitoring after thyroid cancer treatment
–	• Lymphocytic thyroiditis (Hashimoto's): 30%–40% • Atrophic autoimmune thyroiditis (20%–30%) • Graves' disease (10%–20%) • Thyroid carcinoma (30%) • In low concentration: not autoimmune thyroiditis • Healthy: ≤15%

Anti-TSHr Ab; Anti-TR Ab

Antibody against thyroid stimulating hormone (thyrotropin) receptor

Ind	• Suspected Graves' disease • Differentiate between Graves' disease and lymphocytic thyroiditis (Hashimoto's) - In Graves', anti-TSHr is almost always increased; usually normal in Hashimoto's • Evidence of endocrine ophthalmopathy without hyperthyroidism • Myxedema by blocking Ab
↑	• Active Graves' hyperthyroidism: 80%–100% • Graves' hyperthyroidism in remission: 10%–30% • Atrophic autoimmune thyroiditis: 15% • Lymphocytic thyroiditis (Hashimoto's): ≤10%
Note	• Differentiation between stimulating and blocking Ab by immunoassay may be impossible • The level of anti-TSHr does not correlate with the degree of hyperfunction • The level of anti-TSHr is not helpful in the assessment of disease activity or in the detection of recurrence

Anti-PCA	
Parietal cell autoantibodies	
Ind	• Suspected pernicious anemia • Suspected chronic atrophic gastritis type A • Suspected immune endocrinopathy
↑	• Pernicious anemia • Chronic atrophic gastritis type A (30%-60%) • Endocrinopathy (70%-80%) • Normal (≤10%)

Anti-adrenal Ab	
Autoantibodies against adrenal tissue, 70% will be against all three cortical layers; often against enzymes CYP11A1, CYP17, and CYP21A2	
Ind	• Differential of hypocortisolism (Addison's; autoimmune is most common) • Suspected autoimmune polyendocrinopathy • Differential of hypogonadism in polyglandular autoimmune syndrome

↑	• Hypocortisolism with Ab detection
	  - Autoimmune form of Addison's disease
	  - Polyglandular autoimmune syndrome type I (APS)
	• Hypocortisolism without Ab detection
	  - Hypocortisolism after tuberculosis
	  - Adrenal metastases (esp. lung or breast carcinoma or melanoma)
	  - Adrenal hemorrhage (Waterhouse-Friderichsen syndrome, anticoagulant therapy)

Anti-sperm Ab	
Ind	Fertility problems
↑	10-12% of unexplained sterility - IgG or IgA against spermatozoa; Unknown target antigens
Note	Autoagglutination of ejaculate under the microscope

ICA	
Islet cell autoantibodies	
• The most studied serological markers of type 1 diabetes mellitus • IgG autoantibodies directed against several islet cell antigens	
Ind	• Evaluation of the risk for type 1 diabetes (high titer has 20%-50% probability of future development of type 1 DM) • Suspicion of a latent insulin dependent diabetes in adulthood • Differential of diabetes mellitus type 1 or type 2
↑	• Type 1 diabetes (80% at presentation) • First-degree relative of type 1 DM patients (5% - without clinical manifestation) • Gestational diabetes

GADA	
Glutamate-decarboxylase autoantibodies	
Ind	• Evaluation of the risk for type 1 diabetes • Suspected latent insulin dependent diabetes in adulthood • Differential of diabetes mellitus type 1 or type 2
↑	• Type 1 DM (90% at presentation) • First-degree relative of type 1 DM patients (5% - without clinical manifestation) • Normal ≤20 years (0.5%)

IA2	
Tyrosine-phosphatase autoantibodies	
Autoantibodies against 2 proteins from the family of tyrosine phosphatases	
Ind	Evaluation of the risk for type 1 diabetes
↑	• Type 1 diabetics (70% - depending on duration of disease) • First-degree relative with type 1 DM patients (5% - without clinical manifestation) • Normal (0.5%-1%)
Note	Increased titer associated with increased risk for Diabetes mellitus type I, predictive value increased in combination with GADA

IAA	
Insulin autoantibodies	
Antibodies against bovine, porcine, or (rarely) human insulin. Necessitates increasingly higher insulin doses during therapy of diabetes mellitus	
Ind	• Evaluation of the risk for type 1 diabetes • Insulin autoimmune syndrome • Insulin resistance

↑	• High titer: More common in subcutaneous insulin therapy with
	  bovine insulin
	• Lower titer: More common with long term use of porcine insulin or
	  human insulin

Anti-Gliadin	
Gliadin: Partially ethanol-soluble prolamines (3 main types) in **wheat, rye, and barley** that forms **gluten** (along with glutenin)	
Ind	• Suspected gluten-sensitive enteropathy • Suspected dermatitis herpetiformis
↑	• Gluten-sensitive enteropathy (Celiac disease, Celiac sprue): • IgA: sensitivity 75%-90%, specificity 82%-95% • IgG: sensitivity 69%-85%, specificity 73%-90% • Dermatitis herpetiformis: up to 90% of patients have concurrent mild gluten sensitivity
Note	Antibodies to gliadin are not autoantibodies, but they occur together with autoantibodies against endomysium and tissue transglutaminase. The determination of anti-gliadin Ab should be combined with anti- endomysium or anti-tissue transglutaminase for best sensitivity and specificity False negatives: Associated with IgA deficiency; must do IgG; or with strict gluten-free diet
Anti-EMA	
Anti-endomysial autoantibodies	
Endomysium: Layer of connective tissue around a muscle fiber. Contains a specific tissue transglutaminase to which autoantibodies may bind	
Ind	• Suspected gluten-sensitive enteropathy (celiac disease, celiac sprue) • IgA: Sensitivity 85%-98%, specificity 97%-100% • Suspected dermatitis herpetiformis

Anti-EMA (cont.)	
↑	• Gluten-sensitive enteropathy (celiac disease, celiac sprue) • Dermatitis herpetiformis: up to 90% of patients have concurrent mild gluten sensitivity
Note	• Immunofluorescence test - Is "gold standard," but time consuming and expensive • False negatives: Associated with IgA deficiency; must do IgG; or with strict gluten-free diet

ATA/anti-tTG	
	**Tissue transglutaminase autoantibodies**
	Tissue transglutaminase: A Ca^{2+} dependent enzyme that crosslinks amino acids among other functions. Found intra- and extra-cellularly in small intestine (as well as skin, heart and liver). Increased synthesis in cell damage and is essential in wound healing. Contributes to matrix stabilization
Ind	• Suspected gluten-sensitive enteropathy (celiac disease, celiac sprue) IgA: Sensitivity 93%, specificity 99% • Suspected dermatitis herpetiformis (anti-epidermal transglutaminase)
↑	• Gluten-sensitive enteropathy (celiac disease, celiac sprue) - Ab response to TG-bound gluten • Dermatitis herpetiformis: up to 90% of patients have concurrent mild gluten sensitivity
Note	• Enzyme immunoassay - Is relatively easy and inexpensive vs. anti-endomysial testing • False negatives: Associated with IgA deficiency; must do IgG; or with strict gluten-free diet

Anti-GBM	
	**Glomerular basement membrane autoantibodies**
Ind	• Suspected anti-GBM disease (Goodpasture's syndrome) • Differential of rapid progressive glomerulonephritis • Differential of hemoptysis
↑	**Anti-glomerular basement membrane glomerulonephritis (Goodpasture's syndrome):** Type II hypersensitivity disorder with Ab against α3 chain of type IV collagen found in **kidney and lung basement membrane**
False	False positive: SLE, and other diseases with polyclonal immunoglobulin proliferation

Anti-EBM	
Epidermal basement membrane autoantibodies	
Antibodies to hemidesmosomes (IgG, rarely IgA): Causes disruption of the dermal-epidermal junction resulting in subepidermal blister formation; numerous antigens implicated; No acantholysis of Nikolsky's sign (as seen in pemphigus)	
Ind	Suspected pemphigoid - Bullous, gestational (herpes gestationis), mucous membrane (cicatricial)
↑	• Bullous pemphigoid: (70%-80%); type II hypersensitivity reaction, usually IgG against dystonin (BPA1) and/or type XVII collagen (BPA2) • Gestational pemphigoid (Herpes gestationis): usually IgG against BP180 • Mucosal pemphigoid (Cicatricial): usually IgG to BPA1 and/or BPA2 • Linear IgA dermatosis: (10%-30%) IgA against BPA2
Note	Skin biopsy: gold standard - with immunofluorescence positive at DE junction

Anti-LKM	
Antibodies against liver-kidney microsomal antigen	
Ab against cytochrome P450 antigens	
Ind	Suspected autoimmune hepatitis
↑	• Autoimmune hepatitis Type 2 (LKM1) • Chronic hepatitis C (LKM1) • Drug-induced hepatitis (LKM2)
Note	Further work-up in suspected autoimmune hepatitis: ANA, AMA, SLA, anti-HCV

Anti-SLA/LP	
Antibodies against soluble liver antigen/liver-pancreas antigen	
Ind	Suspected autoimmune hepatitis
↑	• Autoimmune hepatitis (type I - 90%, type II - 50%) • Primary sclerosing cholangitis (40%) • Chronic hepatitis C (10%)

Anti-ACHr	
Acetylcholine receptor autoantibody	
Ind	Suspected myasthenia gravis
↑	• Generalized myasthenia gravis: >90% The absolute titer does not correlate with the severity of disease, however, tracking an individual's titer correlates with disease activity • Ocular myasthenia: 70% (women, low titers)

Anti-striated muscle	
Ind	Suspected myasthenia gravis
↑	• Myasthenia gravis; 95% of patients with thymoma; 30% of patients without thymoma; Patients with ocular myasthenia have low titers • Polymyositis • Hepatitis

Anti-SMA	
Anti-smooth muscle autoantibodies	
Heterogeneous group of Ab against intermediate filaments of the smooth muscles	
Ind	• Suspected autoimmune hepatitis • Suspected primary biliary cirrhosis • Suspected chronic active hepatitis C • Suspected polymyositis, post-cardiotomy syndrome, post-myocardial infarction (Dressler's syndrome)
↑	• Autoimmune hepatitis type 1 (50%) • Chronic active hepatitis • Primary biliary cirrhosis • Polymyositis: 30% (determination of CK and LDH important) • Viral infections: Transient anti-SMA

Anti-cardiac muscle	
Ind	Differentiation of infectious and autoimmune etiology of myocarditis or pericarditis
↑	• Cardiomyopathies (myofibrillar type) • Post-cardiotomy syndrome • Post-myocardial infarction syndrome (Dressler's, myofibrillar type) • Viral perimyocarditis (myofibrillar type) • Collagen diseases (sarcolemmal type)

RF	
Rheumatoid factor	
"Classically" IgM directed against the Fc portion of IgG, but there are also IgA, D, E, and G types	
Ind	Rheumatoid arthritis
↑	<ul><li>Rheumatoid arthritis: 70%-80%. High titers are associated with rapid disease progression (must correlate with clinical symptoms for diagnosis)</li><li>Lupus erythematosus (15%-35%)</li><li>Sjögren's syndrome (75%-95%)</li><li>Scleroderma (20%-30%)</li><li>Polymyositis/dermatomyositis (5%-10%)</li><li>Cryoglobulinemia (40%-100%)</li><li>Mixed connective tissue disease (50%-60%)</li></ul>

ADB/anti-DNAse-B	
Antistreptococcal deoxyribonuclease-B Antibody	
In the assay, diluted patient serum is mixed with a defined DNAse-B and a DNA substrate coupled to dye. With normal enzymatic degradation the supernatant becomes colorless. If the patient's serum contains anti-DNAse-B, degradation is prevented, and the solution remains blue	
Ind	<ul><li>Suspected infection with group A beta-hemolytic streptococcus</li><li>Suspected post-streptococcal glomerulonephritis and/or rheumatic fever</li></ul>
↑	Streptococcal infection: high sensitivity for skin infections and tonsillitis; increased after 3-4 weeks. Often done concurrently with ASO

ASO	
Antistreptolysin-O	
"Anti-streptococcal" antibodies: neutralizes streptolysin-O of the beta-hemolytic streptococci of groups A, C and G AST: Antistreptolysin test and Antistreptolysin titer	
Ind	<ul><li>Suspected infection with group A beta-hemolytic streptococcus</li><li>Suspected post-streptococcal glomerulonephritis and/or rheumatic fever</li></ul>

ASO (cont.)	
↑	Streptococcal infection: Increased within 1 wk after infection, max after 4 wks, normalization after 6 wks. Relatively low sensitivity. Preferred single test vs ADB

AH	
Antihyaluronidase test: Detection method for Antihyaluronidase - formed against hyaluronidase produced by group A, B, C, or G hemolytic streptococci. Based on clot formation as a result of an antigen-antibody reaction	
Ind	Suspected infection with Group A Beta-Hemolytic Streptococcus
↑	Streptococcal infection: Increased after 2 wks, normalization within 3-4 wks. High sensitivity for skin infections and tonsillitis

ASTA	
Anti-staphylococcal antibodies	
Ind	Suspected staphylococcal infection
↑	Staphylococcal infection: Increased after 2-3 wks, normalization within 6 months

Anti-red blood cell	
Ind & ↑	Autoimmune hemolytic anemia (AIHA)

Ab	
Warm autoantibodies (IgG)	

	70% of patients with AIHA have warm agglutinins - active at body temperature (37°C)
	• Idiopathic (45%)
	• Secondary:
	  - Non-Hodgkin's lymphomas (eg, CLL)
	  - Systemic lupus erythematosus
	  - Drugs (eg, penicillin, cephalosporins, methyldopa)
	  - Viral infections
	• Steroids (temporary remission in 30% while on medication)
	• High-dose immunoglobulins (temporary blockage of the RES)
	• Splenectomy (for chronic cases, mainly extravascular hemolysis)
	• Immunosuppressants as a last resort

Bithermal autoantibodies (IgG)	
Causes	Very rare autoAb to Donath-Landsteiner: • Idiopathic • Secondary: post-infectious (syphilis, viral infections)
Test	Donath-Landsteiner test: bithermal hemolysins bind at cold temperatures (25°C) and heating (37°C) results in hemolysis

Cold autoantibody (IgM)	

Causes	15% of patients with AIHA have cold agglutinins
	• Idiopathic, monoclonal, very rare
	• Secondary: ("cold agglutinin syndrome")
	  - Acute: Mycoplasma or mononucleosis, polyclonal
	  - Chronic: Non-Hodgkin's lymphoma, monoclonal (Waldenström macroglobulinemia)

Test	• Avoid cold - Most important measure, sufficient in most cases • Therapeutic trial with interferon alpha • Immunosuppressants in pronounced hemolytic anemia • Plasmapheresis in severe cases Note: Steroids are ineffective, as is splenectomy, since RBCs are degraded directly in the periphery

Anti-platelet Ab	
Ind	Suspected immune-related thrombocytopenia
↑	• Acute and chronic immune thrombocytopenic purpura • Lymphoma • Drug-induced thrombocytopenia (heparin, cotrimoxazole) • Evans syndrome (autoimmune hemolytic anemia and immune thrombocytopenia)

Anti-white blood cell Ab	
Causes	• Antibodies directed against leukocytes, especially after the administration of WBC's, blood, or pregnancies • Auto-antibodies to patient's own leukocytes may be found in patients with neutropenia

19.2   Human Leukocyte Antigen (HLA)

A system of the major histocompatibility complex (MHC), located on chr. 6, many alleles and thousands of possible combinations; each person has a specific set of HLAs that allow the immune system to recognize the "self," and that are the major determinant of organ compatibility (along with blood type)

HLA of MHC class I: Major - A, B, C; on all cells; present peptides from inside the cells to CD8+ killer T-cells

HLA of MHC class II: Major - DP, DQ, DR; on antigen presenting cells, present antigens from outside of the cell to CD4+ helper T-cells or B-cells

Certain HLA types are associated with increased risk of specific diseases

HLA-B27	Acute uveitis (10x)
	Ankylosing spondylitis (90x)
	Post-infectious arthritis (20x)
	Reiter's syndrome (40x)
HLA-B47	21-hydroxylase deficiency
HLA-DR2	Systemic lupus
HLA-DR3	Autoimmune hepatitis
	Diabetes mellitus type 1
	Sjögren syndrome
	Systemic lupus
HLA-DR4	Diabetes mellitus type 1
	Gestational pemphigoid
	Hydralazine-induced lupus
	Rheumatoid arthritis

19.3   Hepatitis

General: Laboratory testing in suspected acute hepatitis:
HA-IgM, HBs-Ag, HBc-IgM, HCV, CMV-IgM, EBV-IgM;
With unexplained cases determine toxoplasmosis and leptospirosis antibodies
Accompanying laboratory findings
↑: Bilirubin, iron (often >200 µg/dL), AST, ALT, PTT, lymphocytosis, SPEP: in the later stages increased β- and γ-globulin with normal total protein
↓: PT (no improvement in vitamin K), AT III, fibrinogen, haptoglobin

HAV	HAV-IgM	• Establishes a new hepatitis A infection • Remains positive 3-6 months
	HAV-IgG	• Positive approximately from the beginning of clinical symptoms; remains positive for life • Marker of existing immunity
	Virus RNA in the stool (PCR)	• Only for special situations • Positive before the beginning of clinical symptoms
	Ag in the stool (ELISA)	• Rarely performed since at the beginning of symptoms, about half of the patient's virus (HAV) in stool is eliminated and this number decreases rapidly
HBV	HBs-Ag	• "Surface" antigen • Detectability: weeks before to until after acute illness • 5%-10% of the infections are HBs-negative • Persistence ≥6 months in chronic hepatitis
	HBs-Ab	• Immunity against hepatitis B with titer ≥10 U/mL • Marker of recovery - with HBc-Ab • Parameter for monitoring vaccination - without detectable HBc-Ab
	HBc-Ag	• "Core" antigen (not in the serum, only in hepatocytes) • 3-5 weeks after HBs-Ag and detectable before clinical manifestation • High titer at the beginning of the infection (before anti-HBs and anti-HBc) • Proof of infection (not present after vaccination) • Persistence up to 12 months after infection
	HBc-IgG	• Persistent or previous hepatitis B • Lifetime persistence • Proof of infection (not present after vaccination)

HBV (cont.)	HBe-Ag	• "Envelope" antigen, decomposition of HBc-Ag • Evidence of high infectivity (active viral replication) • Persistence ≥11 months: chronic active hepatitis
	HBe-Ab	• Acute/chronic hepatitis, previous infection • Detectable after reduction of HBe-Ag • Uncertain marker of infectivity (detection at low infectivity)
	HBV-PCR	• Direct viral pathogens • Assessment of infectivity
HCV	HCV-Ab	• Only positive 2-3 months after infection • Not for evaluation of acute infection • In some cases, despite immunosuppression, viremia negative
	HCV-PCR	• Qualitative and quantitative viremia detection • False negative results possible in low viral replication or extra-vascular viral persistence
HDV	All markers	• Order only when positive HBV - required for infection
	HDV-Ag	• For superinfection, co-infection with HBV • Short persistence
	HDV-IgM	• Acute HDV infection • During late acute stage often the only marker positive (HDV-Ag often already negative)
	HDV-IgG	• The most important screening test for the presence of acute HDV infection • False negatives: with immunosuppression
	HDV-PCR	• To differentiate between acute and chronic active Hep D • More reliable than serological markers

HEV	HEV-IgM	• Evidence of a new HEV infection • Detectable around 6-7 weeks, not detectable >3 months after infection • Only ~85% of infected patients will be positive
	HEV-IgG	Usually positive only for a few years
	HEV-PCR	• Evidence of a new HEV infection • Frequently positive in infected patients • Can remain positive up to 3 wks after infection
HGV	HGV-PCR	Evidence of acute or chronic HGV infection

19.4   Syphilis

Principle:
- To exclude syphilis: TPHA sufficient
- To confirm syphilis: TPHA titer, VDRL titers, FTA-Abs, and FTA-IgM (in questionable cases)

Test procedure:

Day	Test	Result	Evaluation
1	TPHA	–	No evidence of antibodies to T. pallidum; possible reasons: • Patient never had infection with T. pallidum • T. pallidum infection, Ab are still not in high enough concentration (Follow-up if clinical suspicion) • Antibody formation is not possible → completed investigation
		+	Acute or resolved infection probable → need for further investigation (see Day 2)

Day	Test	Result	Evaluation
2	FTA–Abs	–	No confirmation of TPHA: → Check serum sample control, new one required if negative → completed investigation
		+	• Confirmation of TPHA: acute or resolved infection • Questionable need for treatment → further testing required
	VDRL	–	"Serological scar" - resolved infection, no treatment required ' completed investigation
		+	Titre >1:16; infection present requiring treatment → completed investigation
		+ weak	Titers 1:2-8 → Further testing needed: follow-up after 14 days or determine specific IgM Ab
3–4	IgM	–	"Serological scar" - resolved infection, no treatment required → completed investigation
		+	New infection, treatment required → completed investigation

Reassess control samples if results uncertain		
After 10–14 days	–	No increase in titer; resolved infection with "serological scar"; no need for treatment
	+	At least 3x increase in titer → new infection, treatment required
Treatment monitoring: VDRL		
After weeks	–	At least 3x decrease in titer → patient successfully treated
	+	No titer change → treatment not successful

Test procedure with a known history of syphilis:
TPHA titer and cardiolipin titer: Cardiolipin unreactive or very low when sufficiently treated

Test procedure for suspected reinfection:
TPHA titer, cardiolipin titer, and FTA-IgM

Syphilis tests in detail:

TPHA: Treponema pallidum hemagglutination assay (screening test):
- Qualitative and, if reactive, quantitative determination (titer)
- Positive 2-3 weeks after infection
- Specificity low: needs to be confirmed by FTA-Abs, cross-reactions are possible - false-positive reactions: Treponema pertenue (Yaws), Treponema carateum (Pinta), Lyme disease, EBV, SLE and others
- Life-long positive if not treated very early ("serological scar")

FTA-Abs: Fluorescent treponemal antibody absorption test (Immunofluorescence test):
- Confirmatory test for positive TPHA
- Positive 2-3 weeks after infection
- Life-long positive if not treated very early ("serological scar")

VDRL: Venereal Diseases Research Laboratories, cardiolipin flocculation test (Flow control test):
- Qualitative and, if reactive, quantitative determination (titer)
- Positive 4-6 weeks after infection
- Active syphilis infection - cardiolipin titers >1:4
- Titers decline during therapy, no life-long titer persistence

FTA-IgM: Fluorescent treponemal antibody absorption test after IgM capture
- Detection of Treponema pallidum-specific IgM antibodies
- Demonstrable in untreated primary and secondary infection (of crucial importance in reinfection)
- Also many patients with inadequately treated infection

20 Vitamins

There are 13 vitamins that the body requires for standard metabolism and development (A, C, D, E, K, and 9 B vitamins). Most vitamins come from diet, though the body can produce vitamins D and K. Vegetarians are at increased risk of vitamin B12 deficiency.

Fat soluble vitamins: A, D, E, K

20.1 Vitamin A

Func: Vitamin A consists of a group of unsaturated hydrocarbons including A1 (retinol), Vitamin A_2, and several other derivatives (retinal, retinoic acid, retinyl esters) as well as several provitamin A carotenoids (see below). They are all yellow in color, **fat-soluble**, and deactivated by oxygen and UV exposure. Vitamin A is important for growth and development of **epithelium** (skin, GI tract, GU tract), **vision** (retina), **embryonic development**, hematopoiesis, bone metabolism, gene transcription, and immune function. The retinol form functions as storage and is reversibly converted to its active form, retinal. Retinoic acid is a metabolite that can be irreversibly synthesized from vitamin A and has only partial vitamin A activity (does not function in the retina)

Ind: Suspected malabsorption; night blindness: twilight interference, increased sensitiveness to glare; suspected overdose (total parenteral nutrition, self-administration [acne, psoriasis])

Prod: Foods of animal origin, primarily as retinyl ester/palmitate, which is converted to retinol in the small intestine

Norm: 50-200 µg/dL

↑ Since it is fat-soluble, may accumulate to toxic levels, usually from excessive intake (TPN, self-medication for acne or psoriasis); Acute ~25,000 IU/kg, chronic ~4,000 IU/kg daily >6 mo, but may occur at lower levels (especially in children [1,500 IU/kg] or the liver of alcoholics)

Nausea, vomiting, anorexia, blurred vision, headache, hair loss, generalized pain and weakness, drowsiness/altered mental status (increased intracranial pressure), and **osteoporosis/fractures**, weight loss, and diarrhea in chronic cases. **Even therapeutic doses can cause neural tube defects**

↓ **Malnutrition:** inadequate intake of meat and dairy (vitamin A) and fruits and vegetables (carotenoids); early breast milk weaning
Malabsorption syndromes: celiac disease, short bowel syndrome, Crohn's disease, giardiasis
Maldigestion syndromes: chronic cholestatic liver and biliary tract disease, bile acid deficiency, exocrine pancreatic insufficiency, lipase deficiency
Deficient vitamin A storage/transport: liver cirrhosis, premature infants, nephrotic syndrome, zinc deficiency, night blindness, xerophthalmia, keratomalacia, epithelial damage of skin and mucous membranes (follicular hyperkeratosis, diarrhea), leukoplakia of the respiratory and urinary tract, squamous metaplasia in salivary, lacrimal, and mucous glands (ear infections, UTIs)

Mat: Serum/EDTA-plasma, protected from light, fasting 12 h

Met: Chromatography

20.2 Beta Carotene

Func:
- Fat soluble provitamin, an inactive precursor of vitamin A (others are α-carotene, β-cryptoxanthin); One β-carotene molecule can be cleaved into 1 or 2 vitamin A molecules depending on the enzyme and coenzyme
- Used to treat **erythropoietic protoporphyria**, and may reduce the risk of breast and ovarian cancer, exercise-related asthma, oral leukoplakia, and age-related macular degeneration.

Ind: Suspicion of malabsorption syndrome

Prod: Found in fruits and vegetables, especially cantaloupe, mangoes, papayas, spinach, carrots, pumpkins, and sweet potatoes; absorption is enhanced if eaten with fats, **absorption restricted to the duodenum;** Predominantly stored in adipose tissue, hence the yellow color of fat in adults, but white color in infants

↑ Metabolic disorders, pregnancy, hypothyroidism, nephrotic syndrome; overdose/excessive self-administration - may lead to **carotenodermia** (orange-tinged skin), and may be associated with increased risk of lung and prostate cancer in smokers
Note: The amount of carotenoids absorbed decreases as dietary intake increases and is inversely proportional to the amount of vitamin A present in the body. Therefore, it is a safe source of vitamin A

↓   Malabsorption, malnutrition, liver disease, OCPs, metformin, neomycin, kanamycin, proton pump inhibitors, cholesterol lowering drugs

Mat: Serum, protect from light

20.3 Vitamin B1 (Thiamine)

Func: Water-soluble, heat-, alkali- and O_2-labile vitamin, essential for carbohydrate metabolism and involved in acetylcholine formation, and is important for enzymes in all organ systems, particularly the nervous system. Requires magnesium for enzyme utilization.

Deficiencies present subacutely and lead to gastrointestinal discomfort, loss of appetite, fatigue, weight loss, tachycardia, small T in the ECG, water balance disorder, and **neurological symptoms** such as paralysis, lack of concentration, and depression. In severe cases: beriberi, Wernicke encephalopathy, Korsakoff syndrome, optic neuroma, coma, and death

Beriberi: A neurological and cardiovascular disease with 3 forms:
- Dry beriberi - peripheral neuropathy consisting of symmetric sensory, motor, and reflex impairment, worse distally
- Wet beriberi - peripheral neuropathy with mental confusion, muscular atrophy, generalized edema, tachycardia, cardiomegaly, and congestive heart failure
- Infantile beriberi - breast-fed by thiamin-deficient mothers, cardiac, aphonic, or pseudomeningitic forms, frequently have a loud piercing cry, vomiting, tachycardia, convulsions, and even death

Korsakoff syndrome: considered a continuum with Wernicke encephalopathy, an amnestic-confabulatory syndrome with retrograde and anterograde amnesia, apathy, lack of insight, and coma

Optic neuropathy: bilateral vision loss, scotomas, and impaired color perception due to optic disk edema and atrophy

Wernicke's encephalopathy: most frequent manifestation of thiamine deficiency in the US, typically due to alcohol abuse, but may be seen with any form of malnutrition, neuro-psychiatric disorder with eye paralysis, abnormal gait, and markedly altered mental status

Ind: Neurological disorders: Wernicke encephalopathy, Korsakoff syndrome, Guillain-Barré syndrome

Prod: Found in grains, beans, nuts, and meat; neither stored nor absorbed in excess

Norm: 15-90 µg/L

↑	Leukemia, Hodgkin's disease, polycythemia vera
↓	• Malnutrition: especially in **alcoholics**, but also **coffee and tea consumption** - prevented by vitamin C, and **raw fish and shellfish**
	• Malabsorption: gluten-sensitive enteropathy, short bowel syndrome, inflammatory bowel disease, HIV
	• Maldigestion: exocrine pancreatic insufficiency, cholestatic biliary tract and liver disease; Increased demand: pregnancy, lactation, extreme exercise; **Areca (betel) nut chewing**

Mat: EDTA whole blood

Met: HPLC; also stimulation >25% during a red blood cell transketolase measurement with thiamine pyrophosphate → deficiency

20.4   Vitamin B2 (Riboflavin)

Func: A fluorescent yellow-green (in solution) or orange-red (solid), alkaline, light-sensitive vitamin important for human health especially in metabolism of carbohydrates, fats, ketones, and proteins. Used as an orange-red food coloring
Continuously excreted in the urine (with healthy kidney function) making deficiencies not uncommon leading to **oral–ocular–genital syndrome: cheilitis/glossitis/stomatitis mouth ulcers, dry eyes with photophobia, dry skin and mucus membranes (scrotal dermatitis)**, iron-deficiency anemia
Used to help **treat neonatal jaundice** along with phototherapy, **prevent migraines** and along with UV light to inhibit replication of pathogens in blood products

Prod: Found in dairy, leafy vegetables, asparagus, bananas, okra, eggs, fish, kidney, liver, beans, mushrooms, and almonds
Note: milk sold in transparent containers may have lower levels due to exposure to light

Ind: No real deficiency or toxicity syndromes; always associated with other deficiencies

Norm: 1–20 µg/L

↓ Malnutrition, malabsorption

Met: Erythrocyte glutathione reductase activity, urinary riboflavin excretion

20.5 Vitamin B3 (Niacin, Nicotinic Acid)

Func: Water-soluble, colorless derivative of pyridine that is a precursor of nicotinamide adenine dinucleotide (NAD) and nicotinamide adenine dinucleotide phosphate (NADP), common coenzymes needed for: NAD - catabolism of carbohydrates, fats, proteins, alcohol, cell signaling, DNA repair; NADP -anabolism of fatty acids and cholesterol. Organs with high metabolic activity (CNS, GI tract, skin) are most susceptible to deficiency
- Mild deficiency: Slow metabolism → cold intolerance
- Severe deficiency: **Pellagra** - 3 D's: diarrhea, dermatitis, and dementia, also "Casal's necklace" neck lesions, hyperpigmentation, skin thickening, inflammation of the mouth and tongue, digestive issues, amnesia, delirium, include irritability, poor concentration, anxiety, fatigue, restlessness, apathy, and depression, and eventually death
- Increases HDL levels when taken in large doses (>1500 mg/daily)

Prod: Found in meats (especially liver, heart, kidney), fish, grains, nuts, beans, and can be synthesized from tryptophan

Norm: 0.5-8.5 µg/mL

↑ Pharmacological doses (>1500 mg/day) cause flushing, itching, rashes, exacerbation of eczema and acanthosis nigricans, hyperuricemia, slightly increased blood glucose, maculopathy, and possibly hepatotoxicity (worse with time-release versions)

↓ Malnutrition (poverty, alcoholism), carcinoid syndrome, Hartnup's disease

20.6 Vitamin B5 (Pantothenic Acid)

Func:
- Water soluble; used to synthesize and metabolize proteins, carbohydrates, and fatty acids as well as coenzyme A
- Deficiencies are rare, may cause fatigue, irritability, depression, cramping, hypoglycemia, and neurological deficits (numbness, weakness), rarely adrenal insufficiency and hepatic encephalopathy
- No known toxicity

Prod: Found in meats, whole grains, legumes, eggs, broccoli, avocado, and yogurt; in many hair and skin products; natural form is protein bound, must be hydrolyzed to free form in intestine for absorption

Norm: 35-150 µg/L

20.7 Vitamin B6 (Pyridoxine)

Func:
- Water soluble, coenzyme involved in amino acid metabolism and synthesis, gluconeogenesis, porphyrin and lipid synthesis
- Deficiency is rare, but leads to a pellagra-like disorder with seborrheic dermatitis, glossitis, cheilitis, conjunctivitis, somnolence, confusion, and normo-to hypochromic anemia (due to inhibition of sideroblast B6-phosphate dependent delta- aminolevulinic acid synthetase, essential for heme synthesis). Infants are at risk of increased excitability, nervousness, seizures and an increased excretion of xanthurenic acid in the urine
- Toxicities are rare due to water solubility and excretion in the urine, but can lead to destruction of the dorsal root ganglia (numbness and pain)

Prod: Found in meats, whole grains, green vegetables, egg yolk, liver, nuts

Norm: 5-30 µg/L

↓ Malnutrition (alcoholics), pregnancy, INH treatment

Mat: EDTA-blood, protected from light

20.8 Vitamin B7 (Biotin, Vitamin H)

Func:
- Water soluble; a coenzyme involved in the synthesis and metabolism of amino acids (isoleucine and valine), fatty acids, and in gluconeogenesis.
- Deficiency is very rare because GI bacteria produce biotin; but may be seen in metabolic disorders or with excessive raw egg white consumption; may cause alopecia, conjunctivitis, **characteristic facial rash** (and genitalia), and neurological issues (depression, weakness, numbness, tingling, hallucination); will have **increased 3-hydroxyisovaleric acid**

Prod: Found in green leafy vegetables, liver, raw egg yolk; found in many hair and skin care products; avidin in egg whites binds biotin and makes it unavailable

Norm: 220-3000 pg/mL

↓ Inherited metabolic disorders (deficient biotin-dependent carboxylases, biotinidase), **excessive egg white consumption (avidin), pregnancy**

20.9 Vitamin B9 (Folic Acid)

Func: Water soluble, important for biosynthesis of nucleic acids, coenzyme in hematopoiesis. If impaired absorption, poor feeding, increased demand (pregnancy, Vitamin-B12-deficiency) as well as in the event of a malfunction of the folic acid metabolism, such as in megaloblastic anemia

Prod: Green leafy vegetables, milk, liver; absorbed in the duodenum and jejunum

Ind: Megaloblastic anemia, long-term anti-epileptic therapy, suspected folic acid deficiencies: pregnancy, dialysis, alcoholics, psoriasis, dermatitis

Norm: >4 µg/L   Serum/plasma
120-800 µg/L Intraerythrocyte

↓   <2 µg/L   Deficiency
2-4 µg/L   Intermediate zone
Malnutrition (poverty, alcoholism), folic acid antagonists, malabsorption (inflammatory bowel disease, gluten-sensitive enteropathy, anti-epileptics, sulfasalazine), increased demand or loss (pregnancy, growth, chronic hemolysis, leukemia, psoriasis, exfoliative dermatitis)

Mat: Folic acid in the serum/plasma: Serum, EDTA-Plasma
Intraerythrocyte: Heparin or EDTA whole blood
Protect from light

Note: • Discontinue methotrexate therapy at least 8 days prior
• Almost always get concomitant vitamin B12
• For anemia associated with folic acid or B12 deficiency, check for iron deficiency

20.10 Vitamin B12 (Cobalamin)

Func:
- Water-soluble vitamin, required for hematopoiesis and normal neural function, as well as DNA and fatty acid synthesis. Obtained from the dietary proteins, is poorly absorbed without the aid of intrinsic factor (IF) from parietal cells of the stomach. No biosynthesis in fungi, plants or animals, formed by bacteria in/on food or in GI tract/liver
- Signs and symptoms: occur after exhaustion of the liver stores; macrocytic anemia, glossitis, peripheral neuropathy, weakness, hyperreflexia, ataxia, loss of proprioception, poor coordination, and behavioral changes (depression, paranoia, hallucinations)
- Serum methylmalonic acid and homocysteine levels are also elevated

Ind: Megaloblastic anemia (MA), peripheral neuropathy (PN), coordination issues, malabsorption syndromes

Norm: 150-915 ng/L
Sufficient B12-inventory: >250 pg/mL
Not evaluable: 150-250 pg/mL
B12 deficiency: <150 pg/mL

↑ Vitamin B supplementation; liver disease (metastases, acute or chronic hepatitis); hematological disease (leukemia, myelofibrosis, polycythemia vera)

↓ <180 ng/L: May cause signs and symptoms of MA or PN
150-300 ng/L: Intermediate zone
Pernicious anemia - macrocytic anemia due to lack of IF secretion (autoimmune/atrophic gastritis, gastrectomy); strict vegetarian diet; diseases or resection of the terminal ileum (malabsorption); drugs (neomycin, colchicine), tapeworm infection

Mat: Serum, EDTA plasma

Met: Competitive immunoassay

20.11 Vitamin C (Ascorbic Acid/Ascorbate)

Func:
- Water-soluble, crystalline powder; used by all cells of the body; important for collagen synthesis (bone health, wound healing, bleeding diathesis), is a strong antioxidant, and vital for many metabolic reactions
- Widely used as a food additive to prevent oxidation
- **Scurvy**: Due to unstable collagen; leads to skin pigmentation, bleeding gums/mucous membranes, scoliosis, open wounds, loss of teeth, and death
- Chronically low levels increase risk of atherosclerosis
- High doses (≥2000 mg) will lead to an **osmotic diarrhea**
- Enhances iron absorption - may lead to iron poisoning in susceptible patients; may cause a hemolytic anemia in G6PD deficiency

Prod: Found in citrus fruits, kiwi, green vegetables; can be made internally by many animals, excluding humans; actively and passively absorbed along the GI tract; stores last 1-6 months depending on previous consumption; excess is rapidly excreted in the urine

Ind: Suspicion of vitamin C deficiency

Norm: 0.4 -1.5 mg/dL

↓ Malnutrition, malabsorption, pregnancy, renal insufficiency

Mat: Serum (hermetically sealed, protected from light)

20.12 Vitamin D (Calciferol)

Func:
- Collective term for fat-soluble, photosensitive, sterol derivatives, especially vitamins D_2 and D_3 (ergocalciferol and cholecalciferol, respectively) and their natural pro-vitamins, ergosterol and 7-dehydrocholesterol, which form vitamin D in skin with UV exposure. Metabolized in the liver to 25-hydroxycholecalciferol (calcidiol - more accurately reflects the body's stores) and in the kidney to 1,25-dihydroxycholecalciferol (calcitriol - the most potent metabolite). Production is regulated by calcium, phosphorus, and parathyroid hormone
- Involved in calcium homeostasis and skeletal mineralization. Often thought of less as a vitamin and more as a calciotropic hormone
- Stimulates calcium absorption in the intestines

Prod: D_3 is found in animal tissues, liver, fish oil, eggs, and dairy. D_2 is found in vegetables. Precursors transformed in the skin upon UV exposure

Ind: Suspicion of vitamin D deficiency, hyper-/hypocalcemia, renal disease

Norm: 25-80 ng/ml

↑ >80 ng/mL - may lead to toxicity
Substitution therapy, **hyperparathyroidism** (primary or secondary due to low calcium), **granulomatous disease** (sarcoidosis, TB), hypercalcemia, vitamin D receptor defects, vitamin D dependent rickets type II, hypothyroidism

↓ <10 ng/mL   Marked deficiency
10-24 ng/mL Deficiency
Hypoparathyroidis, pseudohypoparathyroidism, hypophosphatemia, hereditary vitamin D-dependent rickets type I (1-alpha hydroxylase), malnutrition, malabsorption, renal failure/nephrotic syndrome, hyperthyroidism, cadmium toxicity, anticonvulsants (carbamazepine, phenytoin, phenobarbital, valproic acid), **osteoporosis**

Mat: Serum/plasma, protected from light (prefer morning/fasting; or before dialysis)

Met: Immunoassay
Note: High triglycerides may yield false results

20.13 Vitamin E (Tocopherol)

Func:
- A group of fat soluble vitamins that is involved in endothelial membrane integrity and function, nervous system function, skin, and is an antioxidant
- Promotes prostacyclin and inhibits thromboxane formation decreasing platelet aggregation (deficiency may be related to increased risk of atherosclerosis/thrombosis)
- Been shown to reduce risk and severity of bronchopulmonary dysplasia and retrolental fibroplasia in premature infants on high-oxygen supplementation
- Deficiency leads to motor and sensory neuropathies, especially in children; and abetalipoproteinemia

Prod: Found in seeds, grains, and soybeans; particularly safflower oil, sunflower oil, and wheat germ oil

Norm: 5.5-17 mg/L

| ↓ | Malnutrition, malabsorption (IBD, pancreatic insufficiency, gluten-sensitive enteropathy), cholestasis |

Mat: Serum/plasma; fasting
Note: Nonfasting specimen or vitamin supplementation may lead to falsely elevated levels

20.14 Vitamin K

Func: A group of fat soluble vitamins with a common quinone ring. A cofactor in the carboxylation of glutamate necessary for the activation of numerous proteins involved in coagulation (factors II, VII, IX, and X, proteins C and S), as well as others involved in cell growth and apoptosis, and bone metabolism
- K1 and K2: natural forms, non-toxic; K3, K4, and K5: synthetic
- K1: Phylloquinone, phytomenadion, or phytonadione; found in plants, particularly green leafy vegetables; can be converted to K2 by bacteria in colon
- K2: Menaquinones; main storage form in humans; produced by bacterial anaerobic respiration
- K3: Menadion; synthetically produced, **may cause toxicity**

Prod: Found in green leafy vegetables, avocado, and kiwi

Ind: Warfarin therapy, coagulopathy

↓ Malnutrition, malabsorption (GI tract disease), antibiotics, oral anticoagulation, cholestasis, biliary tract fistulas

Mat: Serum, fasting, protected from light

Met: Liquid chromatography/mass spectrometry
Note: Nonfasting or fatty acid heavy (lipemic) specimens can lead to falsely elevated levels

21 Minerals

- Minerals are needed for many metabolic and synthetic pathways, including protein, hormone, and bone formation
- Macrominerals are needed in larger quantities: calcium (Ca^{2+}), chloride (Cl^-), magnesium (Mg^{2+}), potassium (K^+), sodium (Na^+), and sulfur (S)
- Trace minerals are needed in small amounts: chromium (Cr), cobalt (Co), copper (Cu), fluoride (F^-), iodine (I), iron (Fe), manganese (Mn), selenium (Se), and zinc (Zn)

Note: Gadolinium, iodine and barium contrast dyes will interfere with metals testing, should wait at least 72 h after administration

Several of these are discussed in other sections and will not be repeated here

21.1 Calcium (Ca)

Func:	Essential for muscle and nerve function, bone health, and coagulation. Excessive intake may lead to kidney stones or milk-alkali syndrome
Ind:	Disorders of protein, vitamin D, bone, kidney, or parathyroid
Prod:	Found in dairy products, green leafy vegetables, nuts and seeds, eggshell Note: Some veggies, such as chard, rhubarb, and spinach, as well as many nuts, contain oxalic acid which binds calcium reducing its absorption. ~90% is stored in bones and teeth
Norm:	8.8-10.5 mg/dL Serum 20-300 mq 24 h urine
↑	Hypercalcemia: Increase bone resorption, increased GI absorption, hyperparathyroidism, bone metastasis
↓	Hypocalcemia: hypoparathyroidism, vitamin D deficiency/impairment, chronic renal failure
Mat:	Serum/plasma

21.2 Magnesium (Mg)

Func:
- A major intracellular cation (along with K^+) and cofactor for numerous enzymes (such as anything requiring ATP); ~30% bound to proteins (albumin), citrates, phosphate, etc.
- Hypomagnesemia increases the cell membrane permeability for Na^+, K^+, and Ca^{2+} and increases intracellular Ca concentration causing clinical hypocalcemia and related cardiac disorders (such as ventricular arrhythmias that are not responsive to traditional therapy, digoxin sensitivity, and coronary spasms)
- Hypomagnesemia generally indicates Mg deficiency, but blood Mg levels may be normal even with Mg depletion

Ind: Neuromuscular disorders, arrhythmia, insulin therapy, total parenteral nutrition, preeclampsia treatment with magnesium sulfate (often just use respiratory rate and deep tendon reflexes)

Prod: 98% is intracellular, of which ~60% localized to bone and 35% in skeletal muscle; absorbed in the small intestine, secreted by kidney, regulated in the loop of Henle

Norm: 1.7–2.3 mg/dL Serum
75–150 mg   24 h urine

↑ Hypermagnesemia: acute and chronic renal failure, dehydration, severe untreated diabetic ketoacidosis, Addison's disease, excessive intake (antacids, laxatives)

↓ Chronic renal disease, burns, endocrine disorders (ketoacidosis, hyperthyroidism, hypoparathyroidism, hyperaldosteronism), malnutrition, malabsorption, lactation, alcoholism, total parenteral nutrition

Mat: Serum/plasma, urine

Met: Atomic absorption spectrometry, photometrically

Mg^{2+}↓	Mg^{2+}↑
Clinical:	**Clinical:**
Usually associated with hypokalemia and/or hypocalcemia: Irritability, depression, paresthesia, possibly intestinal spasms Heart: arrhythmias, increased digitalis sensitivity, coronary artery spasms with angina ECG: QT prolongation	Usually associated with hyperkalemia: Muscle weakness, somnolence ECG: Excessive T wave disturbances (intraventricular excitation propagation)
Therapy:	**Therapy:**
• Chronic deficiency: Magnesium-containing foods such as fruits, nuts, vegetables, +/- magnesium salts • Acute deficiency: Symptomatic hypomagnesemia: Magnesium sulfate, 10 mL in 100 mL 20% glucose, over 10-20 min IV, then 10 mm Mg^{2+}/ 24 h continuous infusion	Dialysis

21.3 Cobalt (Co)

Func: Cofactor in vitamin B12 metabolism; no known deficiency, extreme toxicity may lead to nausea, vomiting, hemorrhage, pulmonary edema, and kidney failure; industrial inhalation may lead to interstitial lung disease

Ind: Suspected toxicity

Norm: 1 ng/dL Serum
<2 µq 24 h urine

↑ Toxicity (glass and dye industries), metallic surgical hardware

Mat: Serum, urine

Met: Atomic absorption spectrometry

21.4 Copper (Cu)

Func:
- Required for formation of cytochrome oxidase C; 95% found in ceruloplasmin, rest is albumin bound
- Hypocupremia leads to impaired growth and hematopoiesis
- Wilson disease: Hepatolenticular degeneration; autosomal recessive chr 13q; due to decreased ceruloplasmin leading to increased tissue deposition manifesting in liver disease (bleeding, hepatic encephalopathy, portal hypertension), neuropsychiatric issues (depression, cognitive decline, behavioral changes, parkinsonian features), Kayser-Fleischer rings of the eyes (Cu in Descemet's membrane)
- Ceruloplasmin and copper may be normal during acute phase (fulminant liver failure) due to liver destruction and increased release
- Menkes syndrome: Cu transport disease characterized by kinky steely hair, muscle hypotonia, developmental delay, growth failure, nervous system degeneration; x-linked recessive
- Hypercupremia

Ind: Wilson disease, primary biliary cirrhosis, primary sclerosing cholangitis, Menkes syndrome

Prod: Stored in the liver, muscle, and bone

Norm: 75-150 µg/dL Serum
15-60 µg   24 h urine

↑ Primary biliary cirrhosis, primary sclerosing cholangitis, hemochromatosis, leukemia, thyrotoxicosis, chronic inflammation, pregnancy, OCPs, estrogen therapy

↓ Wilson disease, Menkes syndrome, nephrotic syndrome, malnutrition, malabsorption, excess Fe or Zn intake (interferes with GI absorption)

Mat: Serum/urine

Met: Atomic absorption spectrometry

21.5 Chromium (Cr)

Func: Multiple states from 2- to 6+; most common is 3+ and 6+, the former is found in humans, the latter is used in industry, is a carcinogen, and is transformed to the former in the body

Ind: Long-term total parenteral nutrition, suspected toxicity (steel, dye, glass, and rubber industry)

Norm: <5 µg/L Serum
0-8 µg 24 h urine

↑ Chromium toxicity, metallic surgical hardware, renal disease, peritoneal dialysis

↓ Total parenteral nutrition, infection, stress, pregnancy

Mat: Serum, urine

Met: Atomic absorption spectrometry

21.6 Manganese (Mn)

Func:
- Cofactor for numerous enzymes, particularly those reducing free oxygen radicals
- Toxicity is usually by inhalation and leads to largely irreversible neurologic deficits (weakness, lethargy, headaches, sexual dysfunction, altered mental status, motor function disturbance)

Ind: Suspicion of toxicity (steel and colorant industries)

Prod: Found in fruits and vegetables

Norm: 0.4-2.2 µg/L Serum
0.2-1.0 µg 24 h urine

↑ Manganese toxicity, occasionally with fulminant hepatitis, severe ischemic heart disease, and renal failure requiring dialysis

↓ Long-term total parenteral nutrition, occasionally in epilepsy and postmenopausal osteoporosis

Mat: Serum, urine

Met: Atomic absorption spectrometry

21.7 Selenium (Se)

Func:
- Essential cofactor for glutathione peroxidase which is necessary to breakdown free radicals, ie, is a strong antioxidant
- Heart is most susceptible to deficiencies, cell damage leads to fibroblastic proliferation
- Keshan disease: Rare myofibrillar dystrophy of skeletal and cardiac muscles caused by dietary selenium deficiency and a specific Coxsackie virus, found mostly in China

Ind: Long-term total parenteral nutrition, muscular dystrophy, cardiomyopathy, suspected toxicity

Norm: 7-14 µg/dL   Serum
5-30 µg   24 h urine

↑ Excessive ingestion, occupational exposure (electrical, glass, porcelain industry)

↓ Long-term total parenteral nutrition, muscular dystrophy, cardiomyopathy, liver cirrhosis, Keshan disease

Mat: Serum, urine

Met: Atomic absorption spectrometry

21.8 Zinc (Zn)

Func:
- Essential cofactor for numerous enzymes and proteins including alkaline phosphatase, alcohol dehydrogenase, carbonic anhydrase, and DNA and RNA polymerase. Also required form proper wound healing
- No really toxicity, except hypocupremia
- Acrodermatitis enteropathica: Autosomal recessive; defective zinc uptake; leads to periorificial and acral rash, alopecia, and diarrhea

Ind: Acrodermatitis enteropathica; chronic non-healing wound; secondary zinc deficiency (inflammatory bowel disease, cirrhosis, nephrotic syndrome, penicillamine therapy)

Norm: 60-110 µg/dL Serum
300-600 µg   24 h urine

↑ Iatrogenic, excessive ingestion, polycythemia

↓   Acrodermatitis enteropathica, massive burns, cirrhosis (leads to excessive renal excretion), long-term total parenteral nutrition, inflammatory bowel disease, gluten-sensitive enteropathy, malignancy, nephropathy, alcoholism, excessive Fe or Cu ingestion (interferes with GI absorption)

Mat: Serum/plasma, urine

Met: Atomic absorption spectrometry

Note: Falsely high levels may be seen in hemolysis, venous congestion, Zinc-based heparin therapy

22 Therapeutic & Toxicological Analyses

22.1 Basic Concepts

Three main components: **Therapeutic drug monitoring, screening for drugs of abuse, management of overdose/poisoning**

- **Clearance:** Most drugs are cleared by 1st order kinetics, by the kidneys (renal excretion), liver (metabolized), or both
- **Half-life ($t_{1/2}$):** Time needed in order for a drug's blood concentration to decrease by half (50% of starting point). Medications are typically dosed according to their half-life
- **Bound vs. free:** Like most molecules in the body, many drugs have a proportion that travels in the blood stream "bound" to a protein (often albumin) with the rest being "free". This "free" component is the therapeutically active component. It is also the component responsible for toxicity. This "free" component is inversely proportional to the amount of protein in the blood stream: when protein is low, "free" drug will be high, and vice versa. There is also "competition" for binding sites; hence, certain drugs will be displaced if other compounds are present. Hence it is important to know the patients protein levels and other medications in order to prescribe adequate doses
- **Volume of distribution:** Drugs are variably distributed in the body based on their size and solubility; ie, drugs that are hydrophilic (lipophobic) will stay in vascular spaces, or partially enter the interstitial aqueous fluid, whereas lipophilic drugs can also enter the adipose tissue. The larger a drug's volume of distribution, the more spaces a drug may enter. This value is expressed in liters and is calculated based on the given dose and measured plasma concentration:

$$Vd = Dose/concentration$$

22.2 Therapeutic Drug Monitoring

Many drugs are monitored so that patient response and dosage can be adjusted accordingly. Reasons include: a narrow therapeutic window (highly toxic at levels just above therapeutic or undertreatment), making sure that a patient is taking medications appropriately, patient variation in enzymes may affect plasma concentrations, variable pharmacokinetics, other medications may effect metabolism of drug.

Commonly monitored medications:

- Antibiotics: amikacin, gentamicin, netilmicin, tobramycin, vancomycin
- Anti-epileptics: carbamazepine, ethosuximide, phenobarbital, phenytoin, valproic acid
- Anti-arrhythmics: digitoxin, digoxin, lidocaine, procainamide, quinidine
- Bronchodilators: caffeine, theophylline
- Immunosuppressants: cyclosporine, everolimus, mycophenolic acid, sirolimus, tacrolimus
- Mood stabilizers: lithium
- Antipsychotics: clozapine, pimozide

22.3 Drugs of Abuse

Certain drugs are commonly used for recreational reasons. They may be illegal (cocaine, heroin) or legal drugs that are being abused (ethanol, morphine, codeine, diazepam). Screenings are often performed for professional reasons (employment), in emergency situations, or as part of treatment monitoring.

- **Urine** is the common medium for testing, though **blood, saliva, and hair** may be used. Hair is useful if you need to see a long history of drug use as substances stay in the hair and can be used as a timeline.
- **Screening tests** are designed to have **high sensitivity**, but have a rather **low specificity**. It is for this reason that a positive screen is followed up with a more specific confirmatory test (gas chromatography, mass spectrometry)

Common drugs of abuse

Alcohols:
- Hypopnea, stupor, disorientation, unsteady gait, unconsciousness, usually **metabolic acidosis with increase anion and osmolal gap** (EG or methanol)
- Ethylene glycol - antifreeze, metabolized to oxalate, forms calcium oxalate crystals, envelope-shaped and birefringent, in the urine or in renal parenchyma on biopsy/autopsy
- **Isopropyl alcohol** - rubbing alcohol, metabolized to acetone, **marked osmolal gap and ketones, but no acidosis or anion gap**
- **Methanol** - windshield washer fluid, paint remover, "wood alcohol", metabolized to formaldehyde/formic acid, **blindness**

	Source(s)	Acidosis w/ anion gap	Osmolal gap	Ketones	Metabolite(s)
Ethanol	Beer, wine, liquor	In high doses/chronic use	Yes	In high doses/chronic use	
Ethylene glycol	Antifreeze	Yes	Yes	No	Oxalate
Isopropyl alcohol	OTC rubbing alcohol	No	Yes	Yes	Acetone
Methanol	Windshield washer fluid	Yes	Yes	No	Formaldehyde/formic acid

Ethanol: Altered mental status, respiratory depression. Metabolized by alcohol dehydrogenase in the liver to acetaldehyde which is further converted by aldehyde dehydrogenase to acetic acid. May be measured in the blood (serum, plasma, or whole **blood - must be in sodium fluoride and potassium oxalate** to prevent production of or metabolism of ethanol in order to prevent false results), **breath, or urine**.

Note: ~80% of patients of **Asian descent** have a **variant alcohol dehydrogenase** that converts alcohol to acetaldehyde at a much faster rate, in addition ~50% have a variant acetaldehyde dehydrogenase that is less functional, this results in **better metabolism of alcohol, but an increase in the toxic metabolites, leading to the "flushing" common to these patients**

Clinical effects of alcohol	
BAC (%)	
• <0.05	• Normal
• 0.05–0.1	• Mild euphoria, loss of Inhibition
• 0.1–0.2	• Easily excited (happiness or irritability)
• 0.2–0.3	• Increased confusion
• 0.3–0.4	• Lethargy
• >0.4	• Coma and death
CDT	Levels are raised after 1-2 weeks of heavy consumption; may be increased in liver disease; generally higher at baseline in females

Clinical effects of alcohol (cont.)	
GGT	Levels raised after 4 weeks of heavy consumption; levels will normalize after ~4 weeks of abstinence
MCV	Often increased in heavy consumption of greater than 8 weeks; presumed to be due to vitamin deficiencies (B12, folic acid)

BAC: Blood alcohol concentration; CDT: Carbohydrate-deficient transferrin; GGT: Gamma glutamyl transferase; MCV: Mean corpuscular volume
CDT and GGT used to monitor alcohol abstinence
BAC levels are approximate; those who are chronic drinkers may be able to tolerate higher concentrations

Amphetamines: Hyperpnea, hyperthermia, tachycardia, hypertension, anxiety, irritability, cerebral hemorrhage, seizures. Acts via release of dopamine in the CNS; prolonged use leads to destruction of dopamine-secreting cells and can result in an **irreversible Parkinsonian syndrome**

Barbiturates: Altered consciousness, respiratory suppression, myocardial dysfunction, hypotension, hypothermia, pulmonary edema, respiratory failure. Vary in onset and duration. **Potentially lethal in both toxicity and withdrawal.** CNS depressants that stimulate release of γ-aminobutyric acid (GABA)

Benzos: Drowsiness, dizziness, hypotension, hypopnea, decreased consciousness/concentration, cognitive impairment, memory problem, lack of coordination, decreased libido, **paradoxical aggression, irritability, seizures.** Enhance the effect of GABA in the CNS. Flunitrazepam (Rohypnol), common drug of abuse

Cannabis: Analgesia, antiemetic, disinhibition, lack of initiative, increased appetite, subdued consciousness. Cannabinoid receptor agonist mainly in the CNS and immune system, lead to decreased cAMP via adenylate cyclase inhibition. Lipophilic molecule

Cocaine: Sympathetic nervous system hyperactivity: tachycardia, hypertension, diaphoresis, mydriasis, agitation/irritability. Vasoconstriction/vasospasm w/ or w/o MI → **chest pain** (should be considered in any young person with idiopathic chest pain). Left ventricular hypertrophy with extended use
Note: Myoglobin and CK-MB levels less sensitive in cocaine induced MI due to skeletal muscle defects; **use troponin I**

GHB:
Euphoria, disinhibition, nausea, drowsiness, agitation, hypopnea/apnea, bradycardia, **amnesia, unconsciousness**, death. Decreases elimination of alcohol from the system → increases alcohol effects and toxicity. Naturally occurring CNS depressant. Used in treatment of narcolepsy and cataplexy, increases slow-wave sleep. Common drug of abuse; colorless and odorless, but has salty taste

Ketamine:
Blurred vision, nystagmus, delirium, HTN, tachycardia, hypersalivation, nausea, vomiting, tonic-clonic movements, urinary system problems, cognitive impairment, hallucinations. A NMDA receptor antagonist, also interacts with cholinergic receptors and calcium channels

LSD:
Mydriasis, decreased appetite, alertness, hallucinations, altered sense of time, anxiety, paranoia, delusions. Semisynthetic drug made from ergotamine, a chemical made from a grain fungus that grows on rye (ergot). Activates serotonin receptors. Believed to be mostly non-addictive, not known to cause brain damage, low toxicity. May cause dissociative states in patients on lithium or tricyclics. Tolerance builds quickly and has cross-tolerance with other psychedelics (mescaline, psilocybin)

Mescaline:
Similar to LSD. Naturally occurring in certain cacti (eg, peyote, San Pedro, and Peruvian torch). Can be synthesized from phenylalanine or tyrosine

Psilocybin:
Similar to LSD. Found in over 200 species of mushrooms

Opiates:
Sedation, miosis, hypotension, bradycardia, altered mental status and respiratory failure. Includes morphine, codeine, morphones, codones, fentanyl, heroin, and opium. **Propoxyphene** is a unique opioid no longer available in the US that interferes with Na^+ thereby also causing **myocardial dysfunction and seizures and may not be detected on routine tests**

PCP:
Aggressive or paranoid behavior, **horizontal nystagmus**, hyperpnea, hypertension, tachycardia. Extreme intoxication may show bradycardia, hypotension, hypoglycemia, seizures, hyperthermia and even rhabdomyolysis. Very lipid soluble leading to fluctuating blood levels: variably calm and sedate then bursts of irritability and aggression

Drug	Detectability of drug or metabolite	Main metabolite(s)
Amphetamines		
• Amphetamine	• 3 d	• Amphetamine
• Methamphetamine	• 3 d	• Amphetamine
• MDMA (3,4 Methylenedioxy-methylamphetamine, ecstasy)	• 2 d	• 3, 4 Methylene-dioxy-amphetamine (MDA)
Barbiturates		–
• Pentobarbital/secobarbital	• 3 d	
• Phenobarbital	• 15 d	
Benzodiazepines		–
• Triazolam/flurazepam	• 2 d	
• Alprazolam/lorazepam/Oxazepam	• 5 d	
• Diazepam	• 10 d	
Ketamine	2 d	–
Cocaine	5 d	Benzoylecgonine
Psychogenics		
• Lysergic acid diethylamide (LSD)	• 5 d	• 2-oxo-3-hydroxy-LSD
• Psilocybin	• 7 d	• Psilocin → 4-hydroxy-indole-3-acetaldehyde/ or acetic acid, 4-hydroxytryptophol or bound to glucuronic acid
Methadone	7 d	–
Opiates	3 d	
• Codeine		• Morphine, hydrocodone
• Morphine		• Morphine, hydromorphone
• Codone (Hydro, Oxy)		• Morphone
• Morphone (Hydro, Oxy)		• Morphone
• Heroin (Diacetylmorphine)		• Morphine
• 6-monoacetyle morphine (6-MAM)		• Morphine
• Propoxyphene		• Norpropoxyphene

Drug (cont.)	Detectability of drug or	Main metabolite(s)
Phencyclidine (PCP, Angel dust)	8 d	1-(1-Phenylcyclohexyl)-4-hydroxypiperidine (PCHP), 4-Phenyl-4-(1-piperidinyl)-cyclohexanol (PPC), 5-[N-(1-Phenylcyclohexyl)]-aminopentanoic acid (PCAA)
Cannabis	Single use - 3 d 4x/wk - 5 d Daily - 10 d Chronic Heavy - 30 d	Delta-9-THC-COOH (highly lipophilic)
Gamma hydroxybutyric acid (GHB)	1 d	–

22.4 Poisoning/Overdose

Onset of symptoms:

> **Seconds to minutes:** cyanide, hydrogen sulfide
> **Minutes to hours:** carbon monoxide, carbon dioxide, ammonia, parathion, acids, alkalis
> **Hours to days:** opiates, analgesics, irritant gases (ozone, nitrogen oxides, chlorine, fluorine), methylating agents, hypnotics, methemoglobin
> **Days to weeks:** carbon tetrachloride, trichlorethylene, xylene, metal poisons (arsenic, thallium, mercury), paraquat

Main symptoms:

Pupils:	Miosis: Opiates, barbiturates, phosphate ester, cholinergics Mydriasis: Cocaine, hypoxia, hypothermia, anticholinergics
Salivation:	Dry mouth: Anticholinergic medications Hypersalivation: Cholinergics, anticholinesterases
Abnormal sensations:	Paresthesia, numbness, burning of the mouth: Antiarrhythmics, aconitine

Neuro:
- Reflex loss, quiet coma: opiates, barbiturates
- Motor restlessness: methaqualone, anticholinergics
- Cramps: analgesics, opiates, antiarrhythmics
- Muscle twitching: phosphoric acid esters
- Diaphoresis: cocaine

Heart:
- Congestive heart failure: Beta-blockers, anticholinergics, phosphate esters
- Arrhythmia: Cocaine, cardiac glycosides, anti-arrhythmics, tri- and tetracyclic antidepressants
- Tachycardia/HTN: Cocaine, amphetamines, PCP (acutely), Ketamine
- Bradycardia/Hypotension: Barbiturates, opiates, PCP (marked toxicity)

Breathing: Central/peripheral respiratory paralysis: Hypnotics, sedatives, motor end plate blockers, opiates, barbiturates
Pulmonary edema: Cardiodepressive agents, barbiturates, inhalants

Signs and symptoms of common drug toxicities		
Class	Examples	Signs/symptoms
Anticholinergics: Block the action of acetylcholine	**Anti-muscarinics:** Atropine, Benztropine, Diphenhydramine, Ipratropium, Scopolamine **Anti-nicotinics:** Buproprion, Dextromethorphan, Doxacurium, Mecamylamine	Stimulates **Sympathetics:** Psychosis, dry skin/mouth/eyes, hyperthermia, flushing, altered mental status, (**"mad as a hatter, dry as a bone, hot as a hare, red as a beet"**); mydriasis, tachycardia, constipation, urinary retention
Adrenergics	Albuterol, Amphetamines, Cocaine, Dobutamine, Ephedrine, Epinephrine, Norepinephrine, Phenylephrine, Pseudoephedrine, PCP	Stimulates **sympathetics:** HTN, tachycardia, dry mouth, mydriasis, nausea, vomiting, hyperthermia, anxiety, irritability
Narcotics	Morphine, Codeine, Hydro/Oxymorphone, Hydro/Oxycodone, Heroin, Opium, Fentanyl	Altered mental status, sedation, miosis, respiratory depression/ failure, pulmonary edema

Class (cont.)	Examples	Signs/symptoms
Cholinergics: Stimulate nicotinic and/or muscarinic receptors; either directly or by increasing acetylcholine (promoting release, blocking cholinesterase)	**Direct:** Acetylcholine, Organophosphates (pesticides), Carbachol, Carbamate, Nicotine, Muscarine, Pilocarpine **Indirect:** Atenolol, Cisapride, Clonidine, Donepezil, Caffeine, Edrophonium, Malathion, Metoclopramide, Methyldopa, Neostigmine, Physostigmine, Propranolol, Risperidone, Trazodone	Stimulates **Parasympathetics:** Salivation, lacrimation, urination, diarrhea, GI cramping, emesis (**"SLUDGE"**); diaphoresis, miosis, flaccid paralysis, respiratory failure
Sedatives	Barbiturates, Benzodiazepines, Ethanol, Opiates	Altered mental status, slurred speech, lethargy, respiratory depression/failure
Hallucinogens	Amphetamines (MDMA, Meth), Cocaine, LSD, PCP	Hallucinations, anxiety, hyperthermia

Basic testing in suspected poisoning:
Blood counts, platelets, blood gas analysis, glucose, lactate, PT, PTT, thrombin time, AST, ALT, ALKPhos, cholinesterase, Na^+, K^+, Cl^-, Ca^+, anion gap, osmolar gap, osmolality, creatinine, urea, urine analysis, ethanol screen

Poison elimination methods (Antidotes)	
Acetaminophen	N-acetylcysteine
Acetylcholinesterases	Atropine, pralidoxime
Amphetamines	Ammonium chloride (NH_4Cl) - acidify urine
Anticholinergics	Physostigmine
Barbiturates	Charcoal, sodium carbonate ($NaHCO_3$) - alkalinize urine
Benzodiazepines	Flumazenil
Beta blockers	Glucagon
Carbon monoxide	100% O_2, Hyperbaric O_2
Cyanide ("bitter almonds")	Hydroxocobalamin, amyl nitrate/sodium nitrate/thiosulfate
Digitalis (bidirectional ventricular tachy.)	Charcoal, dialysis, anti-digoxin Ab, give Mg
Heavy metals (Arsenic ("garlic breath"), copper, gold, lead, mercury)	Chelation therapy: CaEDTA, dimercaprol, succimer, penicillamine
Inorganic salts	Dialysis
Iron	Deferoxamine
Isoniazid	Pyridoxamine
Heparin	Protamine
Methemoglobin	Methylene blue, vitamin C
Methanol, ethylene glycol, isopropyl alcohol	Ethanol, fomepizole, dialysis
Opiates	Naloxone, naltrexone
Salicylates	Sodium carbonate ($NaHCO_3$) - alkalinize urine, dialysis
Streptokinase, tPA	Aminocaproic acid
Sulfonylurea	Octreotide
Theophylline	Gastric lavage/charcoal, beta blockers
Tricyclic antidepressants	Sodium carbonate ($NaHCO_3$) - alkalinize plasma
Valproic acid	Carnitine
Warfarin (rat poison)	Vitamin K, FFP

Emergency contact information:
- **Poison control:** 1-800-222-1222
- **American Association of Poison Control Centers:** http://www.aapcc.org/

22.5 Targeted Testing of Blood and Urine

Diabetic coma	B: Excessive glucose U: Excessive glucose
Hypoglycemic shock	B: Ketones, K^+, Lactate, osmolality, acid-base balance U: Ketones
Acute renal failure	B: Urea, creatinine
Uremia with nephropathy	B: Acid-base balance, urea, creatinine
Coma	B: Ammonia, AST, ALT, bilirubin, acid-base balance U: Indole derivatives
Acute intermittent porphyria	U: Porphobilinogen, porphyrins, δ-aminolevulinic acid
Thyrotoxicosis, hypothyroid coma	B: T3, T4
Addison crisis, hypopituitary coma	B: Glucose, Na^+, K^+, Cl^-, Ca^{++}, cortisol, acid-base balance, T3, T4 U: 17-Ketosteroids (Androstenedione, androsterone, estrone, dehydroepiandrosterone)

23 Prenatal Testing

23.1 Human Chorionic Gonadotropin (hCG)

Func: A glycoprotein heterodimer; same α subunit with FSH, LH, and TSH; β subunit on chr 19; maintains the corpus luteum after conception and promotes progesterone secretion
- Highly negatively charged: may aid in protecting fetus from mother's immune response
- May be linked to severity of morning sickness
- Due to similarity to LH, can induce ovulation in women or testosterone production in men

Ind: Suspected pregnancy (intrauterine or ectopic); suspected/post-treatment monitoring of gestational trophoblastic disease and certain germ cell tumors

Prod: Syncytiotrophoblasts

Norm: Serum: <5 mIU/mL

↑
- **Pregnancy (intrauterine or ectopic);** increased above expected in multiple gestation, polyhydramnios, eclampsia, erythroblastosis fetalis, Down syndrome
- Gestational trophoblastic disease (complete moles > partial)
- Germ cell tumors with syncytiotrophoblasts (choriocarcinoma component)
- Doubles ~q 2-3 days in first wks of pregnancy; then q 4 days until peak at end of first trimester; then begins to decline
  - An abnormality may indicate ectopic (↓) or gestational trophoblastic disease (↑)

Positive: >25 mIU/mL
Indeterminate: 5-25 mIU/mL
- Repeat testing suggested in 72 h if indeterminate

↓ During pregnancy levels may be decreased in ectopic pregnancy, smoking, maternal diabetes, or Edwards' syndrome (trisomy 18)

Mat: Serum/plasma - quantitative; urine - qualitative

Note:
- Detectable 6-12 days after conception (serum before urine) to 2-4 wks after delivery/ectopic removal or 10 wks after molar pregnancy removal (no need for intervention as long as serial hCG measurements are declining)
- False urine negatives may be seen in very early pregnancy (before missed period) or in dilute samples (early morning is best); **a negative serum test makes pregnancy highly unlikely**
- False positives may be seen with heterophile antibody interference or those taking hCG medically (eg, weight loss)

23.2 Prenatal Screening

Evaluation of specific markers may aid in diagnosing certain disorders of the fetus

Alpha-fetoprotein (AFP): Principle plasma protein in the fetus; maternal AFP rises during pregnancy; **higher in African Americans and with multiple gestations; lower in overweight patients and those with diabetes**

↑	**Neural tube defects - >2.5x the median ~80% sensitivity** Bowel obstruction/gastroschisis/omphalocele; cystic hygroma; fetal demise; hydrops fetalis; maternal-fetal hemorrhage; renal anomalies; smoking, teratoma; Turner's syndrome; wrong gestational age (most common)
Dimeric inhibin A (dIA)	Glycoprotein produced by the placenta that is increased ~2x in Down syndrome; **relatively constant throughout 2nd trimester limiting effect of gestational age**
hCG:	• ~2x normal in Down syndrome; must consider maternal weight, diabetes, smoking, and multiple gestations • Difficult to evaluate multiple gestations that naturally have increased hCG - sensitivity for Down syndrome 50%-70% (better for monozygotic twins where both fetuses are affected, whereas in dizygotic usually one 1 fetus is affected)
Uncon-jugated estriol (uE):	• Slightly decreased in Down syndrome - low sensitivity; decreased in diabetes and smokers • Better sensitivity for **Trisomy 18** (Edwards' syndrome), 7-dehydrocholesterol reductase deficiency (Smith-Lemli-Optiz syndrome [SLOS] - autosomal recessive disorder for cholesterol synthesis), and steroid sulfatase deficiency

Triple screen: hCG, AFP, uE; best at 18wks - sensitivity for Down syndrome ~70%

Quad screen: hCG, AFP, uE, and dimeric inhibin A (dIA) - sensitivity for Down syndrome ~80%

Integrated screen: hCG measured at 10-13 wks and AFP, uE, and dIA at 18 weeks - sensitivity for Down syndrome ~85%

Integrated screen with nuchal fold thickness: Sensitivity ~90%

Note hCG and uE slightly ↓ in diabetes
In smokers: AFP ↑, uE and hCG ↓

Cause/disorder	AFP	dIA	hCG	uE	Sensitivity	Specificity
Trisomy 21 (Down syndrome)	↓	↑	↑	↓	70%-90%	~90%
Trisomy 18 (Edwards' syndrome)	↓	↓	↓	↓	~80%	10%-30%
Neural tube defects	↑↑	-		↓	~90%	10%-30%
Maternal diabetes	↓	-	↓	↓	-	-
Smokers	↑		↓	↓	-	-

23.3 Preterm Delivery Risk Evaluation

Def: Regular contractions with cervical changes prior to 37 wks gestational age
- Most important cause of morbidity and mortality
- Both serum estradiol and salivary estriol increase slightly before preterm labor, but with limited sensitivity
- Bacterial vaginosis is associated with preterm labor

23.3.1 Fetal fibronectin (FFN)
- Protein normally found at maternal-fetal placental interface; present in cervical mucus in early pregnancy and again before labor
- The absence of FFN in cervical secretions is very sensitive and specific for ruling out impending labor, whereas the presence of FFN is suggestive of the onset of labor, but the time to active labor may be long
- Transvaginal ultrasound to assess cervical length is also a good predictor of labor

23.4 Fetal Lung Maturity Methods

Fetal lungs are developed (mature) enough to function between 34–37 wks; prior to this time the risk of respiratory distress syndrome (RDS) is very high

23.4.1 Lecithin: Sphingomyelin ratio (L:S)

Lecithin production increases with lung maturity whereas sphingomyelin is relatively constant (~2% of total surfactant phospholipid); before 26 wks gestation the ratio is ~1:1

L:S ratio reaches ~2:1 around 35 wks – this is considered the ratio of maturity
L:S >2:1 - <5% will develop RDS
L:S <2:1 - >50% will develop RDS

Ind:	To test for **fetal lung maturity (FLM)**, usually when preterm birth is imminent or necessary for fetal/maternal health
Prod:	Type II pneumocytes produce phosphatidylcholine (major lecithin) and sphingomyelin among others
Norm:	<26 wks: 1:1 **2:1 FLM**
Mat:	Amniotic fluid
Met:	• Not reliable in maternal diabetes → PG better in those patients • Falsely low ratios may be seen with meconium contamination • Blood contamination will yield a ratio of ~1.5:1

23.4.2 Other methods

Disaturated phosphatidylcholine concentration:	Direct measurement used to evaluate FLM; not affected by blood or meconium contamination
Fluorescence polarization assay:	Commonly used method; **<260 = FLM**; affected by blood levels >0.5%, but even in the presence of blood, levels <230 are considered mature
Lamellar body concentration:	Surfactant lamellar bodies are measured using a cell counter (approximately the size of platelets); **>50,000/mL = FLM**
Phosphatidylglycerol (PG):	Production begins around 36 wks gestation; **presence is indicative of FLM; not affected by blood or meconium** → best for contaminated amniotic specimens

Stability test: Measurement of the stability of amniotic fluid to support a substance, typically foam; serial dilutions with ethanol are performed and the highest concentration of stability is measured

23.5 Fetal Hemolysis and Bilirubin Levels:

Fetal hemolysis and amniotic fluid bilirubin levels

Func: Fetal bilirubin levels increase in response to hemolysis

Ind: Suspected alloimmunization with resultant fetal hemolysis; to monitor fetal hemolysis in known cases; aids clinical decision making (eg, delivery, intrauterine transfusion)

Mat: Amniotic fluid - **protected from light**, preferably with minimal blood contamination

Met: Spectrophotometry → Concentration is proportional to absorbance

23.6 Effect of Pregnancy on Certain Laboratory Tests

Analyte	Change	Comment
Albumin	↓	Due to hemodilution
Amylase	↑	Should be considered along with clinical symptoms (pancreatitis)
BUN	↓	Due to increased GFR
Calcium	↓	Declines throughout pregnancy
Creatinine	↓	Due to increased GFR
Fibrinogen	↑	Smaller elevation in preeclampsia
GFR	↑	Believed to be due to increased blood volume
Hematocrit	↓	Due to hemodilution
Hemoglobin	↓	Due to hemodilution
Potassium	NL	-
Sodium	NL	-
TBG	↑	Estrogen effect
Triglyceride	↑	Estrogen effect
Urine protein	↑	Due to increased GFR and GBM permeability

24 Appendix

24.1 Abbreviations

↓	decrease
↑	increase
~	approximate, unchanged
°C	degree celsius
A1AD	alpha-1-antitrypsin deficiency
A1AT	alpha-1-antitrypsin
AABB	American Association of Blood Banks
AAS	atomic absorption spectroscopy
Ab	antibody
ACD	acid-citrate-dextrose
ACE	angiotensin converting enzyme
AChE	acetylcholinesterase
AChr	acetylcholine receptor
ACLA	anticardiolipin antibody
ACT	activated clotting time
ACTH	adrenocorticotropin hormone
AD	autosomal dominant
ADB	antistreptococcal deoxyribonuclease-b
ADH	antidiuretic hormone
ADP	adenosine diphosphate
AFP	alphafetoprotein
Ag	antigen
AH	antihyaluronidase

AHG	anti-human globulin
AIHA	autoimmune hemolytic anemia
AKA	also known as
ALA	aminolevulinic acid
ALL	acute lymphoblastic leukemia
ALP	alkaline phosphatase
ALT	alanine aminotransferase
AMA	antimitochondrial antibodies
AML	acute myeloid/myelogenous leukemia
ANA	antinuclear antibody
ANCA	antineutrophil cytoplasmic antibodies
ANDRO	androstenedione
AP	acid phosphatase
AP	alkaline phosphatase
APA	anti-phospholipid antibody
APC	activated protein C
APLS	anti-phospholipid syndrome
Apo	apolipoprotein
APS	autoimmune polyglandular syndrome
aPTT	activated partial thromboplastin time
AR	autosomal recessive
ASA	acetylsalicylic acid
ASO	anti-streptolysin o

AST	aspartate aminotransferase
AT	antithrombin
ATA	anti-transglutaminase antibodies
ATP	adenosine triphosphate
β2-GPI	beta 2-glycoprotein I
BAC	blood alcohol concentration
BChE	butyrylcholinesterase
BHB	beta-hydroxybutyrate
BM	bone marrow
BMI	body mass index
BPA	bullous pemphigoid antigen
BPH	benign prostatic hypertrophy/ hyperplasia
BSA	body surface area
BUN	blood urea nitrogen
C	coulomb
C	cytoplasmic
Ca	cancer
Ca^{2+}	calcium
$CaCO_3$	calcium carbonate
$CaCl_2$	calcium chloride
CaF_2	calcium fluoride
$Ca(OH)_2$	calcium hydroxide
$Ca_3(PO4)_2$	calcium phosphate
CA	carbohydrate-antigen
CaEDTA	calcium disodium EDTA
CAH	chronic active hepatitis
CAIHA	cold autoimmune hemolytic anemia

CAMT	congenital amegakaryocytic thrombocytopenia
cANCA	cytoplasmic antineutrophil cytoplasmic antibodies
CBC	complete blood count
CBG	cortisol-binding globulin
CCK	cholecystokinin
CDT	carbohydrate-deficient transferrin
CENP-A	centromere protein A
CENP-B	centromere protein B
CENP-C	centromere protein C
CEA	carcinoembryonic antigen
CF	cystic fibrosis
ChE	cholinesterase
CHF	chronic heart failure
Chr	chromosome
CK	creatinine kinase
CK-MB	creatinine kinase-isoenzyme - cardiac muscle subunit
CLL	chronic lymphocytic leukemia
CML	chronic myeloid/myelogenous leukemia
CMV	cytomegalovirus
CNS	central nervous system
CO	carbon monoxide
CO2	carbon dioxide
COPD	chronic obstructive pulmonary disease
Cp	phosphate clearance
CPP	coproporphyrinogen

CPPD	calcium pyrophosphate deposition disease	DVT	deep vein thrombosis
		DPyD	deoxypyridinoline
CREST	calcinosis, Raynaud phenomenon, esophageal dysmotility, skin pigmentation, telangiectasias	DVT	deep vein thrombosis
		EBM	epidermal basement membrane
		EBMA	epidermal basement membrane antibody
CRH	corticotropin-releasing hormone	EBV	epstein-barr virus
CSF	cerebrospinal fluid	ECG	electrocardiogram
CTAD	citrate/theophylline/ adenosine/dipyridamole	ECL	enterochromaffin-like cells
		EDTA	ethylenediamine tetra acetic acid
CTx	type-I collagen telopeptide	eGFR	estimate glomerular filtration rate
CVA	cerebral vascular accidents		
CYFRA	cytokeratin-19 fragments	EIA	enzyme immunoassay
D5W	5% dextrose in water	EICA	epidermal intercellular substance antibodies
DAT	direct antiglobulin test		
DDAVP	1-deamino-8-D-arginine vasopressin	ELISA	enzyme-linked immunosorbent assay
		ELT	euglobulin lysis time
DDT	dithiothreitol	EMIT	enzyme multiplied immunoassay technique
DDx	differential diagnosis		
DHEA	dehydroepiandrosterone	ENA	extractable nuclear antigens
DHEA-S	dehydroepiandrosterone-sulfate	EPO	erythropoietin
		ERCP	endoscopic retrograde cholangiopancreatography
dIA	dimeric inhibin A		
DIC	disseminated intravascular coagulation	ESR	erythrocyte sedimentation rate
		ESRD	end stage renal disease
DKA	diabetic ketoacidosis	ET	essential thrombocytosis
dL	deciliter	F	female
DNA	deoxyribose nucleic acid	FAB	French-American-British
DRE	digital rectal examination		
dsDNA	double stranded deoxyribo-nucleic acid		

FCT	fecal chymotrypsin	GH	growth hormone
FDP	fibrin degradation products	GHB	gamma-hydroxybutyrate
Fe^{2+}	ferric iron	GIT	gastrointestinal tract
Fe^{3+}	ferrous iron	GRH/ GHRH	growth hormone releasing hormone
FFP	fresh frozen plasma		
FFN	fetal fibronectin	GI	gastrointestinal
FLM	fetal lung maturity	Glc	glucose
fMTC	familial medullary thyroid carcinoma	GIT	gastrointestinal tract
		GLDH	glutamate dehydrogenase
Frc	fructose	GnRH	gonadotropin-releasing hormone
HPF	high power field		
FPFH	hereditary persistence of fetal hemoglobin	GRF	growth hormone releasing factor
FSH	follicle stimulating hormone	G6PD	glucose-6-phosphate-dehydrogenase
FSP	fibrin split products		
FT3	free Triiodothyronine	GU	genitourinary
FT4	free Thyroxine	GYN	gynecology
FTA-Abs	fluorescent treponemal antibody	h	hour(s)
		H^+	hydrogen
FTA-IgM	fluorescent treponemal immunoglobulin m	HA	hemagglutination assay
		HAV	hepatitis A virus
Func	function	Hb	hemoglobin
g	gram(s)	HbA1c	hemoglobin A1c
GABA	gamma-aminobutyric acid	HbC	hemoglobin C
GADA	glutamate decarboxylase antibodies	HBc-Ag	hepatitis B core antigen
		HBDH	hydroxybutyrate dehydrogenase
Gal	galactose		
GBM	glomerular basement membrane	HbE	hemoglobin E
		HBe-Ab	hepatitis B early antibody
GFR	glomerular filtration rate	HBe-Ag	hepatitis B early Antigen
GGT	gamma glutamyl transferase	HbS	sickle hemoglobin

HBs-Ab	hepatitis B surface antibody		HMWK	williams-fitzgerald-flaujeac factor
HBs-Ag	hepatitis B surface antigen		HPP	hereditary pyropoikilocytosis
HBV	hepatitis B virus		HRT	hormone replacement therapy
HBV-PCR	hepatitis B virus- polymerase chain reaction		HS	hereditary spherocytosis
hCG	human chorionic gonadotropin		HSP	heat shock proteins
Hct	hematocrit		HTN	hypertension
HCV	hepatitis C virus		HUS	hemolytic uremic syndrome
HDV	hepatitis D virus		HVA	homovanillinic acid
HEV	hepatitis E virus		Hydro	hydrocodone
HGV	hepatitis G virus		IAA	insulin antibodies
HPLC	high performance liquid chromatography		IAT	indirect antiglobulin test
HCG	human chorionic gonadotrophin		IBD	inflammatory bowel disease
			ICA	Islet cell antibodies
HCO_3^-	bicarbonate		ICT	indirect coombs test
HDL	high-density lipoprotein		IDL	intermediate-density lipoprotein
HDN	hemolytic disease of the new-born		IEF	isoelectric focusing
HE	hereditary elliptocytosis		IF	intrinsic factor
HIPA	heparin-induced platelet activation		IFA	Intrinsic factor antibody
HIT	heparin-induced thrombocy-topenia		IgA	immunoglobulin A
			IgG	immunoglobulin G
			IgM	immunoglobulin M
HIV	human immunodeficiency virus		Ind	indications
HLA	human leukocyte antigen		inh	Inhibitor
HMB	hydroxymethyl bilane		INR	international normalized ratio
HMWK	high-molecular-weight kininogen		ISI	international sensitivity index
			ITP	immune thrombocytopenia purpura
			IU	international unit

IV	intravenous
K	potassium
KCl	potassium chloride
kDa	kilodalton
K2EDTA	potassium (K2) ethylene diamine tetraacetic acid
K3EDTA	potassium (K3) ethylene diamine tetraacetic acid
kIU	kallidinogenase inactivator unit
L	liter
L:S	lecithin : sphingomyelin ratio
LA	lupus anticoagulant
LACT	lecithin cholesterol acyl transferase
LAP	leukocyte alkaline phosphatase
LAP	leucine aminopeptidases
LDH	lactic dehydrogenase
LDL	low density lipoprotein
LE	lower extremities
LES	lower esophageal sphincter
LH	luteinizing hormone
LISS	low ionic strength solution
LKM	liver-kidney microsomal
LMWH	low molecular weight heparin
LN	lupus nephritis
LP	lumbar puncture
LPA	liver-pancreas antigen
LPL	lipoprotein lipase
LSD	lysergic acid diethylamide

Lu	lutheran
6-MAM	6-monoacetyle morphine
m	meter(s)
M	male
M	monoclonal
MA	megaloblastic anemia
MA	maximum amplitude
MAHA	microangiopathic hemolytic anemia
MAOI	monoamine oxidase inhibitor
Mat	materials
MCH	mean corpuscular hemoglobin
MCHC	mean corpuscular hemoglobin concentration
MCTD	mixed connective tissue disease
MCV	mean corpuscular volume
MDA	3, 4 methylene-dioxy-amphetamine
MDMA	3,4-methylenedioxymetham-phetamine
MDS	myelodysplastic syndrome
MEN II	multiple endocrine neoplasia type 2
Met	methods
metHb	methemoglobin
mg	milligram
Mg	magnesium
MGUS	monoclonal gammopathy of undetermined significance

MHC	major histocompatibility complex
MI	myocardial infarction
min	minute/minutes
mL	milliliter
mo	month(s)
MOI	mode of inheritance
MPD	myeloproliferative disorders
MPN	myeloproliferative neoplasms
MPO	myeloperoxidase
MPS	myeloproliferative syndromes
MS	multiple sclerosis
MSH	melanocyte stimulating hormone
MTC	medullary thyroid carcinoma
N	nuclear
Na	sodium
NaCl	sodium chloride
NAD	nicotinamide adenine dinucleotide
NADH	nicotinamide adenine dinucleotide-cytochrome
NADP	nicotinamide adenine dinucleotide phosphate
NADPH	nicotinamide adenine dinucleotide phosphate hydrogen
Na_2EDTA	sodium (Na_2) ethylene diamine tetraacetic acid
NaF	sodium fluoride
$NaHCO_3$	sodium carbonate

NAIT	neonatal alloimmune thrombocytopenia
NaOH	sodium hydroxide
NATP	neonatal alloimmune thrombocytopenia
NBT-PABA-test	N-benzoyl-L-tyrosyl-p-aminobenzoic-acid-test
nl	normal
$NH4Cl$	ammonium chloride
NMDA	N-methyl-D-aspartate
N-MID	N-terminal/midregion
Norm	normal
NOS	not otherwise specified
NPT	normal prothrombin time
NPV	negative predictive value
NSAIDS	non-steroidal anti-inflammatory drugs
NSE	neuron-specific enolase
O2	oxygen
OCP	oral contraceptive pill
OGGT	oral glucose tolerance test
OH-proline	hydroxyproline
Oxy	oxycodone
PAF	platelet-activating-factor
PAH	para-aminohippuric acid
pANCA	perinuclear anti-neutrophil cytoplasmic antibodies
Path	pathology
PBC	primary biliary cirrhosis
PBG	porphobilinogen

PC	protein C
PCA	parietal cell antibody
PCAA	5-[N-(1-phenylcyclohexyl)]-aminopentanoic acid
PCH	paroxysmal cold hemoglobinuria
PCHP	1-(1-phenylcyclohexyl)-4-hydroxypiperidine
PCO_2	partial pressure of carbon dioxide
PCP	phencyclidine
PCR	polymerase chain reaction
PCr	phosphocreatine
PCR	polymerase chain reaction
PE	pulmonary embolism
PEG	polyethylene glycol
PEP	phosphoenol pyruvate
PF4	platelet factor 4
PFT	platelet function test
PG	phosphatidylglycerol
PGB	porphobilinogen
PICP	carboxy-terminal propeptide of type I procollagen
PIF	prolactin inhibiting factor
PINP	amino-terminal propeptide of type I procollagen
PID	pelvic inflammatory disease
PK	pyruvate kinase
PM	primary myelofibrosis
PMN	polymorphonuclear
PN	peripheral neuropathy

PNH	paroxysmal nocturnal hemoglobinuria
PO	by mouth
PO_2	partial pressure of oxygen
PO_4^3	phosphate
PPC	4-Phenyl-4-(1-piperdinyl)-cyclohexanol
PP	protoporphyrin
PPP	protoporphyrinogen
PPV	positive predictive value
Prod	production
PS	protein S
PSA	prostate specific antigen
PSI	pounds per square inch
PSS	progressive systemic sclerosis
PT	prothrombin time
PTH	parathyroid hormone
PTP	post-transfusion purpura
PTT	partial thromboplastin time
PTZ	plasma thrombin
PV	polycythemia vera
PyD	pyridinoline
QA	quality assurance
qPCR	real-time polymerase chain reaction
RA	rheumatoid arthritis
RA	refractory anemia
RAAS	renin-angiotensin-aldosterone system
RAEB	refractory anemia with excess blasts

RAEB-T	refractory anemia with excess blasts in transformation
RARS	refractory anemia with ringed sideroblasts
RAST	radioallergosorbent test
RBC	red blood corpuscle
RCMD	refractory cytopenia with multilineage dysplasia
Rco	ristocetin cofactor
RCUD	refractory cytopenia with unilineage dysplasia
RDS	respiratory distress syndrome
RET	rearranged during transfection
RF	rheumatoid factor
Rh	rhesus
RIA	radioimmunoassay
RN	refractory neutropenia
RNA	ribose nucleic acid
ROTI	related organ or tissue impairment
RT	reptilase time
RT	refractory thrombocytopenia
RT-PCR	reverse transcription polymerase chain reaction
RVVT	russell's viper venom time
SCC	squamous cell carcinoma
SCr	serum creatinine
SD	standard deviation
SG	specific gravity
SHARP	mixed connective tissue disease
SHBG	sex hormone binding globulin
SIADH	syndrome of inappropriate antidiuretic hormone secretion
SKM	skeletal muscle
SLA	soluble liver/pancreas antigen
SLE	systemic lupus erythematosus
SLOS	Smith-Lemli-Optiz syndrome
SMA	smooth muscle antibody
snRNP	small nuclear ribonucleic particles
SPEP	serum protein electrophoresis
SPS	sodium polyanethol sulfonate
SRA	serotonin release assay
SRF	somatotropin releasing-factor
ssDNA	single-stranded deoxyribonucleic acid
T3	triiodothyronine
T4	thyroxine
TB	tuberculosis
TBG	thyroxine-binding globulin
TBPA	thyroid binding prealbumin
TC	total cholesterol
TEG	thromboelastogram
TG	triglyceride(s)
TLC	thin layer chromatography
TPA	tissue plasminogen activator
TPHA	treponema pallidum hemagglutination test
TPN	total parenteral nutrition

TPO	thyroid peroxidase
TRAP	tartrate resistant acid phosphatase
TRH	thyroid releasing hormone
TSH	thyroid stimulating hormone
TSHr	thyroid stimulating hormone (thyrotropin) receptor
TT	thrombin time
tTG	tissue transglutaminase
TTP	thrombotic thrombocytopenic purpura
TXA2	thromboxane a2
UCr	urine creatinine
uE	unconjugated estriol
UE	upper extremities
UFH	unfractionated heparin
uPA	urokinase-type plasminogen activator
UPEP	urine protein electrophoresis
URI	upper respiratory illness
URO	uroporphyrinogen
UTIs	urinary tract infections
UV	ultraviolet
Uvol	urine volume
VDRL	venereal disease research laboratory
VKA	vitamin- k antagonists
VMA	vanillylmandelic acid
vWD	von Willebrand disease
vWF	von Willebrand factor

VLDL	very low density lipoprotein
WAIHA	warm autoimmune hemolytic anemia
WBC	white blood cells
WHO	World Health Organization
wk	week
y	year/years
ZZAP	mixture of cysteine-activated proteolytic papain and dithiothreitol
ZES	Zollinger-Ellison syndrome

Numerics

11-Deoxycortisol 290
17-Beta-estradiol 301
17-Hydroxyprogesterone 289
5-Hydroxyindoleacetic acid
  (5-HIAA) 309
5-Hydroxytryptophane (5-HTP) 310

A

Absorption 256
Accelerin 168
Acetaminophen 375
Acetylcholinesterase 375
Acid phosphatase (AP) 107
Acid-Base
- algorithm 317
- compensation 316
- disorders 315
- normogram 318
Acidemia 315
Acidosis 315, 319
- lactic 320
- metabolic 315, 320
- renal tubular 320
- respiratory 315
Acquired (secondary)
  immunoglobulin deficiency 49
Acromegaly 298
ACTH test 288
- long 288
- short 288
Activated partial thromboplastin
  time (aPTT) 172
Acute phase reactants 53
Addison disease 285
Addison's disease 291, 320
Additives 13
Adrenal androgens 289
Adrenergic 373
Adrenocortical insufficiency 285
Adrenocorticotropic
  hormone (ACTH) 286
Agglutination 30
Agranulocytosis 142
- cyclic 142
- infantile hereditary 142
Albumin 381
Albumin quotient 264

Alcohol
- clinical effects 368
Aldosterone 291
Alkalemia 315
Alkaline phosphatase 97, 271
- bone specific 273
Alkalosis 315, 319
- metabolic 315
- respiratory 315
Alpha granules 183
Alpha-1
- acid glycoprotein 42
- antichymotrypsin 42
- antitrypsin (A1AT) 42
- lipoprotein 42
- microglobulin 42
Alpha-2
- antiplasmin 44
- lipoprotein 44
- macroglobulin 43
Alpha-amylase 98
Alpha-fetoprotein (AFP) 69, 305, 378
Amino acid disorder
- hereditary 61
Ammonia 54
Amniotic fluid bilirubin levels 381
Amphetamine 375
Amylase 381
Amyloidosis 162
Anabolism 256
Analytical methods
- chromatographic separation
  processes 34
- electrochemical 27
- electrophoresis 28
- immunological 30
- molecular diagnostics 36
- optical measurement 26
- osmotic pressure 36
Analytical phase 18
- coefficient of variation 19
- control 19
- interpretation of lab values 18
- precision 18
- quality assurance 19
- standard deviation 19
Anamoly
- Alder's 145
- Pelger-Huet 145
Androstenedione (ANDRO) 289

Anemia 114
- aplastic 115
- autoimmune hemolytic 321
- corpuscular hemolytic 116
- disorders of erythropoiesis 114
- dyserythropoietic 115
- Fanconi's 145
- hemolytic 112, 116
- hemorrhagic 115
- hyperchromic 122
- hypochromic 122
- iron deficiency 114
- macrocytic 121
- megaloblastic 112, 114, 355
- microangiopathic hemolytic 113
- microcytic 121
- myelophthisic 112, 115
- normochromic 122
- normocytic 121
- pernicious 112, 322
- refractory 158
- renal 115
- sickle cell 112, 118, 129
- sideroblastic 111
- X-linked sideroblastic 133
Angiotensin converting
  enzyme (ACE) 292
Angiotensinogenase 290
Anion gap 222, 316
- falsely low 317
- increased 317
- normal 317
Anisocytosis 111
Antibody
- acetylcholine receptor 322
- adrenocortical 322
- anti TPO 322
- anti-21-hydrolylase 322
- anti-AChr 338
- anti-adrenal 333
- anti-cardiac muscle 338
- anticardiolipin 323
- anti-centromere 327
- anti-cytoplasmic 328
- anti-DNAse-B 339
- anti-EBM 337
- anti-endomysial 335
- anti-endomysium 321
- anti-erythrocyte 321
- anti-GBM 336

- anti-gliadin 321
- anti-histone 328
- anti-La 327
- anti-LKM 337
- anti-melanocyte 324
- anti-mitochondrial 330
- antimitochondrial 322
- antineutrophil cytoplasmic (ANCA) 330
- antinuclear (ANA) 324
- anti-PCA 333
- anti-phospholipid 323, 329
- anti-platelet 322, 341
- anti-reticulin 321
- anti-Ro 327
- anti-SCL 70 327
- anti-SLA 331, 337
- anti-Sm 326
- anti-SMA 338
- anti-sperm 331
- anti-staphylococcal 340
- antistreptolysin-O 339
- anti-striated muscle 338
- anti-TG 332
- anti-TPO 331
- anti-TR 332
- anti-TSHr 322, 332
- anti-white blood cell 341
- bithermal 341
- cold 341
- CREST 323
- double stranded DNA 325
- glutamate-decarboxylase 334
- IAA 335
- IgA-endomysium 321
- IgA-gliadin 321
- pANCA 321, 322
- single stranded DNA 325
- smooth muscle 321
- tyrosine-phosphatase 334
- warm 340
- warm and cold erythrocyte 321
Anticholinergic 373, 375
Anticoagulants 13
Anticoagulation monitoring errors 173
Antidiuretic effect 295
Antidiuretic hormone 295
Antigen
- carcinoembryonic 63
- prostate specific 68

Antiglobulin test
- direct 31, 217
- indirect 31, 217
Antihemophilic factor A 168
Antihemophilic factor B 169
Antithrombin (AT) 169, 178
Anti-Xa activity 185
Anulocytes 111
Anuria 232
Arterial blood gas analysis 312
Ascites 33, 269
- infection 269
- malignancy 269
- portal HTN 269
Assimilation 256
AST/ALT ratio 104
Atomic absorption spectroscopy (AAS) 27
Auer rods 145
Autoimmune hemolytic anemia
- cold 119
- warm 119

B

Barbiturate 375
Basophil 110, 138
Basophilia 143
Basophilic stippling 111
Bence-Jones proteins 230
Benzodiazepine 375
Beriberi 350
- dry 350
- infantile 350
- wet 350
Beta carotene 349
Bicarbonate 316
Bilirubin 139
- direct 139
- indirect 139
- total 139
Diuret-method 39
Bleeding disorders
- clinical manifestations 184
Bleeding time 166
Blood collection tubes
- color codes 14
Blood gas analysis 311

Blood groups 207
- ABO-system 207
- antibody differentiation 215
- antibody screening testing 214
- cross-match (serological testing) 213
- Duffy 212
- Kidd 212
- MNS 212
- rhesus system 208
Blood loss stages 166
Blood urea nitrogen (BUN) 381
Blot method
- dot blot 37
- southern 37
Bone formation marker 271
Bone marrow differential 137
Bone resorption marker 275

C

Cabot ring 111
Calcitonin 252, 282
Calcium 228, 359, 381
Captopril test 294
Carbaminohemoglobin 124
Carbohydrate 82
- antigen 125 68
- antigen 15-3 66
- antigen 72-4 67
- congenital disorders of metabolism 94
Carbohydrate-deficient transferrin (CDT) 50
Carboxyhemoglobin 124
Carcinoma
- hepatocellular 70
- medullary thyroid 282
- squamous cell 65
Cardiac markers 108
Carotenodermia 349
Carter-Robbins test 297
Catabolism 256
Catecholamines
- plasma 308
- urine 308
- urine metabolites 309
Cerebrospinal fluid 260
- cells 260
- macroscopic examination 260
- protein 262
- rhinorrhea 265

Ceruloplasmin 44
Chloride 227
Cholesterol 76, 77
Cholinergic 374
Cholinesterase 98
Chromatography 34
- affinity 35
- column 34
- displacement 35
- gas 35
- gel permeation 35
- ion exchange 35
- liquid 35
- planar 35
Chromium 363
Chvostek's sign 229, 283
Chylomicron 80, 81
Chyluria 237
Chymotrypsin 253
Circulatory insufficiency 312
Citrate (sodium-citrate) 14
Citric acid cycle 133
Clonidine test 309
Clotting disorders
- algorithmic diagnosis 200
Clotting factors 168
Coagulation
- activation due to vascular injury 168
- cascade 170
- global tests 165
- inhibitors 169
- phase specific tests 166
- specific factor deficiencies 187
- testing 205
Cobalt 361
Codocyte 112
Colloid osmotic pressure 220
Common variable (primary) immunodeficiency (CVID) 49
Complement factor C1-esterase inhibitor 47
Complement factors 45
Complement fixation test 32
Complete blood count (CBC) 133
- left shift 134
- right shift 134
Consumptive coagulopathy 201
Coomassie method 39
Copper 362
Coproporphyria 133

Corticotropin 286
Corticotropin releasing hormone test 287
Cortisol 284
Cortodoxone 290
Coulometry 28
Coumarins 186
C-peptide 90
C-reactive protein (CRP) 46
Creatinine 381
Creatinine clearance 245
Creatinine kinase 99
- macro–CK 100
- MB 100
Crystal
- apatite 271
Crystals
- calcium pyrophosphate 270
- corticosteroid 270
- hydroxyapatite 270
- monosodium urate 270
CSF differentials
- meningitis 261
- normal 261
Cyanide 375
Cystic fibrosis 259
Cystinuria 243
Cytokeratin-19 fragment 65

D

Dacrocyte 112
Danaparoid 185
DDAVP test 296
Deferoxamine test 52
Deficiency
- factor IX 190
- factor V 187
- factor VII 187
- factor VIII 189
- factor X 188
- factor XI 188
- factor XII 188
- factor XIII 188
- fibrinogen 189
Dehydroepiandrosterone (DHEA) 289
- sulfate (DHEA-S) 289
Delta-aminolevulinic acid 139
Deoxypyridinoline 275
Dermatomyositis 322

Desmopressin test 296
Dexamethasone suppression test 286
Diabetes insipidus
- central 295
- renal 295
Diabetes mellitus 82
- classification 82
- diagnosis 83
- gestational 82
- type-1 82
- type-2 82
Diabetic ketoacidosis 83
Digestion 256
Digitalis 375
Disaccharides 96
Disinfection methods 11
Disseminated intravascular coagulation (DIC) 121, 201
Downey cells 146
Drepanocyte 112
Drug metabolites 371
Drug toxicity symptoms 373
Dysfibrinogenemia 204
Dysproteinemia 38

E

EDTA (ethylenediamine tetra acetic acid) 14
Electrophoresis 28
- capillary 29
- gel 29
- hemoglobin 126
- immunofixation 31
- isoelectric focusing (IEF) 29
- isotachophoresis 29
- lipoprotein 80
- serum protein (SPEP) 28, 39
Elliptocyte 112
Encephalopathy
- Wernicke's 350
Enzyme immunoassay (EIA) 33
- Enzyme multiplied immunoassay technique (EMIT) 33
- Enzyme-linked immunosorbent assay (ELISA) 33
Enzymes 97
- half-life 108
- localization 107
- specific laboratory findings 108

Eosinophil 110, 138
Eosinophilia 143
Erythroblastosis fetalis 118
Erythrocyte sedimentation
   rate (ESR) 113
Erythropoiesis 135
Erythropoietic protoporphyria 133
Erythropoietin (EPO) 138
Essential thrombocythemia 156
Ethanol 368
Ethylene glycol 368
Euglobulin lysis time (ELT) 181
Euvolemia 221
Extracellular space 220

F

FAB classification of AML 152
Factor V Leiden 180
Familial hyperlipoproteinemia 79
Fecal chymotrypsin (FCT) 253
Fecal occult blood test 258
Ferritin 51
Fetal fibronectin (FFN) 379
Fetal hemolysis 381
Fetal lung maturity methods 380
Fibrin split products (FSPs) 175
Fibrinogen 45, 168, 175, 381
Fibrin-stabilizing factor 169
Fischer antigen 210
Fitzgerald factor 169
Flame emission spectrometry 27
Flow cytometry 34
Fluorescence anisotropy 27
Fluorescence polarization assay 380
Fluorescent spot test 117
Fluoride 14
Fluorophotometry 26
Follicle stimulating hormone (FSH) 303
fPSA/tPSA ratio 69
Fredrickson classification 79
Friedewald formula 76
Fructosamine 89
Fructosuria 94

G

Galactosemia 94
Gamma glutamyl transferase (GGT) 101
Gastric secretions 250
Gastrin 250
Gastrinoma 251
Gene probes 37
Glanzmann thrombasthenia 177, 182
Globulin
 - alpha-1 42
 - alpha-2 43
 - gamma 46
   retinol binding 43
 - sex hormone binding 307
Glomerular filtration rate (GFR) 244
Glucagon 92
Glucagon test 93
Glucose-6-phosphate-
   dehydrogenase (G6PD) 101
 - deficiency 117
Glutamate dehydrogenase (GLDH) 104
Glycogen storage disorder 95
 - type I (Von Gierke's) 95
 - type II (Pompe's) 95
 - type III (Cori's or Forbes') 95
 - type IV (Andersen) 95
 - type IX 95
 - type V (McArdle's) 95
 - type VI (Hers') 95
 - type VII (Tarui's) 95
 - type XI 95
 - type XII 95
 - type XIII 95
Glycosuria 85
 - hyperglycemic 85
 - normoglycemic 85
Gonadotropin-releasing hormone
   test 304
Granulocyte elastase 57
Granulocytes 138
Granulocytopoiesis 137
Granulocytosis 142
Granulopoiesis 135
Graves' disease 322
Growth-hormone-releasing-
   hormone test 298

H

Hagemann factor 169
Hallucinogen 374
Haptoglobin 44
Haptoglobin complex 43
HCG test 307
Heinz body (Heinz-Ehrlich body)
   101, 112
Helmet cell 113
Hemagglutination assay (HA) 32
Hematocrit 110, 125, 381
Hematology 110
Hematopoiesis 135
Hematuria 238
 - postrenal 239
 - prerenal 239
 - renal 239
Hemoglobin 110, 124, 381
 - A1c 87
 - C 130
 - complex 43
 - E 130
 - fetal 130
Hemoglobinuria 239
 - paroxysmal cold 120
 - paroxysmal nocturnal 117
Hemolytic anemia
 - alloimmune 118
 - autoimmune 119, 120
 - extracorpuscular 118
 - mechanical 120
 - microangiopathic 120
Hemopexin 46
Hemophilia 171, 189
 - factor-inhibitor induced 190
 - mild 190
 - moderate 190
 - severe 190
Hemophilia A 187, 189
Hemophilia B 187, 190
Hemophilia C 188
Hemostasis 164
 - primary 164
 - secondary 165
 - vascular 164
Heparin 14, 184, 185, 375
Heparin-induced platelet
   activation test (HIPA) 196
Heparin-PF4 induced-antibody
   assay (HPIA) 196

Hepatitis, chronic active 321
Hereditary elliptocytosis (HE) 116
Hereditary pyropoikilocytosis (HPP) 116
Hereditary spherocytosis (HS) 116
Hickey-Hare test 297
Hirsutism 289
Homeostasis, acid 316
Homocysteine 56
Homocysteinemia 204
Homocystinuria 57, 243
Homovanillinic acid (HVA) 309
Hormone 278
- adrenal cortex 284
- antidiuretic 290
- catecholamines 308
- growth 297
- parathyroid 278
- prolactin 300
- sex hormones 301
- thyroid 278
Howell Jolly body 112
Human chorionic gonadotropin
  (hCG) 70, 305, 377
Human leukocyte antigen (HLA) 342
Hydroxybutyrate
  dehydrogenase (HBDH) 106
Hydroxyproline 276
Hyperaldosteronism
- primary 294, 297
- secondary 291, 294
Hypercalcemia 229, 283
Hypercortisolism 285
Hyperfibrinolysis 176
Hyperglycemia 84
Hyperimmunoglobulinemia 48
- monoclonal 48
- polyclonal 48
Hyperkalemia 226
Hypermagnesemia 360
Hypernatremia 224
Hyperparathyroidism 283, 284, 320
- primary 277
Hyperphosphatemia 231
Hyperproteinemia 38
Hypersplenism 121
Hypertension
- essential 294
- renovascular 294
Hyperthyroidism
- primary 278
- secondary 278

Hyperuricemia
- primary 56
- secondary 56
Hypervolemia 220
Hypoalbuminemia 317
Hypoaldosteronism
- primary 292
- secondary 292
Hypocalcemia 229, 283
Hypoglycemia 84
Hypoimmunoglobulinemia 49
Hypokalemia 226
Hypomagnesemia 360
Hyponatremia 224
Hypoparathyroidism 357
Hypophosphatemia 230
Hypopituitarism 298
Hypoproteinemia 38
Hypothyroidism 283
- primary 278
- secondary 278
- tertiary 278
Hypovolemia 221

Idiopathic myelofibrosis 156
IgG quotient 264
Immunoblotting 34
Immunodiffusion 30
- agar gel 30
- Ouchterlony double 30
- simple/radial 30
Immunoelectrophoresis 30
- affinity 30
- crossed 30
- rocket 30
Immunofluorescence
- direct 32
- indirect 33
Immunonephelometry 31
Immunoturbidimetry 31
Impaired glucose tolerance 83
Insulin 90
Insulin hypoglycemia test (IHT) 299
International normalized ratio (INR) 172
Interzone
- albumin-alpha-1 43
- alpha-1-alpha-2 43
- beta-gamma 46

Intracellular space 220
Iron 51
Isoniazid 375

J

Jaundice 116
- hepatic 140
- posthepatic 140
- prehepatic 140

K

Kayser-Fleischer rings 362
Keshan disease 364
Ketoacidosis 320
Ketone bodies 86
Kjeldahl method 39

L

Laboratory errors 16
- interference 17
- physiologic 17
- preanalytical 16
Lactate 91
Lactate dehydrogenase (LDH) 105
Lactose intolerance 95
Lactose-load test 257
Lamellar body concentration 380
Latex agglutination test 31
LDH/AST ratio 106
Lecithin sphingomyelin ratio 380
Leucine aminopeptidase (LAP) 107
Leukemia 146
- acute 146
- acute lymphoblastic (ALL) 147
- acute myeloid 149
- chronic 152
- chronic lymphocytic 152
- chronic myeloid 153
- chronic myelomonocytic 158
- hairy cell 276
- myelogenous 149, 153
- T lymphoblastic 148
Leukemic hiatus 134
Leukocyte 110
Leukocyte alkaline
  phosphatase (LAP) 97

Leukocytopenia 141
Leukocytosis 141
Leukopenia 141
Lipase 106
Lipoprotein 81
- beta 45
- pre-beta 44
Lumbar puncture contraindications 266
Luminescence 26
Luteinizing hormone (LH) 302
Lymphocyte 110, 138
Lymphocytopenia 144
Lymphocytosis 144
Lysozyme 58

M

Macroalbuminuria 238
Macrocyte 112
Macroovalocyte 112
Magnesium 360
Mancini method 30
Manganese 363
Maple syrup urine disease (MSUD) 62
March hemoglobinuria 121
May-Hegglin anomaly 199
McArdle's disease 91
Mean corpuscular
    hemoglobin (MCH) 110
Mean corpuscular hemoglobin
    concentration (MCHC) 110
Mean corpuscular volume (MCV) 110
Meconium albumin testing 259
Mediterranean
    macrothrombocytopenia 199
Melliuria 85
Meningitis
- bacterial 262
- tuberculous 262
- viral 262
Metabolic acidosis
- hyperchloremic 317
Methanol 368
Methemoglobin 125, 312, 375
Methemoglobinemia 312
Metoclopramide test 300
Microalbuminuria 238
Microcyte 112
Monoclonal gammopathy 161
Monocyte 110, 138

Monocytopenia 144
Monocytosis 144
Monosaccharides 96
Muramidase 58
Myasthenia gravis 322
Myeloblast 137
Myelodysplasia 151
Myeloma
- asymptomatic 162
- asymptomatic (smoldering) 48
- MGUS 48
- multiple 160
- multiple/plasmacytoma 48
- plasma cell 160
- solitary plasmacytoma 48
Myeloproliferative disorders 183
Myoglobin 58
Myoglobulinuria 239

N

N-acetylmuramide glycanhydrolase 58
Narcotic 373
Natriuretic peptide
- atrial (ANP) 60
- B-type 60
NBT-PABA-test 255
Neonatal alloimmune
    thrombocytopenia 198
Neoplasm
- osteoblastic 277
- osteoclastic 277
Neopterin 53
Nephelometry 26
Neuroblastoma 309
Neuron-specific enolase 64
Neuropathy
- optic 350
- peripheral 355
Neutropenia 143
Neutrophil 110
Neutrophilia 143
Neutrophilic
- bands 138
- metamyelocytes 137
- myelocytes 137
Neutrophils 137
Nicotinic acid 352
Normoblast 138
Normocyte 112
Nucleic acid hybridization 37

O

Oliguria 232
Oncotic pressure 220
Opiate 375
Oral glucose challenge 298
Oral glucose tolerance
    test (OGGT) 85
Orosomucoid 42
Osmolal gap 317
Osmolality 221
- increased (serum) 222
Osmolar gap, increased 320
Osmolarity 221
Osmotic gap 222
Osmotic resistance 124
Osteoblast 275
Osteocalcin 273
Osteoclastoma 276
Osteoid 271
Osteomalacia 277
Osteoporosis 277, 357
Overdose 372
- onset of symptoms 372
- symptoms 372
Oxyhemoglobin 124

P

Paget's disease 273, 276, 277
Pancreatic elastase 254
Pancreatic enzyme secretion test 255
Pancreoauryl test 254
Paraproteinemia 183
Parathyroid hormone (PTH) 283
Pellagra 352
Pemphigoid 322
Pemphigus vulgaris 322
Pentagastrin 252
Pentagastrin stimulation test 252
Peritoneal lavage 269
Phenylketonuria 61
Pheochromocytoma 309
Phosphate 230
Phosphate clearance 248
Phosphatidylglycerol (PG) 380
Phospholipid 80
Plasma cell 138
- disorders 160
- dyscrasia 48

Plasmacytoma 162
Plasmatic coagulation 165
Plasmin 181
Platelet 111
- acquired disorders 183
- aggregation 164
- aggregometry 177
- disorders 182, 184
- monitoring in heparin therapy 197
- storage disorders 182
Platelet function test (PFT) 177
Pleural effusion 73, 267
- chylous 268
- exudate 267
- malignancy 267
- parapneumonic 267
- transudate 267
Poikilocytosis 113
Poisoning 372
- basic testing 374
- cyanide 312
- onset of symptoms 372
- poison elimination methods 375
Polyarteritis nodosa 322
Polychromasia 113
Polycythemia 123
Polycythemia vera 156
Polymerase chain reaction (PCR) 36
Polymyositis 322
Polyradiculitis 262
Polyuria 232
Porphyria 131
- acute intermittent 131
- congenital erythropoietic 132
- cutanea tarda 132
- hepatoerythropoietic 132
- variegate 133
Porphyrinemia 131
Porphyrins 131
Porphyrinuria 131
Postanalytical phase 21
- longitudinal evaluation 23
- plausibility 23
- predictive value 23
- reference ranges 21
- sensitivity 21
- specificity 22
Potassium 225, 381
Potentiometry 27

Predictive value
- negative 23
- positive 23
Prenatal screening 378
Preterm delivery risk evaluation 379
Proaccelerin 168
Procalcitonin (PCT) 52
Procollagen 274
Proconvertin 168
Proerythroblast 138
Progesterone 302
Prolactin 300
Prolonged PTT 173
Promyelocytes 137
Propoxyphene 370
Protein C 169, 178, 204
Protein S 169, 179, 204
Proteinuria
- glomerular 236
- glomerular-tubular (mixed) 236
- orthostatic 236, 237
- physiological 237
- post-renal 237
- pre-renal 236
- renal 236
- tubular 236
Prothrombin 168
Prothrombin time (PT) 171
Pseudogout 270
Psilocybin 371
Pulse oximetry 311
- reflectance 311
- transmissive 311
Punnett square for sensitivity and
    specifity 22
Purpura
- immune thrombocytopenic (ITP) 198
- post-transfusion (PTP) 198
- thrombotic thrombocytopenic
    (TTP) 198
Pyelonephritis 237
Pyridinium crosslinks 275
Pyridinoline 275
Pyruvate kinase (PK) 102

R

Radioimmunoassay (RIA) 33
Recalcification time 174
Refractory cytopenia
- multilineage dysplasia (RCMD) 159
- unilineage dysplasia (RCUD) 158
Refrigerated standing plasma
    test 80
Reiber protein quotient graph 263
Renal perfusion 245
Renin 290
Renin-aldosterone-orthostatic-test 293
Reptilase time (RT) 174
Reticulocyte 110, 113, 123
Rhabdomyolysis 320
Rheumatoid factor 321
Ristocetin cofactor 191
Rosenthal factor 169
Rouleaux formation 113
Russell's viper venom time 329

S

Salicylate 375
Salt loading test 297
Sample
- cerebrospinal fluid (CSF) 16
- extraction method 12
- special considerations 15
- transport 16
- types 12
- urine 15
Schilling test 258
Schistocyte 113
Scurvy 356
Secretin provocation test 252
Sedative 374
Segmented neutrophils 138
Selenium 364
Serotonin 308, 310
Serotonin release assay 196
Severe combined
    immunodeficiency (SCID) 49
Small intestine function 256
Smudge cells 146
Sodium 223, 381
Soluble transferrin-receptor (sTfR) 50
Somatotropic hormone 297
Southeast Asian ovalocytosis 116

Spectrophotometry 26
Spectroscopy 27
Spherocyte 113
Spontaneous clot lysis time 181
Stability test 301
Steatorrhea 256
Stem cells 135
Stomatocytes 113
Stomatocytic elliptocytosis 116
Stool examination 253
Streptokinase 375
Stuart-Prower factor 169
Sulfonylurea 375
Syndrome
 - androgen insensitivity 289
 - anti-phospholipid 329
 - Bartter 291
 - Bernard-Soulier 167, 177, 182
 - carcinoid 309
 - Chediak-Higashi & Hemansky-
   Pudlak 182
 - Churg-Strauss 268
 - Conn's 291
 - Cushing's 285
 - Donath-Landsteiner 120
 - Down 378, 379
 - Dressler's 268
 - Dubin-Johnson 140, 241
 - Edwards' 378, 379
 - Felty's 141
 - Gilbert's 140
 - grey platelet 183
 - Guillain-Barré 350
 - Günther 132
 - Heglin 145
 - hemolytic uremic 199
 - inappropriate ADH secretion
   (SIADH) 295
 - Kelley-Seegmiller 56
 - Korsakoff 350
 - Lambert-Eaton 322
 - Lesch-Nyhan 56
 - McLeod 212
 - Meigs' 268
 - Menke's 362
 - myelodysplastic 115, 157
 - myeloproliferative 155
 - nephrotic 237, 362
 - POEMS 48, 163
 - Schwartz-Bartter 295

 - SHARP 323
 - Sjögren's 141
 - Smith's 144
 - Smith-Lemli-Optiz 378
 - Turner's 378
 - von Willebrand 167
 - Wiskott-Aldrich 145, 167, 183
 - Zollinger-Ellison 250, 251
Synovial fluid 269
Systemic lupus erythematosus 323

T

Tangier disease 76
Tartrate resistant acid
 phosphatase (TRAP) 276
Testosterone 306
Thalassemia 118, 127
 - alpha 128
 - beta (major) 127
 - beta (minor) 127
Therapeutic drug monitoring 366
Three glass test 233
Thrombin time (TT) 174
Thrombocythemia 145
Thrombocytopenia 111, 145, 193
 - algorithmic diagnosis 200
 - alloimmune 199
 - congenital amegakaryocytic
   (CAMT) 199
 - heparin induced 194
 - quinidine-induced 199
 - with absent radii syndrome 199
Thrombocytosis 111, 145
Thromboelastogram 177
Thrombophilia 204
Thromboplastin 168
Thrombopoiesis 138
Thrombotic thrombocytopenic
 purpura (ITP) 120
Thyroid binding globulin (TBG) 280
Thyroid releasing hormone (TRH) 281
Thyroid stimulating hormone (TSH) 278
Thyroid stimulating hormone
 releasing hormone test 301
Thyrotoxicosis 376
Thyrotropin 278
Thyroxine 279
Total complement activity 47

Toxicology 103
 - amphetamine 369
 - barbiturate 369
 - basic concepts 366
 - benzodiazepine 369
 - cannabis 369
 - cocaine 369
 - common drugs of abuse 367
 - GHB 370
 - ketamine 370
 - LSD 370
 - mescaline 370
 - monitored medications 367
 - opiate 370
 - PCP 370
 - psilocybin 370
 - therapeutic drug monitoring 366
Transaminases 103
 - alanine aminotransferase
   (ALT) 103
 - aspartate aminotransferase
   (AST) 103
Transcobalamin 43
Transcortin 43
Transferrin 44
Transferrin saturation 50
Transfusion 207
 - non-planned 217
 - planned 217
 - planning timeline 217
Transthyretin 42
Triglyceride 78, 381
 - endogenous 80
 - exogenous 80
Triiodothyronine 279
Trisomy-18 378, 379
Trisomy-21 379
Troponin, cardiac 59
Trousseau sign 229, 283
Tumor
 - bladder 72
 - breast 71
 - cervix 72
 - colorectal 71
 - hepatocellular 72
 - lung 71
 - ovarian 72
 - pancreas 71
 - prostate 72
 - stomach 71

Tumor marker 63
- clinically relevant 63
- sensitivities for solid tumors 71
- weighting in tumors 74
Turbidimetry 26
Type-I collagen telopeptide (CTx) 277

U

Units of measurement 24
Urea 54
Uremia 320
Uric acid 55
Urinalysis 232
- dipstick evaluation 233
- macroscopic assessment 232
- microscopic examination 234
Urinary calculi 249
Urine
- amylase 242
- bilirubin 240
- concentration 243
- creatinine 245
- cystatin C 247
- cysteine 243
- glucose 235
- homocysteine 243
- ketones 240
- leukocytes 240
- nitrite 242
- phenylketone 243
- protein 236
- sulfite 243
- urea 249
Urine pH 235
Urine protein quotient 237
Urobilinogen 241

V

Vanillylmandelic acid (VMA) 309
Vasoactive intestinal polypeptide (VIP) 61
Vasopressor effect 295
Virilism 289
Vitamin
- A 348
- B1 (Thiamine) 350
- B12 (Cobalamin) 355
- B2 (Riboflavin) 351
- B3 (Niacin) 352
- B5 (Pantothenic acid) 352
- B6 (Pyridoxine) 353
- B7 (Biotin) 353
- B9 (Folic acid) 354
- C (Ascorbic acid) 356
- D (Calciferol) 356
- E (Tocopherol) 357
- K 358
Vitamin B12 absorption test 258
Vitiligo 324
Voltammetry 28
von Willebrand classification 193
von Willebrand factor 169, 191

W

Waldenström's macroglobulinemia
49, 162, 265
Warfarin 186, 375
Water deprivation test 296
Weiner gene 210
White blood cell 136

X

Xanthochromia 260
X-linked agammaglobulinemia 49
Xylose tolerance test 257

Z

Zinc 364